CARE OF THE NEWBORN

by Ten Teachers

CARE OF THE NEWBORN

by Ten Teachers

Edited By

Hilary Lumsden RN RM BSc(Hons) MSC RMT ENB 405

Senior Lecturer in Midwifery,

University of Wolverhampton; and

External Examiner, University of Sheffield

Debbie Holmes RN RM BSc(Hons) PCGE (HE)

Senior Lecturer in Midwifery,

University of Wolverhampton; and

External Examiner, King's College, London

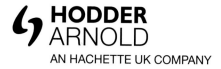

HODDER ARNOLD

AN HACHETTE UK COMPANY

First published in Great Britain in 2010 by
Hodder Arnold, an imprint of Hodder Education, an Hachette UK Company
338 Euston Road, London NW1 3BH

http://www.hodderarnold.com

Whilst the advice and information in this book are believed to be true and accurate at the date of going to press, neither the author[s] nor the publisher can accept any legal responsibility or liability for any errors or omissions that may be made. In particular (but without limiting the generality of the preceding disclaimer) every effort has been made to check drug dosages; however it is still possible that errors have been missed. Furthermore, dosage schedules are constantly being revised and new side-effects recognized. For these reasons the reader is strongly urged to consult the drug companies' printed instructions before administering any of the drugs recommended in this book.

British Library Cataloguing in Publication Data
A catalogue record for this book is available from the British Library

Library of Congress Cataloging-in-Publication Data
A catalog record for this book is available from the Library of Congress

ISBN   978 0 340 968 413
ISBN (ISE)   978 0 340 971 550 (International Students Edition, restricted territorial availability)

1 2 3 4 5 6 7 8 9 10

Commissioning Editor: Naomi Wilkinson
Project Editors: Joanna Silman and Jane Tod
Production Controller: Rachel Manguel
Cover Designer: Lynda King
Indexer: Shirley May

Typeset in 9.5 pt Minion by Phoenix Photosetting Ltd, Chatham, Kent, UK
Printed in India

Cover image © Anna Kern/Etsa/Corbis

What do you think about this book? Or any other Hodder Arnold title?
Please visit our website: www.hodderarnold.com

Contents

The Ten Teachers

Marcia Edwards *RN RM ADM CERT ED (HE) MA*

Senior Lecturer, School of Health, University of Wolverhampton, Walsall

Carole England *RN RM CERT ED (FE) ENB 405 BSc(HONS)*

Midwife Teacher, School of Nursing, Midwifery and Physiotherapy, University of Nottingham

Jane Henley *RN RM ENB 405 DPSN BSc(HONS) ENB A19 MSc*

Advanced Neonatal Nurse Practitioner, Manor Hospital, Walsall

Debbie Holmes *RN RM BSc(HONS) PCGE (HE)*

Senior Lecturer, University of Wolverhampton, Walsall

Hilary Lumsden *RN RM BSc(HONS) MSc RMT ENB 405*

Senior Lecturer, University of Wolverhampton, Walsall

Lynne Paterson *RGN RM ENB 100 405 A19 DIP NEONATAL NURSING SCIENCES BSc MSc AND POST REG DIP ED*

Nurse Consultant, Neonatal Unit, James Cook University Hospital, Middlesbrough

Sandra Sandbrook *BA(HONS) RN RM ADM MTD CERT ED (FE)*

Senior Lecturer, School of Health, University of Wolverhampton, Walsall

Sharon Trotter *RM BSc*

Midwife, Breastfeeding Consultant and Neonatal Skincare Advisor, TIPS Limited

Gillian Warwood *RGN RM ENB 405 A19 AND HIGHER AWARD MSc*

Advanced Neonatal Nurse Practitioner, Neonatal Unit, Sandwell and West Birmingham Hospitals NHS Trust, Birmingham

Linda Wylie *RGN RM BA MN RMT CERT ED (HE)*

Programme Leader BSc Midwifery, University of West of Scotland, Paisley

Preface

The inspiration for this text came from many years' experience of teaching the post-qualifying neonatal nurses' course. It was identified that there are several suitable textbooks to support intensive care of the newborn but very few concentrate on the midwives' role and essentially normal neonatal care. The aim of this book is to inform pre- and post-registration midwives about normal neonatal care in the UK and it is seen to be an excellent addition to the Ten Teachers series. The majority of undergraduate midwifery students will have to study many aspects of newborn care as well as having hands-on experience of neonates in both the community and hospital settings. The book is designed to support both theory and practice.

The aim of *Care of the Newborn by Ten Teachers* is to concentrate on the recognition of common problems associated with newborn babies that student midwives will encounter on a daily basis as well as addressing some of the less common conditions. In-depth knowledge providing theoretical underpinning and contemporary practice is core to each chapter. Professional guidance is underpinned by the rules and code of practice for midwives, which are explicitly referred to throughout.

The contributors were recruited as enthusiastic experts in neonatal and midwifery care and come from wide geographical and practice areas. We see this as being a significant strength of *Care of the Newborn by Ten Teachers* that readers will find invaluable to their studies. The original proposal was made upon individual practitioner contributions and has resulted in a comprehensive collection of chapters by teachers of reputation.

Hilary Lumsden and Debbie Holmes
2010

Acknowledgements

We would like to thank our families, friends and colleagues for their support, time and encouragement during the writing and editing of this book.

Special thanks also goes to student midwives at the University of Wolverhampton who contributed so readily to Chapter 16 by providing their own questions as well as those of parents they have cared for in practice.

Finally to our colleague and friend Pauline Lim for her expert help, support and contributions to Chapter 6.

Hilary Lumsden
Debbie Holmes

CHAPTER 1

PARENTING – ATTACHMENT, SEPARATION AND LOSS

Sandra Sandbrook

OVERVIEW

This chapter explores the attachment relationship parents develop with their baby. Attachment is an interactional process that starts as acquaintance during pregnancy and develops through reciprocal interaction to become an exceptional, enduring and important relationship. Midwives should be aware of the many factors that may affect the developing relationship during pregnancy, childbirth and the early days following birth. The development of the relationship between the parents and their baby has implications for the parents if they are separated from their baby due to illness resulting in admission to a neonatal unit or due to the baby's death.

This chapter will examine the possible psychological implications for the parents when they are separated from their baby due to illness or prematurity and how midwives and nurses can provide support to give the woman or couple confidence in their ability to parent. It ends with a discussion on attachment and loss, the devastation that can result from bereavement at the beginning of life. Grief and mourning will be considered, together with how the midwife can sympathetically facilitate the process of mourning and provide empathetic support.

Attachment

When perinatal and infant mortality rates were high and infant death was the norm, parents did not expect to rear all their children to maturity. Child-rearing practices emphasized discipline and were aimed at promoting survival and moral strength. As mortality rates improved, with the expectation that the majority of children would survive childhood, the emphasis changed from survival to providing sensitive child-rearing practices that would promote the physical and psychological well-being of the child.

Sigmund Freud acknowledged that within successful child-rearing the mother–child relationship was of primary importance. He further identified that early childhood experiences were critical as they could affect the normal psychological functioning of the adult. This was reinforced by John Bowlby's work following the Second World War on the profound emotional and cognitive consequences of maternal deprivation during the early years of a child's life. In his Report for the World Health Organization in 1951, *Maternal Care and Mental Health*, Bowlby stated that essential for a child's mental health is a reciprocal 'warm, intimate and continuous relationship' with a mother or caregiver (Figure 1.1). Bowlby is considered the 'Father of Attachment' and this is the beginnings of attachment theory that has evolved through research in the twentieth and twenty-first century.

The attachment relationship

Attachment describes the unique and enduring relationships each individual seeks to forge with its care-

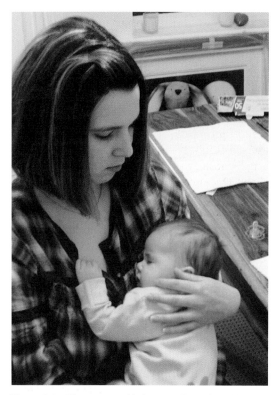

Figure 1.1   The warm and intimate early mother–child relationship

riences: the increasingly strong fetal movements, listening to the fetal heartbeat and visualizing the fetus on ultrasound scans. This is reinforced following birth with powerful sensori-motor interactions activated through embracing, rocking and maintaining prolonged visual contact with her baby. The infant seeks physical and psychological closeness through clinging, following and calling behaviours, and if these are appropriately satisfied both parties experience reciprocal feelings of love, security and joy. In the carer these feelings ensure altruistic commitment to the infant, placing the infant at the centre of his or her life. The reciprocal pleasure and synchronicity of the interaction serves as a catalyst for the continued strengthening of the attachment relationship.

Attachment is very important to the child's physical, social and psychological well-being. The success of the individual's ability to form close attachment relationships is fundamental to his or her ability to develop and sustain all subsequent relationships throughout life. Bowlby suggests that relationship patterns are transmitted through social interaction across the generations. Interactions between child and caregiver are internalized and become almost a blueprint for subsequent relationships. These initial attachment relationships act as a basis for expectation, belief and evaluation of intimate relationships across the individual's lifespan.

Attachment relationships remain important throughout a person's life. In adulthood stressful life events cause individuals to seek their secure attachment figures for help, soothing and safety. As with infants the adults will exhibit anguish if an attachment figure becomes unavailable. The loss of this attachment relationship can be catastrophic at any time during an individual's lifespan, constituting a potent stressor. This suggests that attachment security remains important into adulthood.

Secure attachment

Mary Ainsworth (1963, 1967) through rigorous empirical work identified and explained the concept of secure attachment. She noted the importance of a parent's sensitivity to their infant's cues and that this sensitivity is essential to the successful development of the attachment relationship. Secure attachment is crucial to provide safety and comfort to a child that is tired, distressed or presented with a challenging situation; the lack of opportunity to develop selective attach-

givers and a select group of special individuals. This relationship ensures survival, facilitates both communication and socialization and assists cultural transmission. Initially this intimate relationship begins as maternal–fetal attachment during pregnancy and is then developed through reciprocal interactions between the infant, caregivers and a special group of chosen individuals during childhood. Indeed there is empirical evidence revealing that the majority of children during their first year of life become attached to a small group of familiar people whom the child categorizes into a hierarchy of attachment figures – usually with the child's parents being the most important. In most cultures the child's attachment group consists of parents, siblings, grandparents, aunts, uncles and daycare providers.

Attachment has been described as an interactional process that begins as acquaintance and develops towards the unique and enduring attachment relationship (Goulet et al., 1998). The acquaintance phase begins during pregnancy as the expectant woman seeks to get to know her 'baby' through assigning meanings to the physical and technical signs she expe-

ments may damage the child's social and emotional development. A secure attachment figure provides the child with a safe environment to explore their world and allow them a healthy mental development. Bowlby found that secure attachment facilitated the development of internal working models that socialize the child and allow them to make sense of the world they live in, responding appropriately and safely to the myriad social and environmental cues. These increasingly complex models operate outside consciousness and are formed through continued interpersonal and environmental transactions. Secure attachment also facilitates the development of the child's self-belief. Optimal parenting style, described as responsive, reassuring and comforting, promote the child's autonomy and sense of self-confidence and worth.

Attachment as a developmental process

Attachment is a developmental process that continues throughout the life. For many years it was considered that birth marked the beginnings of the relationship between parents and baby; it is now recognized, however, that the attachment relationship begins during pregnancy.

(i) Maternal–fetal attachment

Maternal–fetal attachment is an emotional response to the growing life within that develops as the pregnancy becomes more tangible. The woman becomes increasingly preoccupied with the physical realities of the pregnancy, actively focusing her attention on the developing life inside her. It would appear that the woman's affectionate behaviour towards her fetus develops with each progressive trimester. Initially women fantasize about their fetus, but as pregnancy progresses they become more actively involved with their 'baby', stroking and talking to their pregnant abdomens, often giving their 'baby' a pet name. As pregnancy advances the woman perceives the fetus in increasingly human terms, attributing characteristics and personality traits to it. The physical reality and experiences of pregnancy appears to positively encourage and intensify maternal attachment. Studies have shown that quickening, ultrasound visualization, the growing pregnant abdomen and progressively strong and distinctive fetal movements enhance attachment.

This developing maternal–fetal attachment throughout the trimesters has been aptly illustrated by Raphael-Leff (2005) as constituting three progressive phases: belief in the pregnancy, belief in the fetus and ultimately belief in a baby who will survive his or her birth.

There are many factors that appear to influence the development of the maternal–fetal attachment: the woman's own experiences of being parented, social support, the support of a compassionate partner and previous personal experiences of pregnancy and childbirth. Personal experiences of being parented fundamentally affect the individual's ability to parent. Once internalized and operating at an unconscious level the working model of attachment becomes a blueprint for future parenting. This constitutes intergenerational attachment. Parenting attitudes, behaviours and models are passed from generation to generation, with early experiences of secure selective attachment being associated with a greater capacity to be well-functioning parents.

Pregnancy is the catalyst that stimulates the woman to explore attachment relationships, particularly evaluating her relationship with her mother. Pregnant women actively seek increased contact with their mothers, particularly in the final trimester. Research has shown that women who have affectionate, loving relationships with their mothers are more able to establish and maintain positive attachment (Siddiqui *et al.*, 2000). It must be acknowledged, however, that individual women will have both positive and negative parenting experiences and it would be over-simplistic to suggest that experiences of poor parenting result in poor maternal–fetal/infant attachment. If a woman has a clear understanding of her experiences of being parented and is able to fully discuss its impact with another attachment figure, supportive partner or within a therapeutic relationship, she will be able to develop maternal–fetal attachment and ultimately provide sensitive and responsive parenting.

Accommodation to pregnancy and subsequent attachment behaviours is influenced by the woman's social, financial and health status. Inequalities and inadequacies may cause the woman to be so preoccupied with her dilemma that she is unable to respond effectively to the developing relationship. The woman's satisfaction with her social networks and economic circumstances can have profound effects on the developing attachment relationship, competing with her ability to focus on her pregnancy and baby.

The transition to parenthood is a critical period in an individual's life, causing substantial lifestyle and role changes. Responsive, sensitive and appropriate social support can have a positive effect and encourage the development of attachment. Social support can be from a variety of people: friends, colleagues, helping healthcare professionals, family and partners. However it is not simply the provision of support, it is the woman's satisfaction with the quality of support provided that is most influential in promoting maternal–fetal attachment. Practical support provided by a partner is especially valued; doing household chores, shopping and generally paying close attention to the pregnant woman's health and well-being, especially if this behaviour is new, is very beneficial for the developing attachment relationship.

It would appear that the most influential social support is from a loving and empathetic partner. Bowlby (1988) noted that expectant mothers had a strong desire to be cared for and supported by their partners. He suggested that the experience of being loved facilitates and enhances the woman's ability to love. It has been found that women with positive and sustained support from their partners adapt more easily to pregnancy. A supportive relationship strengthens and maintains the woman's constructive feelings about motherhood and the fetus. Gjerdingen and Chaloner (1994) found that the partner's sensitive, caring and appropriate practical help strongly impacted on the woman's sense of emotional well-being and self-confidence, which results in a reduction in the incidence of postnatal depression. Siddiqui et al. (1999) found that the woman's partner's attitude and reaction to her pregnancy are powerful contributors to the woman's adjustment to pregnancy, her relationship to her fetus and mothering behaviour. The support of a partner can positively affect the woman's caregiving functions, providing a secure base from which she can explore and rectify any previous experiences of insecure attachment, allowing her to concentrate on her pregnancy and develop attachment to her fetus. This security is provided through loving support and practical assistance during pregnancy, actively participating in some functional caregiving capacity.

It should also be noted that previous childbearing experiences will affect the woman's ability to concentrate on her pregnancy and develop an emotional attachment to her fetus. It would appear that within the first trimester of pregnancy most women are at times ambivalent towards the fetus. It is common knowledge that miscarriage within the first 12 weeks of pregnancy is not unusual; women are sometimes hesitant of becoming emotionally attached to a fetus that may not

be viable. This does not mean they have not developed feelings and aspirations for their pregnancy and will not be bereaved should miscarriage occur. However, if the woman has already experienced a miscarriage her fear of becoming emotionally attached is aggravated and she may attempt to withhold her emotion until viability is confirmed. Any experiences of pregnancy loss will affect the woman's emotional experience of pregnancy: although she will become attached to her fetus, she will be fearful that events will be repeated and anxious until the previous time of loss has past. For some couples who suffered a previous late stillbirth this may mean a very anxious time that could predispose some women to develop antenatal depression. In some women a previous poor obstetric history may result in what Katz-Rothman (1986) identified as a 'tentative pregnancy'. This is particularly pertinent to those women with a history of serious fetal anomaly and subsequent termination for abnormality. These women may withhold attachment until normality is established and the pregnancy viable in an attempt to limit the psychological loss. All women who have experienced loss need sensitive support from their carers. It is important that all the woman's previous childbearing experiences are acknowledged, careful individual care-planning is negotiated and the woman's emotional well-being is given priority.

Difficulties within the current pregnancy may also affect the development of the attachment relationship. It is well documented that pregnancy, the birth of a baby and the transition to parenting are critical developmental phases that involve change and reorganization within an individual's life and relationships. This transition itself has been reported for some couples as resulting in decreased feelings of personal well-being and distress at the considerable adaptations being made. For most this is a transitory and modest phase, reducing with the birth of a healthy baby. However for those couples whose pregnancy is complicated by significant fetal or maternal risk, resulting in a 'high-risk' pregnancy, the fear of losing their baby may result in emotional instability, heightened anxiety, distress and depression. Research has shown that although both prospective parents may experience distress, this is often heightened within the woman. The woman may question her competence to protect her fetus and her capability to successfully mother. Studies exploring the consequences of high-risk pregnancy on developing attachment levels have given wide-ranging results.

Attachment is multifactorial in nature, therefore the effects on the woman of a pregnancy complicated by high risk to her or her fetus is unique and individual. Results of research are inconclusive, ranging from lowered levels of attachment, though no significant alteration to heightened attachment. However the distress and anxiety suffered by the woman or couple should always be acknowledged, ensuring sufficient understandable and contemporary information is given so that the couple are able to respond effectively.

(ii) Following birth

The process of attachment as described by Goulet *et al.* (1998) consists of four interdependent and continuing phases: interaction, proximity, reciprocity and commitment. The interactional stage that begins in pregnancy as the woman forms a mental picture of her fetus in response to physical and technical cues has been discussed earlier within this chapter. This interactional phase that begins as acquaintance and develops into an intimate relationship is facilitated by gaining and maintaining proximity. Extensive contact between the parents and the baby allows the parents the full sensory experience of their baby, fostering the continued development of affectional ties. Seeking and maintaining proximity arouses pleasurable feelings of intimacy. The ability of the parents and infant to communicate is important to the development of the relationship. Parents communicate through touch, cuddling and prolonged visualization; while the baby communicates through crying, grasping and visual contact. Babies are genetically programmed to respond to human interaction in order to provoke nurturing behaviour in their caregivers; within 16 hours of birth the newborn responds to human voice with coordinated, rhythmical movements. At two days old a baby can identify its mother's face and odour; by three days the baby will demonstrate a clear preference for its mother's voice.

Mothers make great efforts to establish eye contact with their babies; indeed women in all cultures instinctively interact with their babies at a distance of approximately 30 cm, which is the optimal distance to facilitate the newborn's developing vision. When the baby reciprocates eye contact, the mother exaggerates her facial expressions, maintains visual contact, slows her speech patterns and raises her voice one octave, all of which is thought to be an instinctive adaptation to the infant's developing visual and auditory ability. Reciprocity is the adaptive process that leads parents

and infant to mutually satisfying behaviours. The parents adapt their behaviour to the signals from their baby. Parents who become sensitive to their baby's needs and appropriately satisfy their baby are rewarded through the positive development of their own sense of their successful parenting ability. Parents place their infant at the centre of their life, developing a stable and permanent relationship in which they feel responsible for and committed to their baby. This commitment becomes an integral part of the relationship, ensuring the safety, growth and development of their child.

It was suggested by Klaus and Kennell (1976) that there is a critical period immediately following the birth, during which it is essential for continued contact in order that attachment can be instigated and developed. However this assumption was based on research that has been criticized for its questionable methodology and has been successfully refuted. The original research was conducted on only 28 women (14 having traditional care and 14 having extra time with their baby), results were not reported objectively and subsequent attempts to replicate the research have not been successful.

While some parents may find immediate and continued physical 'skin to skin' contact with their baby pleasurable and fulfilling, this is by no means universally experienced by all new parents and has no significant benefit to the development of the attachment relationship. Unfortunately this critical period has passed into midwifery folklore and many couples may feel pressurized into having prolonged contact with their baby at a time when they may be tired and preoccupied with their own well-being and not yet ready to establish contact. It should be remembered that all couples are unique and should be asked as labour progresses whether they want 'skin to skin' contact with their baby immediately following birth. Attachment is developmental in nature and does not operate within a limited timeframe.

Factors that may affect attachment

There are many factors within the multifactorial construct of attachment that can affect the developing relationship. Experiences of being parented, economic status, social support and perceived or actual threats to the viability of the fetus or health of the woman can have detrimental affects on the developing attachment relationship. Fundamental to the development of attachment is whether the pregnancy was planned or wanted. This does not mean that an unplanned pregnancy will result in poor attachment as the support of a special attachment figure or therapeutic counselling can facilitate the progressive development of attachment. The mother's good physical and mental health is also important to the developing relationship. A mother who is preoccupied with her own debility will be unable to initially invest the time or commitment necessary to facilitate the development of this special relationship; the attachment relationship may take longer to develop. The woman's birthing experiences can affect her ability to attach, as can the appearance, gender and perceived personality of the baby. Any prolonged separation from the baby in the early postnatal days will lead to anxiety, distress and potential feelings of inadequacy as a parent.

The birth of a sick or premature baby

The birth of a sick or premature baby is an acute emotional crisis for the woman/parents. Many parents feel anxious and guilty, blaming themselves for their baby's plight. In very preterm infants parental anxiety is often heightened by the appearance of the tiny, underdeveloped and vulnerable baby, very different from the image of their term baby they had developed during pregnancy. Parents have lost the expectation of a strong and healthy baby; as a result they initially suffer the shock and disbelief that is associated with a grief process. The potential uncertainty regarding the survival and ultimate health of very sick babies leads to intense distress, with the level of neonatal risk closely associated with the degree of emotional distress and depression experienced by the parents. This uncertainty regarding survival can result in anticipatory grief and the withdrawal of emotional attachment as the parents seek strategies to cope with the potential loss of their infant. Studies have found that mothers often feel useless and helpless when they are separated from their babies.

The care of the baby is determined by the infant's condition and the practices of the neonatal intensive care unit (NICU). As a result the women often report a lack of control over their baby's continued health and survival. Women have stated that they feel powerless, unable to protect or help their baby. The mother goes from being the sole protector of her fetus to an onlooker, watching skilled professionals provide the care, support and protection she cannot give.

In studies women reported a feeling that their babies were not theirs; that they belonged more to the nursing staff who were more adept and skilled at providing therapeutic care to the sick baby. Although research has shown that the separation caused by admission to the NICU results in disruption to the woman's attachment relationship with her baby, it has also shown that the attachment relationship continues its development once the woman has taken her baby home and is competently providing appropriate care.

In the early days of NICU development the care provided was controlled by medical needs, parental visiting was severely restricted and parents were not allowed to touch, hold or feed their babies. This has now changed and the importance of the family within care is acknowledged, as is the particular importance of maintaining mother–infant proximity and interaction. Care provided within the NICU has evolved to become receptive to the needs of the parents, with the development of family-centred care and empowered decision-making for parents. Family-centred care aims to overcome the barriers that previously disempowered the parents. It allows the parents full 24-hour access to their baby, participation in clinical decision-making and education to facilitate appropriate parenting and caring skills. Neonatal staff actively empower parents through teaching and assessing parenting skills and through the provision of appropriate information to help parents make decisions regarding their baby's medical care.

The shock of their baby's admission to NICU may result in the parents being unable to accept their parenting role and responsibility. It is therefore important to provide psychological care at this stressful time. Parental control can be facilitated by the inclusion of the parents in decision-making at an early stage, emphasizing their responsibility and providing a sense of empowerment. Parents need to be prepared before they see their baby; it can be very frightening to see a tiny, vulnerable baby hooked up to machines and covered by tubes and sensors. Simple non-medicalized explanations of the equipment being used, the baby's condition and prognosis will facilitate understanding and allow the parents to participate in decision-making. During the early stages of intensive care professional expertise is required, but as the baby's medical and care needs become less intense the parents can be taught to participate in their infant's care, providing them some degree of control and parental skill.

As the baby gets stronger it is important to provide some quiet time to promote the attachment relationship. During this time medical intervention is at a minimum so that the parents and baby can spend time getting to know each other through reciprocal interaction: touching, cuddling and continued eye contact. The provision of accommodation on NICUs allows the family to spend time getting to know the new family member and facilitates the transition to care at home.

Parents may benefit from the psychological support of parents who have previously experienced the trauma they are currently facing; this can be provided by voluntary organizations that specifically focus on offering practical and emotional support to parents and families of babies who need special or intensive care. National Information for Parents of Prematures: Education, Resources & Support (NIPPERS) and BLISSLINK (BLISS Baby Life Support Systems) are proactive groups that provide information and put parents in touch with support networks. Various forms of support can be provided to suit individual needs, with one-to-one and group support offered. NIPPERS also have a bereavement group that offers on-going support to parents whose baby has died. As the support is offered by individuals that have 'walked the same path' there is an empathy borne from experience that facilitates understanding and effective communication. Carers should be aware of local groups that offer continuing support to parents and should be able to give them information on how to contact the specialized voluntary groups.

Loss and bereavement

It is only within the last 30–40 years that childbearing loss has been acknowledged and bereaved parents have been allowed to grieve. Every year approximately 6500 babies are stillborn or die within four weeks of their birth in the UK. This equates to the death of 18 babies each day of the year. Childbearing loss, whether this occurs early in pregnancy or following the birth, is unique and painful. The parents have lost their child, their hopes, aspirations and dreams for their future family. Most couples will have made plans to incorporate the baby into their life; they may have considered their ideal birth, their preferred method to feed their baby, chosen names and made a special place in their life for their baby. Even in early pregnancy the couple will probably have already shared their news with those close to them. The loss of the child will result in a special bereavement. When those we have got to know, our family, friends and acquaintances die, they leave us with cherished memories that allow us to remember them in our own inimitable way. However when a pregnancy is lost, a baby is stillborn or dies within the first few weeks or months of life, there will have been very little time for memories to be made. The woman/couple may be afraid they will forget their baby as they have very few tangible memories to facilitate their remembrance.

It is important that those caring for the bereaved family acknowledge the death and facilitate the family's grief. Mourning is a process that takes time and psychological energy. It is important that the midwivery staff recognize that they are caring for the family at the beginning of this difficult and painful

Support groups

For bereaved parents

During early pregnancy

- Miscarriage Association www.miscarriageassociation.org.uk/
- Antenatal Results & Choices (ARC) www.arc-uk.org

Following birth

- The Stillbirth & Neonatal Death Society (SANDS) www.uk-sands.org
- The Child Bereavement Trust www.childbereavement.org.uk
- The Compassionate Friends www.tcf.org.uk
- CRUSE – Bereavement Care www.crusebereavementcare.org.uk

For specific bereavement

National Information for Parents of Prematures: Education, Resources & Support (NIPPERS) 17–21 Emerald Street, London WC1N 3QL Tel: 020 7831 9393

Twins and Multiple Birth Association (TAMBA) – Bereavement Support Group www.tamba-bsg.org.uk

Heart Line Association – for parents with a child heart defect www.heartline.org.uk

Foundation for the Study of Infant Deaths – for those parents who have suffered a cot death www.fsid.org.uk

journey. The family may need support long after the midwife's role ends.

It may be useful to some women/families to have contact numbers for voluntary organizations that will continue to provide compassionate support for as long as it is needed (see box on page 7).

Attachment and loss

Attachment is fundamental to grief. During early life experience of attachment relationships provide the individual with security and safety. Should the attachment figure disappear the child becomes distressed and angry, they search for their attachment figure and when the attachment figure returns the attachment is restored, the grief countered and the distress alleviated. Over time the individual is conditioned to expect attachment to be restored, we expect those we love to remain with us forever. When that figure dies and restoration cannot occur, the individual suffers severe loss and grief takes over.

Attachment begins in pregnancy or even earlier. Mary Ainsworth (1963, 1967) suggested that the attachment relation begins when a couple start to plan for a pregnancy, long before conception. Certainly during early pregnancy the majority of women/parents will be developing an attachment relationship with their baby, about whom they will be forming cognitive pictures, apportioning physical and behavioural characteristics based on family likenesses, idiosyncrasies and the fetus' intrauterine behaviour. The loss of this baby will inevitably result in psychological trauma and a period of mourning will be necessary to facilitate the grief process and regain psychological equilibrium. Grief is the personal experience of loss, the price paid for loving. Mourning is the process that occurs after loss that helps the individual come to terms with their loss and eventually allows them to continue with their personal journey through life. Essential to the understanding of bereavement and fundamental to the provision of care and support is an understanding that all loss is personal, individual and unique.

Normal grief reactions

Worden (2008) states that grief affects the whole person, affecting their feelings, thoughts, physical sensations and behaviour. The individual may feel sad, anxious, shocked and numb. Very often the bereaved parents become angry because they could not prevent loss and as a result of not being able to protect their child feel helpless and powerless. The woman may feel angry at being left alone; it is only she that felt her baby move within, now her womb is empty and she is alone. The individual may also feel guilty that they in some way caused the death. Certain thought patterns are common to those that mourn. The loss results in disbelief and confusion, particularly within the early days. The individual may become preoccupied with the dead baby to the exclusion of everything and everyone else. This may cause friction within a relationship. Some bereaved parents may hear their dead baby crying; some parents have stated that their arms ache to hold their baby. The loss may also cause physical symptoms that may cause concern to the bereaved. They may experience extreme fatigue, breathlessness, hollowness of the stomach and muscle weakness.

Some specific behaviours, crying for example, are frequently demonstrated by the bereaved. Most are usually transitory and resolve over time. Crying is the behaviour most associated with loss. It has been shown that tears from psychological distress are chemically different from physiological tears and may possess healing properties. The bereaved parent often becomes restless, absentminded and withdrawn, finding it difficult to sleep or eat. It should always be remembered that these reactions are individual and will take time to resolve.

The grief process

Mourning is the process that facilitates grief, it is the process that occurs following loss and gradually allows the acceptance of loss in order that the bereaved can continue their journey through life. The process is unique to each individual and has no time limits. The process has been described as being in stages or phases. However all theorists agree that the process is not sequential: the bereaved will pass through the process at their own pace, in their own sequence and may become stuck or revisit certain stages/phases. In general, the bereaved will experience disbelief, shock and numbness; yearning, anger and guilt; disorganization, depression and loss of self-esteem and finally acceptance, resolution and reorganization. Worden (2008) suggests the process of mourning is active and that the bereaved can influence their progress through grief. This model accepts the individuality of each person and allows for intervention if grief becomes protracted or abnormal. Worden describes this model as the 'tasks of mourning'. This model empowers the bereaved to move at their on pace through the painful mourning process.

> ### Tasks of mourning (Worden 2008)
>
> - Task I – To accept the reality of the loss
> - Task II – To work through the pain of grief
> - Task III – Adjust to an environment in which the deceased is missing
> - Task IV – To emotionally relocate the deceased and move on with life.

Caring for bereaved parents

For the parents the death of a baby is an intensely painful experience. There is little anyone can do to help alleviate the pain. It is a time no parent ever forgets, a time of unbearable sorrow and psychological suffering. Nevertheless, the way the parents' bereavement is managed can affect the severity and length of parental grief. Midwives, nurses and medical staff have a great responsibility to react sensitively and practically to the parents' loss. Parents will remember what was said to them and how their baby was handled. It is important to choose the words used carefully and sensitively, avoiding medical terminology that could be open to misunderstanding or misinterpretation. It is also important that other healthcare workers involved within the care are aware of the situation to avoid insensitivity or the need for parents to explain their loss, which could result in further distress.

The midwife should ensure she has all the necessary information and should answer the parent's questions honestly and fully. Remember that in the first instance the parents will be shocked and may take in only part of the information offered. Patience is important as the information may need to be repeated on several occasions. The baby should be handled sensitively and tenderly with all the care that would be afforded a healthy baby. He or she should be called by the name the parents have chosen in any communication with the parents and family. Most of all, the parents should be given the privacy, time and space to be with their baby.

The parents should be treated with respect and dignity and the significance of their loss should be acknowledged. For the health professionals it is painful to witness the suffering of the bereaved that they may feel impotent to help, but the acknowledgement of the parents' loss and the expression of sympathy will facilitate the beginning of the mourning process. Grief is intensely personal and private; care should be non-intrusive to allow the parents time and privacy to express their grief. The health professional should be working to a timescale determined by the parents' needs: some may want to spend many hours alone with their baby in the hospital setting, while others may feel more secure in their own homes, coming back later to spend time with their child. Some may even prefer to take their baby home.

It is important to enquire about the parents' beliefs. Each individual comes from a culture – national, religious and family. Each culture has its traditions and personal beliefs that need to be respected and honoured. The parents should be well informed so that they can, if they wish, participate in the management of their loss, providing them with some control over events.

Parents need accurate and comprehensive information that is communicated clearly, sensitively and in an understandable manner. The parents need to know in a factual and unbiased way about the circumstances surrounding their baby's death, the statutory and practical procedures and arrangements that must be made and the choices they have. This information is best given to the parents together. If the woman is single she will benefit from the support of trusted family or friends. Information should be consistent, coordinated and factual. If the parents do not speak fluent English, interpreters should be sought to facilitate the parents' understanding. The provision of written material in the appropriate language will reinforce the information given and allow the bereaved to revisit the information as and when they need. Effective communication is fundamental. Sufficient time should be allowed for lengthy and unhurried discussion, questions should be encouraged and all questions answered honestly.

Death at the beginning of life is a particularly difficult bereavement: the parents are saying hello and goodbye to their baby at the same time. Memories are essential to facilitate mourning, so it is important to help the woman/parents to create memories to provide a focus for their grief. The most evocative memories will be gained by allowing the parents to spend uninterrupted time with their baby, getting to know him or her. The bereaved parents may also want their family and children to meet the baby. Some parents may wish to bathe their baby and dress them in the special clothes they had chosen to take them home. A memory box can be initiated with keepsakes of their baby: sensitively taken photographs of the baby and family, ultrasound scan photographs, a lock of hair, footprints and handprints. The creation of memories will acknowledge the existence of the baby and in so doing gives permission for the woman/couple/family to grieve. Do not forget, however, that the parent's permission must be sought first; some parents may find it distressing to discover that the baby they could no longer protect was touched without consent.

Key Points

- Attachment is a unique, powerful and enduring relationship.
- The success of the individual's ability to form close attachment relationships is fundamental to the individual's ability to develop and sustain all subsequent relationships throughout their life.
- Attachment is an interactive process that begins in pregnancy and develops throughout life, it has no critical period.
- Many factors may affect the development of attachment.
- The baby will develop attachment relationships with a few important individuals, including parents, siblings, grandparents, uncles and aunts, consistent carers
- Secure attachment is crucial to provide safety and comfort to a child that is tired, distressed or presented with a challenging situation – lack of opportunity to develop selective attachments may damage the child's social and emotional development.

- The birth of a sick or premature baby which results in separation threatens the attachment relationship and necessitates sensitive, family-centred care to encourage the development of parenting responsibility and skills.
- Attachment and loss are intrinsically linked – it is attachment that causes distress when the attachment figure is lost. Therefore the loss of the 'baby' will result in psychological trauma; a period of mourning will be necessary to facilitate the grief process and regain psychological equilibrium.
- Death at the beginning of life is a particularly difficult bereavement – the parents are saying hello and goodbye to their baby at the same time.
- Sensitive, thoughtful and evidence-based care is essential to support the bereaved parents.

References

Ainsworth MDS (1963) The development of infant-mother interactions among the Ganda. In Floss BM (eds) *Determinants of Infant Behaviour.* New York: Wiley, pp. 67–112.

Ainsworth MDS (1967) *Infancy in Uganda: Infant care and the growth of love.* Baltimore: Johns Hopkins University Press.

Bowlby J (1951) Maternal care and mental health. World Health Organization Monograph (Serial No 2).

Bowlby J (1988) *Attachment and Loss*, Vol. 3: *Loss: Sadness and Depression.* London: Hogarth.

Gjerdingen DK and Chaloner K (1994) Mother's experience with household roles and social support during the first postpartum year. *Women and Health* **21**: 57–74.

Goulet C, Bell L, St CyrTribble D, Paul D and Lang A (1998) A concept analysis of parent-infant attachment. *Journal of Advanced Nursing* **28**: 1071–1081.

Katz-Rothman B (1986) *The Tentative Pregnancy: Prenatal Diagnosis and the Future of Motherhood.* New York: Viking Penguin.

Klaus MH and Kennell JH (1976) *Parent–Infant Bonding.* St Louis: Mosby.

Raphael-Leff J (2005) *Psychological Processes of Childbearing*, 4th edn. London: Chapman and Hall.

Siddiqui A, Hagglof B and Eisemann M (1999) An exploration of prenatal attachment in Swedish expectant women. *Journal of Reproductive and Infant Psychology* **17**: 369–380.

Siddiqui A, Hagglof B and Eisemann M (2000) Own memories of upbringing as a determinant of prenatal attachment in expectant women. *Journal of Reproductive and Infant Psychology* **18**: 67–74.

Worden JW (2008) *Grief Counselling & Grief Therapy: A handbook for mental health practitioners*, 4th edn. New York: Springer Publishing.

Further reading

Schott J, Henley A and Kohner N (2007) *Pregnancy, Loss and the Death of a Baby: Guidelines for professionals*, 3rd edn. London: SANDS.

CHAPTER 2

TRANSITION TO EXTRAUTERINE LIFE

Debbie Holmes

OVERVIEW

This chapter looks at fetal development, the birth process and the early days of the infant's life in relation to the transition from life as a fetus to that of a newborn infant. Care by birth attendants is described. Newborn resuscitation procedures as recommended by the Resuscitation Council (UK) are included.

Introduction

The transition from fetal life to the life of a neonate is, for most infants, a relatively straightforward process. The complexities involved, however, mean that some infants experience a delay or, in some cases, major problems related to their anatomy or physiological status. Those infants who show serious signs of not adapting to extrauterine life may have a severe problem such as a complex cardiac abnormality. A difficulty with transition can have a negative effect on subsequent development. It is imperative that midwives, nurses and doctors are alert to signs that the transition may not be progressing normally to enable intervention and optimize the infant's chance for normal development.

The miraculous move from intrauterine to extrauterine life is reliant on anatomical and physiological processes during fetal development, the birth process and the early days of life as a newborn infant. 'Parents to be' should wherever possible consider their own health prior to conceiving, so as to give the fetus optimum conditions to begin normal development. The mother then needs to take care of her health in pregnancy and attend for antenatal care as soon as possible. This will not guarantee a smooth transition, but will increase the chances and enable detection of those fetuses who may be at risk of experiencing a problem.

Cardiovascular system

Fetal development

The cardiovascular system develops early as the embryo has increasing needs for nutrition and oxygen. The development may be influenced by both genetic and environmental factors. Malformations of the heart and vessels are possible as the cardiac development is such a complex process (Moore and Persuad, 2007). The fetal circulatory system differs from that of the adult (Figure 2.1). The cardiovascular system, including the temporary structures, the ductus venosus, the foramen ovale and the ductus arteriosis, allow blood to be diverted from the lungs and allow for placental oxygenation to take place. The temporary structures have specific functions (Table 2.1).

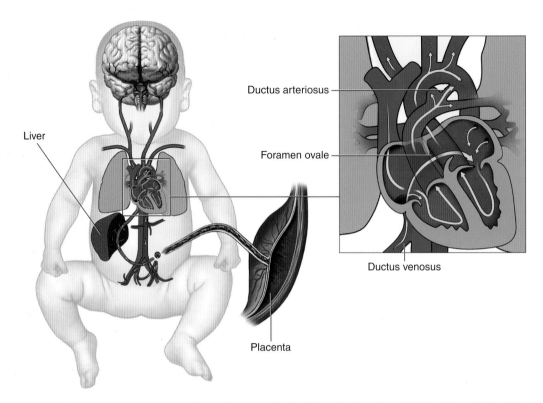

Ductus arteriosus

Foramen ovale

Liver

Ductus venosus

Placenta

Figure 2.1 Diagrammatic representation of fetal circulation. (Medical Illustration Copyright © 2009 Nucleus Medical Media, Inc., all rights reserved. www.nucleusinc.com)

Table 2.1 Functions of the temporary structures

Structure	Function before birth	Following birth
Ductus venosus	Shunts blood away from the liver	Sphincter close to umbilical vein constricts and ductus venosus closes
Foramen ovale	Shunts blood from the right to the left atrium of the heart	Closes due to negative pressure in right atrium
Ductus arteriosus	Shunts blood from the pulmonary artery to the aorta	Constricts and closes

Oxygenated blood from the placenta reaches the fetus via the umbilical vein which has two main branches, one that carries blood to the portal vein of the liver and one (the ductus venosus) that takes blood to the inferior vena cava. The blood in the ductus venosus is under high pressure because it has a narrow diameter; the blood does not mix thoroughly with the blood in the vena cava and is therefore still rich in oxygen when it arrives in the right atrium. Most of this blood is shunted directly from the right atrium into the left atrium via the foramen ovale, mixing with a small amount of deoxygenated blood from the lungs. (The fetal lungs provide no oxygen at this point, but they do utilize oxygenated blood for growth and development.) The blood then enters the left ventricle and is pumped to the body through the aorta. The most oxygenated blood supplies the vital organs: the brain, the heart and the liver. The remainder of the blood from the ductus venosus passes from the right atrium to the right ventricle and is pumped into the pulmonary artery. The majority of the blood is diverted away from the lungs via the ductus arteriosus into the aorta.

At birth

The newborn's circulatory system has to move from a placental exchange of oxygen and carbon dioxide to a pulmonary exchange of gases. Some of these changes are immediate, but some can take longer. Following birth and the cessation of blood flow in the umbilical cord the pressure in the right atrium falls as the blood in the ductus venosus ceases to flow and the sphincter close to the umbilical vein constricts. As the lungs expand, pulmonary vascular resistance falls and blood flows to the lungs which then become the organs of gas exchange. The foramen ovale and ductus ateriosus both close.

Cord clamping

There has been debate on whether or not there should be a delay in the clamping of the cord to enable the newborn to receive as much fetal blood via the umbilical cord as possible to improve iron levels. This does carry a small increased risk of jaundice and polycythemia (McDonald and Middleton, 2008). There is some evidence from high-income countries (where anaemia in babies is less prevalent than in low-income countries) that delayed cord clamping reduces the chance of an anaemic infant. This also applies to the evidence that delayed cord clamping could increase the risk of hyperbilirubinaemia known as jaundice (see Chapter 9).

In the UK, however, active management of the third stage (delivery of the placenta and control of haemorrhage) is recommended by the National Institute for Health and Clinical Excellence (NICE) (2007). This includes early clamping and cutting of the cord following administration of a drug to contract the uterus. It is recognized, however, that a physiological third stage may be preferable for some women and this includes no drugs and no clamping of the cord until pulsation has ceased. Many women will choose this option and anyone doing so should be supported by the professionals caring for her.

Pulmonary system

Fetal development

The development of the lungs is dependent upon the presence of adequate amniotic fluid and fetal breathing movements. Although the lungs are mostly inactive during fetal life and are not responsible for gaseous exchange, fetal breathing movements do occur and contribute to fetal development. These movements increase in frequency as term approaches. While the fetus is in the uterus, the fetal lungs are filled with alveolar fluid. At birth this is no longer required and it ceases to be produced, a process thought to be under the influence of adrenaline.

Production of surfactant is another important part of the successful transition for the fetus. The alveoli in the lungs are lined with surfactant, phospholipids that prevent the alveoli collapsing during expiration by lowering surface tension. The more mature the fetus, the more chance it has of having sufficient quantities of surfactant. A deficiency of surfactant in premature infants can be responsible for respiratory distress syndrome (see Chapter 11). The production of surfactant may be influenced by cortisol, growth restriction of the fetus or ruptured membranes. Steroids are sometimes given in the antenatal period to mothers at risk of preterm birth to increase the production of this vital substance. Current evidence suggests a single course of two injections of corticosteroids to the mother 12–24 hours apart at between 28 and 34 weeks' gestation may be helpful (Royal College of Obstetricians and Gynaecologists, 2004).

At birth

During a normal labour with a healthy fetus the amount of oxygen in the fetal blood decreases and the level of carbon dioxide increases. This is due to strong contractions of the uterus temporarily interrupting the flow of oxygenated blood to the fetus. The cord is also compressed during the descent of the fetus, again reducing oxygen. This is further exaggerated when the cord no longer supplies oxygenated blood after being cut or upon cessation of blood flow naturally at the time of birth. This gaseous status stimulates the respiratory centre in the brain.

Other factors affect the first inhalation at birth. One is the compression of the chest wall of the fetus during descent through the birth canal. As the body of the newborn is delivered the chest wall expands and this encourages inspiration, expanding the alveoli, which, in the presence of sufficient surfactant, will stay inflated. This process will also force out any remaining alveolar fluid which will subsequently be reabsorbed by lymphatics and the pulmonary capillaries. Some fluid will have been expelled as the chest wall has been compressed during the journey through the pelvis.

The neonate who is born by caesarean section will not have undergone the 'physiological' squeeze through the birth canal and if there has been no labour preceding the surgery the newborn will also not have experienced the stimulation of a rising carbon dioxide level in the blood. Stimuli from the external world such as touch, temperature, noise and light also play a part in eliciting the first inhalation.

Neurological

At birth

The respiratory effort and the movement of the muscles of the respiratory system are reliant on the respiratory centre in the brain which, if transition has been normal, has been stimulated into action by the carbon dioxide and oxygen ratios in the fetal blood and external stimuli such as the change in temperature and touch. As breathing becomes established the cells in the medulla respond to the circulating carbon dioxide levels in the blood. If a newborn has been subjected to severe hypoxia during labour the respiratory centre in the brain may not function to stimulate respiration. These newborns will require life support from trained professionals. Certain drugs such as pethidine and heroin can also have this effect by crossing the placental site during labour and depressing the respiratory centre.

It is possible for the newborn infant to tolerate a longer period of hypoxia than a child or adult, but the ability to do this is dependent upon the experience of the fetus in the uterus during the labour. An already hypoxic newborn will have less capability than a baby born following a normal labour.

Placenta

Normal placental development is required for the transition to be normal. The placenta is responsible for exchange of substances between the fetal and maternal circulations during pregnancy. Abnormalities in development of the placenta or pathology arising in pregnancy can result in placental insufficieny compromising the process of transition. A poorly functioning placenta will present an already compromised fetus to the birth process, which may further exacerbate hypoxia, leading to a newborn requiring resuscitation to assist transition.

The placenta is an amazing fetal organ. It is responsible for gaseous exchange of oxygen and carbon dioxide and maintains the acid–base status. The chorionic villi (finger-like projections of placental tissue) bathe in maternal blood that fills the intervillous spaces and by processes of diffusion (gases moving from an area of high concentration to an area of low concentration) take up the oxygen and supply the fetus with this via the umbilical vein. Carbon dioxide is transported back to the placenta via the umbilical arteries to the intervillous spaces around the chorionic villi and through the process of diffusion goes back to the maternal circulation for excretion. Nutrients for the fetus are also supplied in this manner and waste products transported back to the maternal circulation.

The placenta also forms a protective barrier to some substances and it also excretes hormones.

When abnormal placentation occurs the trophoblast invasion in early pregnancy fails or only partially occurs. The maternal circulation plays an important role in supplying oxygen-rich blood to the placental site and to the fetus. Large amounts of maternal blood fill the intervillous spaces and 500–600 mL of blood pass over the area per minute (Holmes and Baker, 2006). If the placentation has not occurred under optimum circumstances the fetus may receive suboptimal oxygen and nutrient supplies for development. Abnormal placentation can result in conditions such as pre-eclampsia, a condition associated with high blood pressure in the mother. When the blood passing over the placental site is under pressure the uptake of oxygen and nutrients can be affected, resulting in a fetus that is small for gestational age. The maternal spiral arteries that supply the chorionic villi are narrowed in this condition and blood flow is restricted due to the absence of normal developmental changes. Normally the spiral arteries undergo a transformation that reduces resistance and increases blood flow to the placenta.

Intrauterine growth restriction can also occur when the placenta has not developed sufficiently or has been subjected to damage by an antepartum haemorrhage and is unable to supply adequate nutrients and oxygen for normal growth. Abruptio placentae, a condition in pregnancy where part of the placenta becomes detached from the uterine wall, can also result in poor growth and development because the detached placenta does not supply adequate nutrition and oxygen. Smoking in pregnancy may also reduce the optimum blood supply and uptake of nutrients, resulting in a fetus with restricted growth. Other maternal conditions associated with reduced placental size and functioning include severe diabetes mellitus, antiphospholipid syndrome and chronic hypertension (Holmes and Baker, 2006).

Examining the placenta post birth can often reveal some answers as to why a newborn has experienced difficulty with transition. Areas of infarction (lobes of the placenta which have had no blood supply) are sometimes seen, explaining why a fetus was already compromised before undergoing the birth process.

Antenatal detection of abnormal fetal growth is important. The height of the uterus can be palpated and measured during the antenatal period and some regions of the UK have adopted customized growth charts to identify the fetus at risk. Attempts to detect abnormal fetal growth by abdominal measurements of the mother have had limited success (Neilson, 2000) but technologies such as ultrasound scanning and Doppler techniques are commonly used to identify the fetus at risk of a complicated transition.

Metabolism

Healthy newborns utilize glucose to assist with their transition. This provides the energy to tolerate the birth process and the effort of initiating the first breaths. When the available glucose has been used, metabolism produces energy in the form of ketones and lactates (Cornblath et al., 2000). This is similar to the way athletes can produce energy when running a marathon. It is a protective measure and if the newborn is short of glucose it can assist to produce more energy prior to the liver taking over the function. A newborn who cannot use this type of metabolism may have difficulty during transition as low blood glucose in a compromised newborn can cause other problems. This type of metabolism can also assist during the establishment of milk production in the mother. Around day 3–4 newborns can begin to utilize the fat they are born with to process into ketones which are a form of energy. Ketones in the neonate

rise on days 2–3 even in a neonate who is able to benefit from a good lactation (Cornblath et al., 2000)

Hypoglycaemia

Healthy term babies are capable of managing their energy requirements and breastfed newborns do not need to be routinely monitored for blood glucose levels. Some newborns are more at risk of developing hypoglycaemia than others and do require the monitoring of their blood glucose as part of early care:

- Intrauterine growth-restricted newborns: these babies will have utilized protein breakdown in their adaptation to extrauterine life but will have little fat to convert to ketones as protein breakdown slows.

- Newborns whose mothers are diabetic: these babies have become accustomed to higher levels of blood glucose during uterine life and are at risk of hypoglycaemia as they begin to regulate their own glycaemic status.

- Preterm newborns undergo 'stress' to be born and utilize readily available stores of glucose. Their reserves of brown fat are depleted as these are laid down in the latter weeks of fetal development. Preterm babies can rapidly become hypoglycaemic as it takes large amounts of energy to maintain their transition to extrauterine life.

- Newborns who have experienced fetal distress: these babies may have used readily available stores during their transition to extrauterine life; they may well also have undergone varying degrees of resuscitation which also utilizes glucose energy.

Gastrointestinal

The normal term neonate who has made a successful transition to newborn life will usually have a digestive system ready to receive and digest breast milk. If the mother chooses to breast or artificially feed it is good practice to observe the baby feed initially.

Most newborns pass meconium (first stool) in the first 24 hours and this may happen at or around the time of birth. This initial bowel movement should be recorded to exclude anal atresia (absence of the anal opening). Meconium is composed of the contents of the gastrointestinal tract that were acquired during fetal life in the uterus. It contains amniotic fluid, vernix, lanugo and other secretions. Once a newborn begins to digest milk the bowel movements will change from the dark, sticky, black/green meconium to a changing stool that is often brown in colour.

Newborns also often pass urine at the time of birth and if observed this should be recorded. It can be quite difficult to detect once the newborn is wearing disposable nappies.

Cognitive development

Those newborns who make a successful transition will from an early stage begin to display evidence of their growing cognitive development that began during intrauterine life. Newborns who have experienced a normal transitional period are often very alert immediately after the birth and will have their eyes open and be responsive to smell which will help them seek out the nipple for food.

Immediate care for babies experiencing normal transition

Signs of normal transition

- The newborn infant cries or gasps within seconds.
- The infant rapidly becomes pink but may be born blue.
- Heart rate 120–150 bpm.
- Breathing adequately by 90 seconds (Resuscitation Council (UK), 2006).
- It is normal for peripheral circulation to be delayed, resulting in 'blue' hands and feet.
- It is normal for the newborn to lose heat through evaporation and conduction if not prevented.

Immediate care requires the neonate to be dried to prevent heat loss as this can quickly lead to hypothermia and a cascade of problems affecting adaptation to extrauterine life (see Chapter 8). While drying the newborn the birth attendant will be stimulating inspiration by touch if this has not already occurred. The birth attendant will also be assessing the condition of the newborn with the Apgar score, a standardized assessment record to identify a baby who may or not be making a smooth transition (Table 2.2). The Apgar score should be awarded at 1 and 5 minutes with a healthy neonate. If the newborn appears at birth to have made a smooth transition and is mostly pink, breathing and maybe crying, he or she is passed to the mother. Skin-to-skin contact is preferable to prevent further heat loss and regulate heartbeat. The room must be warm and draught free, and exposed parts of the newborn's body not in contact with mother's skin may need to be covered with a blanket to prevent further heat loss. Any wet towels should be discarded and replaced with a warm, dry towel or blanket.

If the mother does not wish to have skin-to-skin contact or is unable to provide it her partner may provide it or the baby is dried and wrapped in a blanket. All mothers should be offered skin-to-skin contact with their newborn regardless of intention of feeding choice. If the transition has been normal the newborn infant is mostly alert, so this is a good time to encourage the first feed.

The newborn will continue to be monitored for normal transition. Following a period of skin-to-skin contact that should last as long as the mother wishes or until the first breastfeed, the birth attendant should ensure an initial top to toe examination is performed. If this initial assessment is normal the newborn is weighed and transferred with the mother to the postnatal ward, if in hospital.

Table 2.2   The Apgar score

	0	1	2
Heart rate	Absent	Below 100	Above 100
Respiratory effort	Absent	Gasping or irregular	Regular or crying
Muscle tone	Limp	Some flexion	Active, good tone
Response to stimulation	Nil	Grimace	Cry or cough
Colour	Pale or blue	Body pink, extremities blue	Pink all over

Observations of the newborn's condition should continue and the mother should receive advice from the midwife and healthcare workers on what is normal for the baby and what should alert her to seek help.

Delayed or abnormal transition

Healthcare professionals in attendance around the time of birth and the early neonatal period need to be aware of risk factors that may lead to delayed transition (Table 2.3).

Other possible causes of delayed transition

Congenital heart defects (CHD)

These may not always be obvious at birth and the neonate may appear to make an initial transition that appears relatively smooth. Approximately 4600 babies are born each year in the UK with congenital heart defects and they are responsible for significant infant morbidity and mortality (Petersen *et al.*, 2003). In the light of improved treatments and prognosis it is crucial that these babies are identified early to optimize chances of survival and long-term development. Some hospitals in the UK are using pulse oximetry in trials to detect babies who may have heart defects early in their neonatal life as up to half can be missed even with ultrasound in pregnancy and clinical examination after birth. This could become a valuable screening tool.

Newborn life support

If risk factors are identified and considered significant then someone with advanced neonatal resuscitation skills should be available for the birth. In all cases (including the absence of any risk factors) the birth attendant has a responsibility to be up to date with basic life support. An otherwise normal pregnancy followed by a normal birth can still leave a newborn with problems making the transition to extrauterine life. The following guidelines are not intended to replace a recognized training course such as the Newborn Life Support Course (NLS) or trust-approved mandatory training.

Table 2.3   Risk factors that may lead to delayed transition

Antepartum risk factors	Pregnancy-induced hypertension
	Chronic hypertension
	Pre-eclampsia
	Eclampsia
	Diabetes
	Renal disease
	Sickle cell anaemia
	Severe anaemia
	Pulmonary disease
	Epilepsy
	Severe maternal infections
	Rhesus isoimmunization
	Placental conditions: pre-eclampsia, eclampsia insufficiency (may be known as result of Doppler studies)
	Post mature >42 weeks
	Antepartum haemorrhage
	Multiple pregnancy
Intrapartum risk factors	Malpresentations and their management
	Instrumental deliveries
	Caesarean section
	Maternal sedation or analgesia
	Anaesthesia
	Maternal substance misuse including tobacco and alcohol
	Prolonged or precipitate labour
	Prolonged rupture of membranes
	Hypertonic uterine contractions
	Placental abruption
	Cord compression or prolapse
Fetal risk factors	Birth injury
	Prematurity
	Postmaturity
	Small for gestational age
	Large for gestational age
	Infection
	Metabolic disorders
	Fetal distress
	Meconium in the amniotic fluid

Occasionally babies will need some assistance at birth if transition to extrauterine life is delayed. It is not always possible to anticipate when babies might need some intervention, therefore midwives should be aware of potential problems and call for suitable help to support them with a baby who may need resuscitation. It is usual to call for the help of another midwife, an advanced neonatal nurse practitioner (ANNP) or a paediatrician. It is better to call for help early rather than once the baby has been delivered, when the help could be held up or late arriving. It should be noted that the strategy for resuscitation is based upon Resuscitation Council (UK) (2006) guidelines. Midwives should have yearly mandatory training on newborn resuscitation and should adhere to their trust policy on resuscitation. It should be noted that newborn resuscitation discussed in this chapter varies slightly from how parents will be taught to resuscitate their baby (see Chapter 15), although some of the main principles are the same.

Equipment

A standard resuscitaire should be available in every high-risk delivery room and theatre. Low-risk rooms and planned deliveries in the home should have some basic resuscitation equipment available. The midwife will usually check the equipment when the woman is in established labour. However, anyone who is called to delivery to resuscitate the baby should not assume that the equipment has been checked and should test it themself before it is used.

Resuscitation equipment list

- Firm stable surface
- Clock
- Radiant heater
- Light
- Dry warm towels
- Plastic bags for preterm babies
- Hats
- Face masks (various sizes)
- Self-inflating bag (500 mL) with pop-off valve
- 'T' piece attached to a gas supply with blow-off valve
- Laryngoscope
- Stethoscope
- Guedel airways (various sizes)
- Wide-bore suction catheter
- Drugs

The single most important thing the midwife can do is dry the baby thoroughly, remove the wet towel and wrap the baby in dry warm towels and put the baby onto a pre-warmed resuscitaire or other firm surface. It is good practice to turn the clock on when resuscitation begins to allow for accurate handover and contemporaneous documentation. If the midwife has any concerns about the baby's condition at birth she should call for help using the accepted trust method of contacting further support. Once the baby has been dried and covered the midwife can make an assessment of the baby's condition. Handling and drying the baby will be sufficient stimulation; it is not appropriate to apply any painful stimuli. The four elements to the assessment are colour, tone, breathing and heart rate (Table 2.4).

Table 2.4   Four elements of assessment

Colour	White	Blue	Pink
Tone	Floppy	Flexed	
Breathing	Apnoeic	Gasping/ irregular breaths	Regular breathing
Heart Rate	Absent	<100	>100

Colour, tone and breathing can all be easily assessed by observation. The heart rate, however, needs to be assessed with a stethoscope placed over the apex beat and listened to for a short time to identify whether the heart rate is slow or fast. It is not necessary to listen to the heart for a full minute for an accurate heart rate, an estimate of whether it is over 100 bpm will be sufficient. If a stethoscope is not available, palpating the apex or the base of the umbilicus will also give the midwife an indication of the heart rate although this is less reliable than listening with a stethoscope. It is important to assess the heart rate before any steps of resuscitation are taken, since an increase in heart rate is an excellent indicator that the intervention that has been used has been effective.

Airway

The baby's head should be put in a neutral position to open the airway (Figure 2.2). In a floppy baby the airway will be occluded because of a loss in pharyngeal

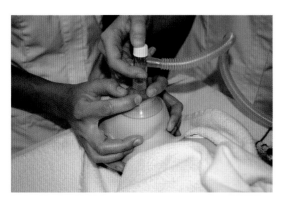

Figure 2.2 Neutral position and position of face mask

tone. The large occiput will force the head into a flexed position and will prevent the baby from breathing. Establishing a neutral head position will allow the airway to open. If the baby is still not breathing, five *inflation* breaths need to be given using an appropriately sized face mask, which should fit over the nose and mouth but should not cover the orbits of the eyes. Applying downward pressure of the mask onto the face makes a good seal.

The inflation breaths should last for 2–3 seconds at a pressure of 30 cmH$_2$0 for a term baby; these inflation breaths will push the lung fluid out of the alveoli and replace the fluid with air. If the baby is not breathing, the inflation breaths will attempt to move the fluid from the lungs. Therefore the chest may not rise with the first few inflation breaths as the fluid is being moved from the lungs but chest movement should be seen by the fourth or fifth breath if the technique is correct and the airway is open. If the inflation breaths are successful, chest movement will be seen and, on reassessment, an increase in the heart rate will be heard. In severely asphyxiated babies the heart rate may not respond as quickly to inflation breaths.

Concentrating on the airway and taking time to ensure that the airway is open is crucial since the baby's condition will not change and the resuscitation cannot progress until an airway is established and chest movement is seen. There are two other airway manoeuvres that can be used if the neutral position is not successful. They are either a jaw thrust (single or two handed) or insertion of an oropharyngeal airway. A jaw thrust will lift the tongue from the back of the throat and open the airway. The resuscitator can do this using one hand or, if a helper is present, two hands may make the manoeuvre more secure and

inflation breaths can be given using either of these techniques.

Alternatively, a Guedel airway will pull the tongue forward out of the oropharynx. The size of the Guedel airway should be carefully measured in order for it to be an effective method of airway control. The flange of the airway should be placed at the centre of the lips and the end should reach the angle of the jaw. The Guedel airway should only be inserted using direct vision with the aid of a laryngoscope. Once a clear airway has been established and the five inflation breaths have been successful the midwife should reassess the baby's colour, tone, breathing and heart rate.

Breathing

If the baby is still not breathing but the heart rate has increased, *ventilation* breaths can be given. These breaths are quicker and should be given at a rate of 30 per minute, reassessing after 30 seconds. If the baby is still not breathing but the heart rate is over 100 bpm, a further 15 ventilation breaths should be given until the baby starts to breathe independently.

Circulation

The aim of cardiac compressions is to move the oxygenated blood from the pulmonary veins to the coronary arteries, to effectively 'bump start' the heart. Following the successful five inflation breaths (as shown by chest movement), on reassessment, if the heart rate has not increased cardiac compressions should be commenced.

The midwife should encircle the chest with both hands with the thumbs placed on the sternum, 1 cm below the inter-nipple line. The thumbs press down on the sternum firmly and quickly approximately one-third of the anterior–posterior (AP) diameter. The ratio of compressions to respirations is 3:1 and this needs to be performed for 30 seconds, after which reassessment takes place. The quality of the compressions cannot be overemphasized, with the relaxation phase being as important as the compression phase, since this is when the ventricles will refill with blood. There should be about 90 compressions and 30 respirations in a minute, which is sometimes difficult to achieve. However, the quality is more important than the quantity. Reassessment should take place every 30 seconds and once the heart rate is rising and is above 100 bpm cardiac compressions can be stopped.

Table 2.5   Drug doses used in resuscitation

Drug	Preparation	Dose	Route
Adrenaline	1:10 000	10 µg/kg (0.1 mL/kg)	UVC
Sodium bicarbonate	4.2%	1-2 mmol/kg (2–4 mL/kg)	UVC
Dextrose	10%	250 mg/kg (2.5 mL/kg)	UVC
Volume (rarely)	0.9% Saline	10 mL/kg	UVC

UVC, umbilical venous catheter.
Resuscitation Council (UK) (2006).

Drugs

If a baby has not responded to the above interventions, it is usual to consider administrating some drugs. If the baby's condition is such that drugs are needed, the outlook is poor. However, it is worthwhile giving drugs via an umbilical venous catheter to try to improve the outcome. A peripheral venous cannula and the intramuscular route of administration of drugs will not be effective in such babies since the peripheral circulation will be shut down and drugs will pool in the tissues rather than circulating effectively.

A catheter or feeding tube can be inserted into the umbilical vein and the drugs and doses listed in Table 2.5 can be administered. Note that volume is rarely given to babies in resuscitation although the dose is indicated above.

When to stop

The decision to stop the resuscitation is usually made by a senior doctor. It is not within the remit of the midwife to make the decision alone. The doctor may wish to do some further tests on the baby before the resuscitation is ended and for this reason sometimes the baby is transferred to the neonatal unit for further treatment and investigations. The general outlook is poor for those babies who still have an absent heart rate after 10 minutes of good-quality resuscitation.

Special circumstances

The algorithm for resuscitation is the same for all situations but some other considerations need to be adhered to in certain cases.

Preterm babies

Babies born before 30 weeks' gestation will get cold very quickly. The head should be dried and a hat placed on the head, the baby's body should not be dried and the baby should be put into a plastic bag. It is essential that the radiant heater is switched on to full power: the heat will warm the baby in its plastic bag and will prevent heat loss. The airway manoeuvres are the same as for the term baby, but because the lungs are fragile the pressure of the inflation and ventilation breaths should commence at 20–25 cmH$_2$O to prevent over-inflation and trauma.

Meconium

If meconium is present at delivery the baby should be carefully assessed. The majority of babies will not have inhaled any particulate matter into the lungs, so if the baby is born crying, no resuscitation is required, the baby simply needs drying, covering and given to mum. If floppy and not breathing, however, the baby should be dried and covered, the head put into the neutral position and the larynx inspected using a laryngoscope. Any meconium that is visible must be sucked out using a wide-bore sucker. Once the meconium has been cleared, five inflation breaths can be given at pressures of 30 cmH$_2$O and the algorithm can continue as above.

Congenital abnormality

Most abnormalities are detected by ultrasound scan antenatally, however, occasionally babies are born with unexpected problems. The resuscitation algorithm should be adhered to even when there is an abnormality present. However, if there is a facial abnormality such as cleft lip/palate or Pierre Robin Sequence it may be difficult to achieve a good seal and the airway could be compromised. In such cases a Guedel airway is recommended to keep the airway patent.

Communication and documentation

The midwife should endeavour to communicate with the parents, as the mother at least will be in the room whilst the resuscitation is taking place and will be worried, even if their baby is only on the resuscitaire for a short time. An explanation of what is happening and keeping them up-to-date using jargon-free language will help to alleviate their fears. However, if the baby is unresponsive and the resuscitation prolonged realistic information from a senior practitioner will be required. The information given to the parents should be checked for understanding because stressful situations can alter their comprehension.

Communication with other professionals is also important and a verbal handover should be given to anyone who comes to help with the situation. All documentation should be written in chronological order with objective facts. The terms 'anoxia', 'hypoxia' and 'asphyxia' should be avoided (Resuscitation Council (UK), 2006) as these are vague terms and cannot be substantiated.

Care following resuscitation

Most babies will recover quickly once they are put on the resuscitaire and the airway is opened. These babies can be given to the mother for skin-to-skin contact and normal postnatal care can resume. Some babies may need subsequent care on the neonatal unit and will need to be transferred either on the resuscitaire or in a transport incubator. The midwife should make sure that baby is correctly labelled before it leaves the delivery room. A post-resuscitation temperature and blood glucose would also be useful prior to admission to the neonatal unit.

CASE HISTORY

The community midwife is called to a woman in labour at home with her first baby. It is planned to have the birth in hospital with the community midwife supporting. On arriving at the house Sarah is already in the advanced stages of labour and is beginning to have the urge to push her baby out. Due to the distance for travel and the normality of the pregnancy a decision is made between the mother and the midwife to birth the baby at home. A second midwife is called.

The birth is normal and the baby makes his first gasp within seconds and his colour is a healthy pink; a beautiful drug-free normal birth. As the midwives are attending to post-birth duties and the mother and baby are experiencing 'skin to skin' the midwife notes that the baby has mild cyanosis of the lips, warmth is assured and the baby is encouraged to breastfeed. As the baby breastfeeds the colour turns once again to pink. Respirations, temperature and pulse rate are all within normal limits. After breastfeeding the colour of the baby once again changes, but appears to resolve almost immediately. The GP is called and informed of the concerns and he visits to perform a neonatal examination.

The GP finds no abnormalities and leaves the midwives to continue their duties; the baby at this time is pink. The pattern of colour changes persists and the midwife decides to call the local special care baby unit to admit the baby who is now over an hour old. The ambulance is called and as a precaution facial oxygen is commenced although the baby continues to act normally in every other way and even has another feed at the breast.

The baby and mother are transferred via ambulance and the midwife follows. On arrival the baby is examined and oxygen saturation measured; the oxygen levels are suboptimal. The baby is quickly examined and investigations performed. The baby is diagnosed with transposition of the great arteries and transferred to a unit where surgery is performed. The baby recovers well and is sent home shortly afterwards.

In this case it was the midwives' visual skills and intuition that were able to facilitate appropriate referral and allow early diagnosis and treatment to be administered.

Transposition of great arteries

In this condition the pulmonary artery may leave the left ventricle instead of the right and the aorta arises from the right ventricle. When this occurs oxygenated blood goes back to the lungs and poorly oxygenated blood circulates around the body. If the ductus arteriosis remains open or there is a septal defect these newborns can compensate and appear to make an initial transition that is normal but will show symptoms soon after birth.

Key Points

- Most babies make a smooth transition to extrauterine life.
- Fetal and placental development are complex and can affect the transition to extrauterine life.
- The birth process is challenging for the fetus and can compromise transition.

- Midwives and health professionals working with neonates must be trained to observe for deviations from normal transition.
- Neonatal resuscitation techniques require training and regular updating.

References

Cornblath M, Hawdon J, Williams A, Aynsley-Green A, Ward-Platt M, Schwartz R and Kalhan S (2000) Controversies regarding definition of neonatal hypoglycaemia: suggested operational thresholds. *Paediatrics* **105**: 1141–1145.

Holmes D and Baker P (eds) (2006) *Ten Teachers in Midwifery*. London: Hodder Arnold.

McDonald SJ and Middleton P (2008) Effect of timing of umbilical cord clamping of term infants on maternal and neonatal outcomes. *Cochrane Database of Systematic Reviews* (**2**): CD004074.

Moore K and Persaud T (2007) *The Developing Human: Clinically oriented embryology*, 7th edn. Philadelphia: Saunders.

Neilson JP (2000) Symphysis–fundal height measurement in pregnancy. *Cochrane Database of Systematic Reviews* (**2**): CD000944.

NICE (National Institute for Health and Clinical Excellence) (2007) *Intrapartum Care. Care of healthy women and their babies during childbirth*. London: Royal College of Obstetricians and Gynaecologists.

Petersen S, Peto V and Rayner M (2003) *Congenital Heart Disease Statistics*. London: British Heart Foundation.

Resuscitation Council (UK) (2006) *Newborn Life Support*, 2nd edn. London: Resuscitation Council (UK).

Royal College of Obstetricians and Gynaecologists (2004) *Antenatal Corticosteroids to Prevent Respiratory Distress Syndrome*. Clinical Guideline No.7. London: RCOG.

CHAPTER 3

NEWBORN SCREENING AND IMMUNIZATION

Linda Wylie

OVERVIEW

Infant mortality rates were very high only a century ago, yet today in the UK women and their families expect and usually have healthy babies with a good life expectancy. Even babies with life-threatening conditions have a greatly improved quality of life. Factors that have contributed to these improvements are better living conditions, good nutrition and major advances in medical treatments. Two areas that have had a huge impact on the improvement in infant mortality rates are the introduction of neonatal screening and major immunization programmes. This chapter will examine these areas within the UK today.

Neonatal screening tests

The blood spot test

Every mother has come to expect her newborn infant to undergo a heel prick test within a few days of birth and she looks forward to this with a mixture of apprehension and reassurance: apprehension that her baby has to go through what appears to be a painful test but at the same time reassurance that the test will identify congenital disorders that her infant may have in order for treatment to be initiated quickly.

Newborn screening began in the 1960s after Dr Robert Guthrie developed a simple blood test for phenylketonuria. The newborn blood spot screening test, once known as the Guthrie test, is offered to all mothers between the fifth and eighth day after the baby's birth and identifies relatively rare conditions which, if not identified early, can have a serious effect on the infant's health. The majority of babies will be found to have none of these conditions, but for those who do, treatment will often prevent severe mental and/or physical disability.

The blood spot test is undertaken by obtaining specimens of blood on special filter paper (Figure 3.1) which then undergo tandem mass spectrometry. Over 150 disorders can be detected in this way (Frye, 2007)

but many of these disorders are unsuitable for neonatal screening as they do not fulfil the UK criteria for screening (UK National Screening Committee, 2003) (see box on page 24). To summarize these criteria, only those conditions that can be treated, can be reliably detected and are economically viable are routinely screened for in all babies.

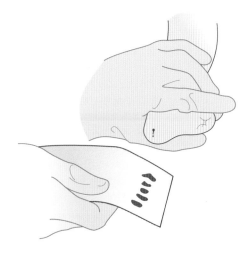

Figure 3.1 Undertaking the blood spot test

Criteria for appraising the viability, effectiveness and appropriateness of a screening programme

Ideally all the following criteria should be met before screening for a condition is initiated:

The condition

1 The condition should be an important health problem.

2 The epidemiology and natural history of the condition, including development from latent to declared disease, should be adequately understood and there should be a detectable risk factor, disease marker, latent period or early symptomatic stage.

3 All the cost-effective primary prevention interventions should have been implemented as far as practicable.

4 If the carriers of a mutation are identified as a result of screening the natural history of people with this status should be understood, including the psychological implications.

The test

5 There should be a simple, safe, precise and validated screening test.

6 The distribution of test values in the target population should be known and a suitable cut-off level defined and agreed.

7 The test should be acceptable to the population.

8 There should be an agreed policy on the further diagnostic investigation of individuals with a positive test result and on the choices available to those individuals.

9 If the test is for mutations the criteria used to select the subset of mutations to be covered by screening, if all possible mutations are not being tested, should be clearly set out.

The treatment

10 There should be an effective treatment or intervention for patients identified through early detection, with evidence of early treatment leading to better outcomes than late treatment.

11 There should be agreed evidence-based policies covering which individuals should be offered treatment and the appropriate treatment to be offered.

12 Clinical management of the condition and patient outcomes should be optimized in all healthcare providers prior to participation in a screening programme.

Policies and standards for blood spot screening

The UK Newborn Screening Programme Centre (2008) regularly publishes updates on the guidelines for the completion of the blood spot test. These guidelines aim to:

- achieve early detection, referral and treatment of babies thought to be affected by the conditions;
- support midwives and nurses in gaining consent for the blood spot test;
- support midwives and nurses in obtaining good-quality samples, reducing the need for repeat samples;
- support midwives and nurses in obtaining a valid screening sample for all conditions;
- reduce pain during the heel puncture;
- support parents and encourage the uptake of newborn blood spot screening through evidence-based information;
- provide a consistent approach to newborn blood spot sampling.

Guidance is given on the technique of completing the blood spot test which is undertaken on the fifth to eighth day after birth, irrespective of prematurity and the taking of milk feeds.

Neonatal screening tests vary throughout the developed world but in the UK the blood spot test screens for:

- phenylketonuria
- hypothyroidism
- cystic fibrosis

and in some areas

- galactosaemia
- unusual haemoglobins
- medium-chain acyl CoA dehydrogenase deficiency (MCADD).

Phenylketonuria (PKU)

Phenylketonuria is an inborn error of metabolism (i.e. a condition in which an enzyme deficiency in a metabolic pathway prevents the conversion of one substance to another within a metabolic process). The resulting accumulation of substrate leads to toxic levels of that substance in the body and can lead to life-threatening imbalances. Inborn errors of metabolism are rare, inherited disorders occurring in approximately 1 in 10 000 births. During fetal life the placenta effectively removes most metabolic toxins, allowing the fetus to grow normally and be born in good condition, but soon after birth and separation from the placenta toxic levels can build up and, if undetected, cause serious mental and physical morbidity.

Aetiology

Absence of the enzyme phenylalanine hydroxylase prevents the conversion of the amino acid phenylalanine to tyrosine. The condition is inherited as an autosomal recessive genetic defect. Phenylalanine accumulates in the bloodstream and produces a build up of phenylpyruvic acid, which causes brain damage and severe learning difficulty.

Signs and symptoms

Many untreated babies will develop normally for many months before problems emerge. Symptoms that then arise may include hyperactivity, projectile vomiting, cerebral palsy or convulsions. Over time the infant will fail to achieve early developmental milestones and will develop microcephaly. The infant will also be blonde and fair skinned as phenylketonuria prevents normal pigmentation. The baby's sweat and urine will smell musty due to the accumulation of phenylacetate.

Treatment

There is no cure for this condition but it can be treated effectively with a diet low in phenylalanine and high in tyrosine if diagnosed early. Foods high in phenylalanine include breast milk, meat and other protein foods, and dairy products. Bread, potatoes and pasta can be enjoyed in moderation. Specialist dietary advice is required and many types of foods have been developed for children with this condition. Regular blood spot tests are carried out to monitor the levels of phenylalanine in the blood.

Prognosis

Early diagnosis will allow most babies with this condition to grow up normally provided they adhere to the diet. Once brain development has ceased, around the age of 12 years, the diet can be relaxed to some extent. However women with phenylketonuria will be advised preconceptually to return to the diet when considering pregnancy to prevent congenital defects in their babies due to high levels of phenylalanine in the intrauterine environment. These defects can include mental disability, microcephaly, congenital heart disease and growth restriction.

Hypothyroidism

Hypothroidism is a relatively common disorder in the newborn with an incidence of around 1 in 3500 births. The blood spot test looks for the presence of high levels of thyroid-stimulating hormone (TSH) caused by low levels of thyroid hormones stimulating the pituitary gland in an attempt to increase production by the thyroid gland.

Aetiology

A variety of factors may result in hypothyroidism in the newborn infant. There may be a congenital absence of or abnormality in the development of the structure of the thyroid gland. The thyroid gland may be present but there may be a problem with the production of the thyroid hormones. Rarely, there may be a problem within the pituitary gland itself. This last will not cause an increase in TSH and therefore will not be detected by neonatal blood spot screening.

Signs and symptoms

Infants with hypothyroidism are often postmature with coarse facial features and a large posterior fontanelle. The infant may present with an umbilical hernia.

Treatment

Treatment is with thyroid hormones to replace those that are not being produced.

Prognosis

Early treatment is essential for best outcomes. If treatment is delayed, however, the infant may have difficulty both neurologically and intellectually. Untreated infants will display serious physical disability, growth failure, impaired hearing and a low IQ.

Cystic fibrosis

Screening for cystic fibrosis has been offered to all neonates in Scotland since 2003 and has recently (2007) been introduced throughout England. Screening is undertaken by the blood spot test. The immunoreactive trypsinogen (IRT) assay identifies high levels of IRT and further tests can confirm the diagnosis. Early testing is essential as babies only demonstrate high levels of IRT in the blood during the first eight weeks after birth.

Cystic fibrosis is the most common autosomal recessive genetic disorder found in the UK, affecting 1 in 2500 people in the white population. About 1 in 25 of the population carries the gene that causes the condition (Figure 3.2). Since the discovery of the gene

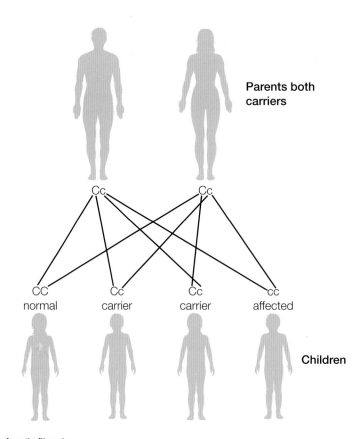

Figure 3.2   Inheritance of cystic fibrosis

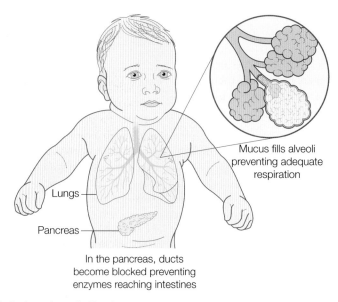

Figure 3.3   Changes in the lungs in cystic fibrosis

responsible for cystic fibrosis, the quality of life of sufferers has improved considerably. Early diagnosis of the condition aids successful management as relevant therapies can be introduced early in the infant's life.

Aetiology

A mutation in the gene that encodes a protein that regulates chloride transport across cell membranes is responsible for cystic fibrosis. In essence sodium and thus water transportation across cell membranes is affected. As a consequence the mucous glands of the lungs, liver, pancreas and intestines are particularly affected (Figure 3.3). Thick mucus builds up in these areas, leading to frequent lung infections and dysfunction of the gastrointestinal system.

Signs and symptoms

In the newborn infant with cystic fibrosis, up to 20 per cent present with meconium ileus. Small bowel obstruction may occur in older children and adults.

Respiratory infection is the most apparent and life-threatening complication of cystic fibrosis. Irreversible lung damage occurs over time. Damage to the pancreas due to impaired secretion of pancreatic enzymes manifests as poor nutrition, weight loss, abdominal pain and flatulence. Liver and biliary cirrhosis may be found in some individuals. Most males with cystic fibrosis are infertile due to a congenital absence of the vas deferens.

Treatment

There is no cure for this condition; treatment with drug therapy and physiotherapy is aimed at reducing the symptoms caused by the build-up of mucus. Nutritional supplements are used to correct the deficits that arise as a result of the lack of digestive enzymes that are prevented from entering the gastrointestinal tract by the thick mucus blocking ducts. Experimentation with gene therapy is currently being undertaken designed to replace the defective gene and correct the condition.

Prognosis

Life expectancy from this disorder is greatly increased nowadays and individuals with this disease can expect to live until early adulthood. Prenatal screening is now offered to couples who are at increased risk of having a baby with cystic fibrosis.

Galactosaemia

This is an autosomal recessive genetic defect that occurs in around 1 in 45 000 babies in the UK, although this again varies with ethnic origin.

Aetiology

In this condition the enzyme galactose-1-phosphate uridyltransferase is missing or severely lacking. This enzyme converts galactose to glucose. Both breast milk and formula milk contain galactose and thus the infant will quickly build up toxic levels of galactose within the body. Galactose thus accumulates in the blood, causing damage to the liver, kidneys, brain and lens of the eyes. Liver failure may occur in those with a severe form of the condition and this carries a high mortality rate.

Signs and symptoms

Babies with galactosaemia will appear normal at birth although cataracts may be present. After commencing milk feeds the infant's condition may deteriorate rapidly. The baby will become reluctant to feed and develop vomiting and diarrhoea with weight loss and dehydration. The infant will be hypoglycaemic and may show evidence of bleeding disorders. Many babies present first with septicaemia and on examination hepatomegaly will be present and the baby may develop jaundice.

Diagnosis is made by testing urine and blood; increased levels of galactose will be found in the urine and confirmation of the diagnosis will be by a deficiency or lack of galactose-1-phosphate uridyltransferase in red blood cells.

Treatment

The main source of galactose is from lactose which is found in milk and milk products. A diet free of these substances will quickly reverse many of the symptoms that have developed in the infant.

Prognosis

Despite introducing a milk-free diet early, many children develop speech and learning difficulties. The reason for this is not known although it has been suggested that galactose is produced in small amounts in the baby and this causes a degree of brain damage despite compliance with the diet. Many women with galactosaemia also develop infertility due to the condition affecting the production of oestrogen.

Sickle cell disease and the haemoglobinopathies

Newborn screening for sickle cell and related disorders (e.g. thalassaemia) is gradually being introduced throughout the UK through the blood spot test. Sickle cell disorders are inherited blood disorders in which there is an abnormality of the structure of the haemoglobin molecule in red blood cells. Sickle cell disorders are found in 1 in 3000 people but this is very dependent on ethnic group. The blood spot test aims to detect both those infants who have the disease and those who carry the genetic defect.

Aetiology

Sickle cell diseases are so termed because the abnormal haemoglobin within the red blood cells prevents them from maintaining their normal round and flexible shape when oxygen levels are low. Even when oxygen levels increase, the red blood cell cannot regain its normal shape. The cells become sickle shaped and can no longer move easily through the narrow capillaries of the circulatory system. The red blood cells become trapped in the smaller blood vessels, preventing blood flow and leading to pain. In addition, the cells become damaged and are destroyed, leading to anaemia.

Signs and symptoms

Symptoms are unlikely to occur in the first few months of life as the infant will continue to produce fetal haemoglobin. Subsequently however, sickle cell disease can lead to a variety of both acute and chronic conditions. Pain will be experienced wherever the sickled cells obstruct blood vessels and the obstruction will lead to organ damage due to lack of blood and the nutrients it carries. This is particularly likely in the spleen, which has the additional function of removing damaged red blood cells. Anaemia and jaundice are likely due to the increased breakdown of the damaged red blood cells.

Treatment

There is no treatment for sickle cell disease. However if the condition has been detected by screening, symptoms can be kept to a minimum by good nutrition and avoidance of situations in which sickling is more likely to occur. A good, well-balanced diet containing foods that contain folic acid will encourage an adequate production of red cells to replace those lost and damaged. Iron is not normally required as the anaemia is caused by excessive breakdown of the red blood cells not by iron deficiency.

Prevention of infection, including the uptake of immunizations against the normal childhood infections and influenza, will be advised to minimize a sickling crisis. Adequate hydration, especially if unwell, will also help to prevent obstruction of blood vessels. Extremes of temperature should be avoided as well as any situations where the infant is likely to become stressed, as this uses up oxygen more quickly and thus predisposes to the red blood cells becoming sickled. Penicillin will be prescribed prophylactically to prevent infection.

Prognosis

Sickle cell disease affects people differently. Some people will experience persistent complications and life expectancy is reduced. Others lead full and normal lives. There is good evidence that early detection of sickle cell disease followed by prophylactic penicillin substantially reduces the risk of serious infections during the first few years of life.

Medium-chain acyl CoA dehydrogenase deficiency (MCADD)

Screening for medium-chain acyl CoA dehydrogenase deficiency is currently being piloted in a number of areas in England with a view to implementing the programme throughout England in 2009. Scotland, Wales and Northern Ireland are currently debating introduction of this screening programme also.

MCADD is an inborn error of metabolism and is inherited as an autosomal recessive disorder. It occurs in 1 in 10 000 babies and is a disorder of fatty acid oxidation. Fatty acid oxidation is crucial to the body's ability to generate energy whilst fasting, infection with fever or during surgery. In an infant a fasting state can occur in as little as 4 hours.

Aetiology

MCADD prevents the oxidation of fatty acids and causes hypoketotic hypoglycaemia and tissue damage due to accumulation of toxic levels of unoxidized fatty acids.

Signs and symptoms

There is no typical presentation in MCADD and it may occur as early as the first day of life or some time later. Any infant or child who has hypoketotic hypoglycaemia or Reyes-like symptoms must be considered as having this condition. Typically the infant will display agitation, lethargy and persistent vomiting, mimicking encephalitis.

Treatment

Treatment is to prevent the development of a fasting state. The introduction of appropriate feeding regimes, supplemented during periods of stress or surgery, will prevent the condition occurring. Supplements of carnitine may be required to remove the toxic levels of unoxidized fatty acids.

Prognosis

Provided diagnosis predates the first episode of severe hypoglycaemia, and therapy prevents the accumulation of toxins, the infant will develop normally. In some infants the condition may develop rapidly soon after birth and this may lead to a high mortality rate.

Storage and further utilization of blood spot specimens

Blood spot cards are retained in the regional laboratories to enable further tests to be carried out should the infant develop symptoms that require further investigation. The newborn blood spot test can also be used to anonymously carry out population surveillance and for research and development. When possible, one blood spot is removed from the card and is tested for human immunodeficiency virus (HIV) to allow the health services to plan services. Left over blood spots can be used to develop new tests and procedures. Parents are asked to inform the midwife if they wish their infant's blood spots not to be utilized in this way.

Newborn hearing screening

Before leaving hospital the majority of babies in the UK receive a hearing test. Congenital hearing loss is estimated to affect 1–3 in every 1000 newborn babies although in areas where universal screening is in place the incidence appears to be at least double this estimate. The causes of hearing loss can be conductive or neurological in origin. In the majority of newborns hearing loss is found to be genetic in origin but cytomegalovirus infection and preterm birth are also known risk factors.

A universal programme of newborn hearing screening has been available throughout the UK since 2005. Early diagnosis and intervention is essential as late identification of deafness has a major effect on language development. Deafness prevents good communication with the young child resulting in long-term social and intellectual difficulties. If deafness is detected before six months and early intervention and support is put into place, language may keep pace with hearing children of similar age.

Before the advent of universal hearing tests for babies, only those babies at increased risk received early tests. These risk factors included a family history of deafness, cranio-facial abnormalities and spending time in the neonatal intensive care unit. However 30–40 per cent of babies with deafness had no known risk factors and therefore were not detected within the first six months.

Early intervention and support can involve a range of professionals, including audiologists, teachers of the deaf, and speech and language therapists. It can also include contact with other parents and deaf adults.

Screening for hearing loss

Screening is normally completed before the infant leaves hospital but can be carried out in the home. The test is carried out by specially trained hearing screeners or health visitors.

Two quick and simple screening tests – the otoacoustic emissions test (OAE) and the automated auditory brainstem response test (AABR) – are used to identify if there is a need for further investigation. Both of these tests accurately diagnose moderate to profound sensorineural hearing loss in newborns and both are painless for the babies.

Otoacoustic emissions test

The OAE test works on the principle that the healthy cochlea (found in the inner ear) produces a faint echo in response to sound waves. A small earpiece is placed within the baby's ear preferably when he or she is settled (Figure 3.4). The earpiece contains a speaker and a microphone and generates a clicking sound which is detected as an echo if the cochlea is functioning correctly. A computer records the findings and identifies if there is a need for a further test. If the test records a strong response from the inner ear there will be no need for further tests.

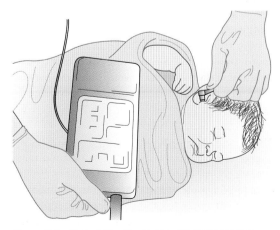

Figure 3.4   Undertaking the otoacoustic emissions test

The advantage of this screening test is that it gives an immediate result. If there is a need for a further test this does not necessarily mean that the baby has a hearing loss, particularly if the baby was unsettled during the test or there was noise in the room in which the test is carried out. The presence of fluid in the ear from the birthing process may also prevent a good result. Only about 15 per cent of babies will require a further hearing test in the form of the AABR.

Automated auditory brainstem response test

The AABR tests the auditory pathway between the external ear and the brainstem. Sound waves enter the outer ear and once they reach the cochlea are converted into electrical signals which are transmitted to the brain where they are interpreted. The AABR test sends a series of clicking sounds through headphones covering the baby's ears. Sensors on the baby's head and neck detect the response to these sounds. A computer compares brain activity with normal response templates. Most babies will show a strong response in the brain but for those who do not a further referral is made for a full diagnostic assessment of their hearing. Around 3 per cent go on for further investigation.

Diagnostic assessment of hearing

About 0.5–1 per cent of babies have some hearing loss in either one ear or in both ears. Therefore those babies who have not shown a good response to the two screening tests will be referred on for a full assessment. This is undertaken either at home or within the local audiology department.

One drawback of the newborn screening for hearing test is the large number of false-positive results. This increases parental anxiety. However good education of parents before screening can keep anxiety to a minimum.

Use of newborn screening of hearing has been shown to reduce the age at which deafness is treated by around eight months, thereby encouraging the development of good language and communication skills.

The midwife's role in neonatal screening tests

The midwife is the primary caregiver in the majority of births across the UK and therefore must supply all women with information during pregnancy so that they can make an informed decision about neonatal screening tests. Leaflets are available covering all the above screening tests and their purpose and these are available in many different languages.

Ideally the leaflets should be given to the women who should have time to read them before the midwife offers them an opportunity to discuss the screening tests. Life is hectic after the baby is born and therefore the woman should be given this opportunity during the prenatal period. Although the midwife does not need to describe fully each individual condition for which screening is offered, she or he must have a good knowledge of these conditions in order to answer any queries and worries the family may have.

Postnatally the midwife's role is to remind the woman and family of the screening tests available to her and her newborn infant. Timing is critical and the midwife must be aware of the optimum time for the tests to be completed. The midwife must again fully explain the purpose of the screening tests and obtain informed consent before carrying out the procedures.

Having completed the tests, the woman and her family should then be informed when they can expect to receive feedback on the findings. They should be reassured that the majority of infants are found to be free of any of the conditions for which screening is offered and also that a positive result may not necessarily mean that her infant has a condition but may indicate further investigation. They should also be informed that in the rare case that an infant has one of the conditions for which screening has been undertaken, early treatment will in many cases ensure that their infant will grow up normally.

Support groups

- Children Living with Metabolic Disorders (CLIMB) www.climb.org.uk
- National Society for Phenylketonuria www.nspku.org
- British Thyroid Foundation www.btf-thyroid.org
- Cystic Fibrosis Trust www.cftrust.org.uk
- Galactosaemia Support Group www.galactosaemia.org
- Sickle Cell Society www.sicklecellsociety.org

Immunization

Many childhood infections which commonly resulted in high mortality and morbidity rates only 50 years ago are rare in the UK today. This is the result of a comprehensive immunization programme available throughout childhood and the early teenage years. Immunization has resulted in dramatic improvements in health, and diseases such as diphtheria, tetanus, whooping cough, measles and poliomyelitis are rarely seen in the UK and developed countries. Some immunizations are offered to all babies and young people while others are available for those at high risk of contracting the infection. Hepatitis B immunization, for example, is advised for all healthcare workers who are regularly exposed to blood and other body fluids.

At birth newborn infants have a passive immunity to many of the infections to which they are exposed as a result of the antibodies passed through the placenta from the mother. However passive immunity only lasts a few weeks or months and thus immunization must be initiated before passive immunity is lost.

Immunization can be achieved either actively or passively

Active immunization, or vaccination, is achieved by giving a vaccine which contains an inactive or attenuated form of a bacterium or virus, or of the toxin that is produced by the infective organism. As the vaccine is inactive it cannot cause the infection but provokes the body to produce antibodies and/or immune cells which will therefore be immediately available on exposure to any infection. After first exposure to an infection it normally takes the body a few days to develop these antibodies and immune cells, by which time the infection has taken a firm hold of the body and the infant or child may be seriously ill as a result. After immunization the antibodies/immune cells are immediately available to remove the foreign cells as soon as they invade the body, thus preventing the illness ever occurring.

Passive immunization involves injecting the antibodies themselves into the body. The body therefore does not have to go through the process of producing these antibodies and immunization occurs very rapidly. However these antibodies are naturally broken down over time and thus passive immunization is short lasting. Passive immunization is useful during the outbreak of a disease or as an emergency treatment for toxins produced by some infective agents such as tetanus.

The childhood immunization programme

Immunization is achieved by giving a vaccine by injection into the arms or legs of infants or children at optimal times in their lives. Diphtheria, tetanus, pertussis, polio and *Haemophilus influenzae* are given as one vaccine: DTaP/IPV/Hib.

Immunizations offered to all infants and children

- Two months – diphtheria, tetanus, pertussis, polio, *Haemophilus influenzae* type B, pneumococcal infection
- Three months – diphtheria, tetanus, pertussis, polio, *Haemophilus influenzae* type B, meningitis C
- Four months – diphtheria, tetanus, pertussis, polio, *Haemophilus influenzae* type B, meningitis C, pneumococcal infection
- One year – *Haemophilus influenzae* type B, meningitis C
- 13 months – measles, mumps and rubella, pneumococcal infection
- Three years and four months – diphtheria, tetanus, pertussis, polio, measles, mumps and rubella
- Twelve years – human papilloma virus types 16 and 18
- 13–18 years – diphtheria, tetanus and polio.

Immunizations offered to those at risk

- At birth – tuberculosis, hepatitis B

Features of the diseases

Diphtheria

Diphtheria is a contagious disease spread by personal contact and droplet infection. The infection causes an upper respiratory infection characterized by sore throat and fever. Typically a membrane forms over the tonsils causing acute breathing difficulties. Complications may occur in the form of cardiac damage and progressive deterioration of the myelin sheaths of the nervous system, resulting in neurological damage. Before the introduction of the vaccine, the infection was common, affecting around 70 000 people a year. It carried a high mortality rate of around 5000 children every year.

Tetanus

Tetanus is an infection which usually enters through an open wound. Typically the infection is caught from the soil or manure which harbour the spores of the bacteria *Clostridium tetani*. The symptoms of the infection are initially caused by a neurotoxin which is produced by the bacteria. Muscular spasm occurs initially in the jaw (lockjaw) and subsequently in the rest of the body. The infected person may have serious breathing difficulties and death is not uncommon.

Pertussis

Pertussis or whooping cough is a highly contagious infection common in childhood until a vaccine was developed. It is characterized by a dry hacking cough followed by a sharp intake of breath sounding like a whoop and can last for several months. It is not usually serious in older children but can kill infants under one year old. Over 100 000 reported cases were identified each year in the UK before the present immunization programme.

Poliomyelitis

Poliomyelitis or infantile paralysis is caused by an acute viral infection transmitted by the faecal–oral route. Most cases cause no symptoms in the infected person but for a very small minority of cases it causes a devastating and permanent paralysis and can kill.

Haemophilus influenzae

Haemophilus influenzae is an infection distinct from influenza and can cause a number of major illnesses such as meningitis, septicaemia and pneumonia. It is an opportunistic infection in that the bacteria are commonly present in the body but only cause problems when the individual has a viral infection or is immunocompromised.

Measles, mumps and rubella

Measles, mumps and rubella are three common viral infections of childhood. Measles is endemic in the world and carries a high mortality rate in areas of poor nutrition. Measles is a highly virulent infection spread by droplet infection and causes acute symptoms of cough, coryza (runny nose) and conjunctivitis. A high fever is present and within a few days a characteristic rash appears. Mumps develops as a swelling of the salivary glands with occasional inflammation of the testicles in boys. Infertility may rarely result. Rubella or German measles is a mild infection that may pass unnoticed. Infection during the first 20 weeks of pregnancy may, however, be devastating to the unborn fetus. Congenital heart disease, deafness and eye abnormalities are common.

Human papilloma virus

Human papilloma virus (HPV) immunization is a recent addition to the routine immunization programme. HPV is spread by sexual contact and has been strongly associated with cervical cancer. HPV vaccination does not protect against all forms of cervical cancer and regular screening must be continued.

The midwife's role

Although the midwife will no longer be involved in the care of women and their babies at two months when the immunization programme commences, she or he has an important role in promoting and educating these women and their families. Before concluding visits and passing responsibilities over to the public health nurse, the midwife can encourage the women to access the child clinics and participate in the immunization programme. Additionally the midwife can ensure that the woman herself is up to date with her immunizations, particularly rubella, so that this vaccination can, if necessary, be administered before conception.

Useful addresses

- UK Newborn Screening Programme Centre
  www.newbornbloodspot.screening.nhs.uk
- NHS Newborn Hearing Screening Programme
  http://hearing.screening.nhs.uk/
- NHS Immunisation Information www.immunisation.nhs.uk

CASE HISTORY

Sarah comes for her booking visit. She was diagnosed with phenylketonuria at birth and has developed normally due to compliance to her diet. Sarah and her husband have planned this pregnancy and were delighted to receive a positive pregnancy test after only two months of trying. Sarah sought the advice of her doctor and returned to her low phenylalanine diet for six months prior to her planned conception. Sarah now wants to know if her condition will harm her unborn baby and if she will need special treatment during her pregnancy and birth. How would you advise Sarah?

Key Points

- Newborn screening tests are available to detect and, where necessary, treat early conditions that are present at birth.
- The blood spot test screens for phenylketonuria, hypothyroidism and cystic fibrosis.
- The NHS plans to introduce screening for galactosaemia, sickle cell disorders and medium-chain acyl CoA dehydrogenase deficiency throughout the UK within the next two years.

- Screening is also available for deafness and these tests are carried out within a week of birth.
- A comprehensive immunization programme is available to every baby in the UK.
- The midwife's role in both screening and immunization programmes is to give the parents the appropriate information and be available to answer any queries they may have.

References

Frye A (2007) *Understanding Diagnostic Tests in the Childbearing Year*. Oregon: Labrys Press.

UK National Screening Committee (2003) Criteria for appraising the viability, effectiveness and appropriateness of a screening programme.

http://www.screening.nhs.uk/criteria#fileid9287 [accessed 9 July 2009].

UK Newborn Screening Programme Centre (2008) *Standards and Guidelines for Newborn Blood Spot Screening*. London: UK Newborn Screening Programme Centre.

CHAPTER 4

EXAMINATION OF THE NEWBORN

Hilary Lumsden

OVERVIEW

Most parents will want confirmation that their baby is perfect as soon as it is born. It is part of the midwife's role to identify any major anomalies and to confirm normality following delivery. This is the beginning of the child health surveillance programme and should be conducted with the importance it deserves (Hall and Elliman, 2006). Following on from the immediate assessment a further, more in-depth examination takes place usually before the mother and baby are discharged home. In some instances this may be around six hours after delivery. This used to be the role of the junior doctor, but in many maternity units now the midwife or an Advanced Neonatal Nurse Practitioner (ANNP) takes on this responsibility. Following the completion of an approved course to attain skills that were previously the remit of the junior doctor, the midwife is in an excellent position to complete holistic care to both mother and her baby. This chapter will discuss all aspects of the physical examination of babies in the early neonatal period. All systems will be described and analysed within a holistic framework.

At delivery

The midwife should make a general assessment of the baby at birth. This comprises initially colour, tone, breathing and heart rate. In assessing these four parameters the midwife can then make a judgement on whether the baby requires any resuscitation. If resuscitation is needed the midwife should call for help and follow the Resuscitation Council (UK) (2006) and hospital guidelines for resuscitation of the newborn. The baby should be observed for any obvious dysmorphic features and any gross abnormalities that are apparent. Assuring the parents that their baby has the requisite number of limbs, eyes, ears, fingers and toes is good practice and reassuring. However, where a problem is identified it is usual to call for medical assistance at the earliest opportunity. The parents will need to be informed if there is a problem.

Physical examination

The newborn infant should have a full assessment before being discharged home unless the community midwife is able to perform this task. The ideal time of assessment is not agreed upon but between 24 and 48 hours would seem the optimum time; however the standard set by the National Screening Committee (NSC) (2008) states that all babies should be examined within 72 hours of birth by a trained healthcare professional. This is because the turbulence of the blood flow in the lungs and heart will have settled and full transition to extrauterine life will be more or less complete. However, it is usual for many mothers to go home before this time and the value of the assessment at such an early stage is questionable. It is still opportune, though, to examine the baby before discharge since it could prove problematic getting the baby examined at a later stage.

Other systems are in place whereby the GP or community midwife can assess the baby. This service is very patchy and there are some areas where GPs have opted out of providing this service to their patients. Some hospitals offer provision whereby mothers can take their baby back to a discharge clinic for the examination. Again, this can be logistically difficult for some mothers if they have other children or transport problems. As a result the two-day examination is fraught with difficulties and conducting the assessment before the mother and baby leave hospital means that at least some aspects of the child health surveillance programme have been addressed.

The newborn's weight, length and head circumference should be measured and plotted on the centile chart appropriate to their sex. This provides a baseline from which to calculate whether all parameters are in proportion and that they fall between the 10th and 90th percentiles.

The examination should be performed in the presence of one of the parents who will be able to answer any questions the midwife asks as she or he carries out this procedure. The EMREN study (Townsend *et al.*, 2004) found that mothers were more satisfied with the midwife performing the assessment than the senior house officer (SHO) because more information about feeding, health promotion and skincare were given. Although a top-to-toe approach is a logical sequence and means that aspects of the examination are not forgotten, it makes more sense to assess the heart and eyes while the baby is quiet and relaxed rather than trying to do them once the baby has had their hips examined and is crying.

A review of maternal history, particularly antenatal and intranatal, should be carried out before the baby is examined. Anything of significance should be documented but it is usual for the midwife to ask the mother to clarify some points that are not clear in the notes.

General observation

Before undressing the baby, the midwife should observe the baby in the cot, at rest before the examination takes place. This is probably the most important aspect of the assessment since many abnormalities can be identified at this stage, particularly around the head and neck area. The baby should be quiet, with normal regular respirations, with no expiratory grunt, nasal flaring and should be pink in colour. The position should be relaxed and fairly well flexed. The mother should be asked whether her baby is feeding well, sleeping in between feeds, appears contented and whether he or she is passing urine, when meconium was first passed and if normal stools are now being seen.

Skin

Assessment of the skin forms an essential component of the newborn examination and in the first instance the skin should be observed for lacerations, bruises and abrasions. Other common marks are:

- Mongolian blue spot
- pigmented naevi
- haemangiomas
- stork bite marks
- port wine stains
- strawberry marks.

Head and neck area

Head

The shape of the neonate's head often relates to the type of delivery. Moulding occurs as a result of the effects of pressure on the head: the sutures and fontanelles allow the skull bones to overlap as they pass through the pelvis. The head should be examined for any swelling or bruising as discussed further in Chapter 13.

The size of the head is significant and any macrocephaly (greater than the 97th centile) or microcephaly (below the 2nd centile) should be noted. This is done most easily by plotting the head circumference on the appropriate growth chart in the child health record. In a baby with asymmetrical intrauterine growth restriction, the head may appear large for the neonate's body size. Asymmetrical growth restriction usually occurs in the third trimester and results from disorders of the placenta or maternal problems. These babies exhibit 'head-sparing growth' in which the head has grown at the normal rate but the body has been deprived of nutrients and is therefore small for gestational age. A large head is also associated with hydrocephalus and other congenital syndromes. Further investigations and specialist referral are essential if a large head is identified.

Microcephaly may be associated with conditions such as fetal alcohol syndrome (FAS) or congenital infection and will also require further investigation and attention.

The anterior fontanelle is a soft, diamond-shaped structure where the parietal and frontal bones meet. It is slightly concave and it is normal to see slight pulsation. The examiner should look carefully for a tense or bulging fontanelle as this indicates raised intracranial pressure, whereas a sunken fontanelle indicates dehydration.

Palpation of the skull will reveal if there are any abnormalities to moulding. If the suture line feels rigid or immobile it could be an indication of premature fusion of the skull bones or craniosynostosis. This leads to an abnormal head shape and may be detected at birth, although it is more likely to be picked up at a later examination. Craniosynostosis are associated with Apert's and Crouzon's syndromes.

Palpation may also detect craniotabes, an abnormal softening of the skull, in which the skull bones give the sensation of pressing on a ping-pong ball. Again this requires further investigation.

While palpating the skull it is important to observe the pattern of hair growth, including the texture and quantity. Abnormal patterns such as low hairline and more than two hair whorls (crowns) can be indicative of a congenital abnormality. A low hairline is associated with Down's syndrome, Klippel–Feil syndrome and Cornelia de Lange syndrome.

Face

The face should be observed as a whole and likenesses to either or both parents should not be discounted. Any unusual features should be identified. They could be familial and therefore of no real concern, but they could also suggest a congenital syndrome, Down's syndrome being the most well-known. Although many chromosomal and congenital syndromes are detected antenatally, it is still crucial to look carefully at the facial features to rule out any such problems.

The symmetry of the face should be observed; any asymmetry may be suggestive of nerve damage and this will become more apparent when the infant cries.

Milia (milk spots) are small papules seen around the nose and are caused by a collection of sebaceous gland secretions. They will usually resolve spontaneously within a few weeks.

Mouth

Examination of the mouth is a simple procedure and should be performed to rule out abnormalities. General observation will identify any major obvious abnormalities. If not diagnosed antenatally, a cleft lip will be apparent as soon as the baby is born and can be unilateral or bilateral and can extend into the palate. A cleft palate, however, is sometimes less obvious and requires thorough assessment in order to confirm its presence. To do this a gloved finger should be inserted into the baby's mouth, eliciting a suck reflex. By palpating the palate, it should be possible to feel if a large cleft is present; smaller clefts in the soft palate are more difficult to locate and the roof of the mouth needs to be examined using a pen-torch. This is best done when the baby is crying.

Clefting of the lip or palate (Figure 4.1) affects around 1:700 babies in the UK and can occur in isolation or together: 50 per cent are cleft lip and palate together, 25 per cent are cleft lip alone, 25 per cent are cleft palate alone (Fletcher, 1997). There is often no specific cause, it can be familial and it can be associated with chromosomal disorders such as Down's, Patau's and CHARGE syndromes. For isolated clefts

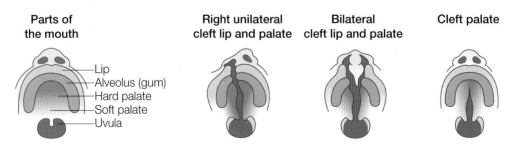

Figure 4.1 Cleft lip and palate. (From Cleft Lip and Palate Association, www.clapa.com, with permission)

midwives should give reassurance that the problem can be corrected, avoid any separation of the mother and baby and encourage skin to skin contact (Bannister, 2008). Babies with a cleft lip or palate will require urgent referral to the regional team for relevant specialist assessment. The cleft lip and palate team have structured care pathways and will be able to offer reassurance, support and information regarding this problem, particularly in relation to feeding and treatment.

Ankyloglossia or tongue-tie occurs when the lingual frenulum, which attaches the tongue to the floor of the mouth, is unusually short. If undetected, ankyloglossia can cause dental, speech and eating difficulties later in infancy and childhood (Hogan *et al.*, 2005). There seems to have been an increase in the diagnosis of ankyloglossia in recent years, which could be attributed to the increase in breastfeeding initiation rates. Where mothers are presenting with cracked or sore nipples or the baby is not feeding well, it is important for the midwife to assess the baby for tongue-tie. A frenulotomy may be required, which is a simple, very quick, safe procedure that divides the frenulum. Following frenulotomy improved feeding for both mother and the baby will usually be seen (Hogan *et al.*, 2005). There are national variations regarding who performs the procedure, the cost and the referral process. The midwife should be aware of the practice for the referral of a baby with tongue-tie.

Some babies are born with natal teeth; if present they are usually seen in the lower incisor region of the gums. Natal teeth are generally very mobile and bring the risk of inhalation and aspiration if not removed. They can also cause ulceration of the tongue. Removal is normally recommended for these reasons and referral to the orthodontic team is needed. Flat, white nodules on the gums known as Epstein's pearls are the same as milia and although they are sometimes confused with natal teeth they require no treatment and parents should be reassured that they will disappear in time.

Eyes

On examination of the eyes the midwife should note any discharge (see Chapter 10) or birthmarks. Bruises and forceps marks are easily identified and reassurance about these should be given to the parents.

The eyes should be symmetrically positioned on the face. The outer canthal distance can be divided

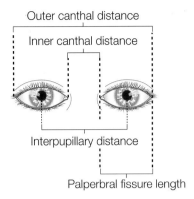

Figure 4.2 Eye measurements. (Reproduced from Aase JM (1990) *Diagnostic Dysmorphology*. New York: Springer)

equally into thirds, with one eye width fitting into the inner canthal space (Figure 4.2). Abnormal placement or small eye openings (palperbral fissues) may indicate a syndrome or abnormality, as may widely or closely spaced eyes. An epicanthal fold is a vertical crease that extends from the nose to the medial angle of the eye. These are common in Down's syndrome and are a normal finding in some ethnic groups.

Examination of the eye is much easier if the baby spontaneously opens his or her eyes and is best done when the infant is in an alert state. Very little information can be gained if the eyes are forced open. Getting the mother to hold the baby in an upright position may be helpful and often results in spontaneous opening of the eyes. The ophthalmoscope should be adjusted and the light shone from a distance of 15 cm onto the baby's lens until a clear red reflex from the retina is reflected back. Any opacity of the lens or cornea will prevent the light being reflected. Absence of the red reflex could mean a congenital cataract and will require referral to an ophthalmologist. Pale or pink reflexes are common in babies from Asian and African ethnic backgrounds and should not be of concern.

Some neonatal eye abnormalities and their treatments are listed in Table 4.1.

Ears

The ears may initially appear asymmetrical due to unequal uterine pressure. This is a temporary condition. In normal placement the upper edge of the ear is

Table 4.1   Neonatal eye abnormalities

Problem	Clinical feature	Treatment
Strabismus	Muscular weakness resulting in appearance of cross-eyes	May improve over next few weeks but needs medical assessment and may require ophthalmologist referral
Ptosis	Drooping eyelid	Medical assessment and may require ophthalmologist referral
Brushfield spots	White specks on the iris	Could be normal but is associated with Down's syndrome
Microphthalmia	Abnormally small eyes	Associated with congenital abnormality particularly rubella and cytomegalovirus infections
Macrophthalmia	Abnormally large eyes	Associated with congenital glaucoma and requires urgent referral

in line with the outer canthus of the eye. Using this as a baseline the midwife can detect abnormally placed ears. The size and shape should also be assessed along with variations in the shape of the helix and lobe. These could, of course, be familial.

Pre-auricular skin tags can sometimes be seen around the tragus. Again these can be familial but may need referral to a plastic surgeon. Pre-auricular sinus is often missed on the first examination. The sinus can be blind or it may be connected to the inner ear and requires an ENT referral. The ears should be examined to ensure that the auditory canals are present and patent. Some ear problems and associated syndromes are listed in Table 4.2.

Table 4.2   Ear problems

Clinical presentation	Association
Low set ears	Normal, Edwards' syndrome, Noonan's syndrome, Apert's syndrome
Misplaced pinna	Goldenhar's syndrome
Abnormal ear attachment	Trisomy 17, 18, Edwards' syndrome
Malformed	Trisomy 17, 18, Treacher Collins syndrome, Noonan's syndrome, Beckwith–Wiedemann syndrome
Darwinian tubercle	Normal variant on the upper helix

Nose

The nose should be symmetrically placed on the midline of the face. The shape and size will be familial, but a flattened or low nasal bridge can be associated with Down's syndrome.

Babies are nose breathers. If there appears to be any obstruction or difficulty with nasal breathing further investigation may be needed. On examination the midwife should observe the patency of the nasal passages. Choanal atresia is a condition in which the posterior nasal passages are blocked, preventing the baby from breathing properly through the nose. The baby with this condition will be cyanotic at rest, but pink when crying and breathing through the mouth. Babies with bilateral or unilateral choanal atresia need urgent referral to an ENT surgeon.

Sneezing can be quite common in newborns, but excessive sneezing may indicate neonatal abstinence syndrome (NAS).

Parents often worry about excessive nasal secretions and 'snuffly' babies. The midwife should give reassurance and no medication is required.

Neck

Babies tend to have relatively short necks but there should be full mobility. The midwife should observe for any webbing of the neck or excess skin, which is associated with Turner's syndrome.

Palpating around the sternomastoid muscle can identify a sternomastoid tumour. The baby may also be holding his or her head over to one side. This tumour is not noticeable at birth but will develop in the days and weeks following delivery. The history may reveal a delivery that required traction to the head and this has altered the circulation to the muscle. A physiotherapy referral is required to treat a sternomastoid tumour but further investigation may be needed to confirm the diagnosis (see Chapter 13).

Gastrointestinal examination

Umbilicus

The position and condition of the umbilical cord should be noted at birth as well as during later examinations. There should be three vessels identifiable in the cord: two arteries and one vein. The arteries are thick walled and protrude slightly from the cord, the vein is thinner walled but has a larger opening. One single umbilical artery occurs in about 1 per cent of babies and may signify renal disease. The cord contains Wharton's jelly and should have a clear, shiny gelatinous appearance. A very thin cord may indicate some placental insufficiency. Any bulging around the cord should be noted since this could be an umbilical hernia. The cord will dry out and should separate by 10 days of age.

Abdomen

Observation of the abdomen while the baby is settled should reveal well-perfused skin and it should appear soft and rounded. Depending on whether the baby has recently been fed, the abdomen will be either flat or slightly rounded. If the abdomen is very distended, if there is tension or obvious abdominal masses the midwife needs to investigate this further since it could reveal an obstruction or underlying gastrointestinal problem. Medical assessment should be sought.

Auscultation of the abdomen should precede palpation. The midwife should listen to the abdomen with a stethoscope. Bowel sounds will be heard in all four quadrants and it is usual to hear breath sounds when auscultating the abdomen. This is quite normal and is due to the close proximity of the lungs.

Palpation of the abdomen will begin with noticing the muscle tone. Hypertonic muscles may indicate pain, whereas hypotonicity could be caused by maternal medication, neuromuscular disease or rare conditions such as 'prune belly' syndrome. Using the pads of the fingers rather than the fingertips the midwife

Signs of gastrointestinal obstruction

- Vomiting – especially bilious
- Abdominal distension
- Poor feeding
- Bowels not opened
- Visible loops of bowel and/or peristalsis
- Crying
- Signs of pain
- May be dehydrated.

Causes of gastrointestinal obstruction

- Duodenal atresia
- Pyloric stenosis
- Malrotation
- Imperforate anus
- Necrotizing enterocolitis
- Hirschsprung's disease
- Delayed passage of meconium syndromes.

Causes of hepatosplenomegaly

- Congenital heart disease
- Congenital infection
- Metabolic conditions
- Heart failure
- Haemolysis
- Trauma
- Intrahepatic haemorrhage.

should gently palpate the organs in the abdomen, starting with the superficial structures before continuing to the deeper organs. The liver in the newborn extends from 1 to 3 cm below the right costal margin depending on the size and gestation of the baby. Therefore the liver edge should always be palpable. In a continuous caudal manner and commencing at the iliac crest and without taking the hands off the abdomen the midwife will be able to feel the edge of the liver. It should feel smooth and firm. When palpating the spleen the normal finding is that no spleen will be palpable. Any organomegaly should be noted. Further investigation and referral is required.

It can be difficult to palpate the kidneys and because deeper palpation is required it may cause discomfort to the baby. With one hand under the baby's back and the other pressing down on the abdomen, the kidneys may be felt in the flanks, with the right kidney slightly lower than the left. Each kidney should feel smooth, firm and not depressible. The midwife should not be too concerned if the kidneys cannot be palpated providing urine output is good and the baby is feeding well. Enlarged kidneys may be easily palpable, in which case the possible causes are:

- hydronephrosis
- nephroblastoma
- cystic dysplastic kidney
- Wilms' tumour
- renal vein thrombosis
- bladder neck obstruction.

The final part of abdominal palpation is to assess the bladder. This can be found 1–3 cm above the symphysis pubis. Starting at the umbilicus the midwife should palpate the bladder, which will feel smooth. Any distension of the bladder may be caused by urinary tract obstruction and requires further attention.

Groin

Any swelling in the groin should be noted and could be either a femoral or inguinal hernia. An inguinal hernia is a weakness in the muscle wall that has allowed bowel to protrude through into the scrotum in boys and soft tissue in girls. A femoral hernia is where bowel is protruding into the femoral area. If the hernia is reducible the baby will need to be followed up by the GP. In all cases a surgical referral is needed. If the hernia is not reducible, an urgent surgical referral is required. Assessment of femoral pulses are discussed later in this chapter.

Anus

The placement and patency of the anus should be checked and an anal wink will be seen. An obvious absence of an anus is a surgical emergency requiring urgent assessment followed by surgery at the neonatal surgical centre. Some babies have what appears to be a perforate anus but there is an underlying defect in the anorectal canal. It is therefore important to confirm with the mother not only the passage of meconium

but also the quantity. Small amounts of meconium can be passed through the urethra if there is a rectourethral fistula or vaginally if there is a rectovaginal fistula. If the baby is not feeding well and if there are any signs of abdominal distension, further investigation is warranted.

Genitalia

The labia majora in the female and scrotum in boys may appear large in newborns, particularly if there is any oedema caused by breech presentation/delivery. Ambiguous genitalia are where it is not clear whether the genitalia are male or female and is usually identifiable at birth although it can be missed at the first examination. With ambiguous genitalia there is usually an underlying condition such as congenital adrenal hyperplasia which will need urgent referral and treatment.

Female genitalia

The female genitalia should be inspected and any major anomalies noted. In preterm babies the labia minora and clitoris are often much more prominent. In term babies the labia majora should cover the labia minora. There is no need to palpate these structures unless the labia majora seems abnormally large and this will be to detect the presence or absence of palpable gonads in the labioscrotal folds. Descended gonads will always be testes because ovaries will never descend below the inguinal ring. Occasionally a hymenal skin tag may be present. Parents should be reassured that this will normally disappear within a few weeks. Vaginal discharge occurs in many female infants and is due to withdrawal from maternal hormones. The discharge is most commonly thick and white, occasionally there will be slight vaginal bleeding. It may persist for up to 10 days and again parents should be reassured that it is normal and will disappear.

The urinary meatus is situated between the clitoris and vaginal opening. If urine is seen to be dribbling from any other position the baby should receive further assessment and possible referral.

Male genitalia

Inspection of the male genitalia should give an indication of gestational age. Rugae develop from 36 weeks' gestation, babies with smooth scrotum are either preterm or there are no testes in the scrotum. The pigmentation of the scrotum is dependent upon the ethnic background of the parents. Any swelling of the scrotum could be a hydrocele and transillumination with a bright light will help the midwife to rule out a hernia. The male genitalia should be palpated to confirm the absence of cryptorchidism (undescended testes). The incidence of cryptorchidism is 3 per cent in term neonates and up to 20 per cent in babies less than 2500 g and 6 per cent of males have one or both testes undescended (Hall and Elliman, 2006). However, about 98 per cent of testes will descend spontaneously by about six weeks of age. It is important to identify undescended testes and this should be documented in the child health record in order for the baby to be followed up at six weeks by the GP or health visitor. Occasionally the testes will be retractile and again this should be noted and pointed out to the parents for follow-up.

Later problems associated with undiagnosed/untreated cryptorchidism can be malignancy and/or infertility in adulthood.

It is essential that the position of the urethral meatus should also be identified because hypospadias and epispadias will require surgical treatment. Hypospadias is where the urethral meatus opens on the ventral surface (underside) of the penis and should be differentiated from a hooded penis, where the foreskin is abnormally shaped. Epispadias is where the urethral opening is situated on the dorsal surface of the penis. The parents should be advised not to have their baby circumcised for religious or cultural reasons because the surgeon will normally need to use the foreskin in the repair of the defect.

Musculoskeletal

Upper extremities

The bones of the newborn are mainly cartilaginous and therefore soft, allowing for delivery through the birth canal. Occasionally damage is caused at delivery resulting in fractures or bruising (see Chapter 13). Nevertheless the musculoskeletal system needs to be assessed thoroughly to rule out any other abnormalities. Observation of the baby as he or she lies in the cot can tell the midwife a great deal about the range and symmetry of movement, posture, position as well as size, shape and length of limbs. The term baby will lie in a slightly flexed position with the head in the mid-

line or turned slightly to one side. The hands are also flexed with the thumb lying underneath the fingers in a fist. If the baby has been in the breech position, the legs are likely to remain in an extended attitude for some time. Hypotonic babies will also have an extended posture and will be ragdoll-like in appearance and behaviour.

Palpation of the muscles will elicit any weakness or hypotonia and should not be mistaken for a sleepy or immature baby. Muscles should feel smooth and should resist pressure very slightly. Palpation will also determine the range of movement, tightness or contractures. It is not essential to be specific about the range of motion and the midwife should not use excessive force.

Attention should be paid to the clavicle and humerus to assess for fractures, particularly if there has been evidence of cephalopelvic disproportion or shoulder dystocia (see Chapter 13). The hands must be assessed for shape, size and number of digits. Accessory digits may be seen at the base of the little fingers and any missing or extra digits (polydactyly) should also be noted. Syndactyly is where there is fusion of the fingers. It may be that only the soft tissue is involved, however an X-ray will confirm complete fusion. A single transverse palmer crease (simian crease) may be a normal feature or in the presence of other typical features be associated with Down's syndrome.

Deformities of the hands and feet

- Syndactyly: fusion of two or more digits with soft tissue involvement
- Polydactyly: excess digits, tends to be hereditary
- Clinodactyly: incurved digit
- Camptodactyly: flexed digit
- Amniotic bands: range can be from superficial indentations of the soft tissue to complete amputation of digit or limb.

Lower extremities

The midwife should palpate the baby's legs to confirm the existence of the femurs, tibia and fibulas. Fractures would be suspected if there is a history of a difficult delivery, particularly a vaginal breech. Fractures are rare but if present, the baby will demonstrate signs of pain on examination, there will be crepitus or mass felt on palpation, the baby will not move the affected limb, swelling or bruising may also be visible. The lower extremities should both be assessed for length and shape. The legs will remain flexed for several days following birth and it may not be easy to extend them from the knees at examination. By placing both the baby's feet on the bed, keeping the knees bent and in alignment, the midwife will be able to detect any difference in femoral length if one of the baby's knees is higher than the other. This test is called the Galeaizzi sign and if positive could also be indicative of developmental dysplasia of the hips (DDH).

As with the hands, the feet need to be examined for the correct number of digits and spacing between them. Overlapping toes are likely to be hereditary and may need stabilizing in the correct position.

The feet should be examined to ensure correct alignment. Talipes is a condition where there is an abnormality of the position of the feet, commonly known as clubfoot. This can be unilateral or bilateral. The incidence of a bilateral deformity is 30–50 per cent and it should be noted; if unilateral, the affected foot is likely to be smaller.

Positional talipes is relatively common, 1:1000, and is often due to malposition *in utero* and can be associated with reduced amniotic fluid, although strong family history and smoking in pregnancy make the condition more common. Positional talipes differ on assessment from true talipes as it should be possible to gently manipulate the feet/foot back into the correct position. In true fixed talipes this reduction will not be achievable and will cause pain to the baby if manipulation is attempted. If the feet/foot are easily manipulated no further diagnostic test is required.

There is a slight male predominance in this condition. It can be diagnosed antenatally on ultrasound scan but to confirm the diagnosis a plain X-ray should be taken of the feet if fixed talipes is suspected. Positional talipes is treated by physiotherapy to the feet. Stretching exercises can be taught to the parents who can conduct the procedure several times a day. If the position of the foot cannot be corrected easily and without force an orthopaedic referral is required.

The most common form is talipes equinovarus. In this condition the forefoot is adducted and the toes point downwards and inwards. In talipes calcaneovalgus the deformity is opposite to that in talipes equinovarus, so the feet or foot is dorsiflexed, turning upward and outwards. Treatment should be started as soon as possible and the Ponsetti regime of manipulation and casting is recommended. Correction is usually established by three months of age. Following this, holding casts are used for a further 3–6 months.

About 20 per cent of confirmed talipes will require surgical intervention. Talipes is also associated with developmental dysplasia of the hips and because severe bilateral talipes is strongly associated with neuromuscular problems these should be ruled out during assessment.

Hips

Assessment and identification of any hip abnormality needs to be completed very early in the postnatal period. The importance of this examination cannot be overemphasized since missing a congenital hip problem can leave the child with walking difficulties that will require complex medical and surgical treatment later in life. Developmental dysplasia of the hip (DDH) is where there is an abnormality of the hip joint. The femoral head is not stable in the acetabulum and it is usually because the acetabulum is not fully formed or is shallow.

Dysplasia can refer to a joint that is subluxatable, dislocatable or currently dislocated. Developmental dysplasia of the hip is the most common childhood disorder, affecting about 20 per 1000 at birth. Although most hips stabilize spontaneously, those that persist require early intervention as already mentioned to prevent long-term damage. The disorder underlies up to 9 per cent of all primary hip replacements and up to 29 per cent of those in people 60 years and under.

There is often a familial tendency or a genetic component, but in 40 per cent of cases no predisposing factors are found. The left hip is the most commonly affected (60 per cent), with the right hip accounting for 20 per cent of cases and 20 per cent affecting both hips. Developmental dysplasia of the hip is more common in girls (80–85 per cent) and is thought to be due to muscles and ligaments being relaxed by female hormones.

Normal development of the hip joint depends upon balanced growth of the cartilages and a well-located, centred femoral head. This is usually achieved by the 11th week of pregnancy where the hip joint is fully formed into its separate components. Malposition *in utero* can affect the developing hip joint, particularly if the fetus is in the extended breech position.

It is common practice in the UK to perform an ultrasound scan on all babies who have been in the breech position from 34 weeks' gestation. Hip position and free hip movement remain important during the first months after birth. This is when the hip continues to develop and forms a deep socket and stable joint.

There are cultural differences that can affect the ongoing development of the hip joint. For example developmental dysplasia of the hip has been reported to be more common in Japanese, Turkish, Native American and Lapp populations where swaddling of infants and the use of papooses/cradle boards tends to hold the hips in extension and adduction. Likewise in modern Western society, putting infants for long periods in baby and car seats as well as the use of very slim disposable nappies which do not abduct the hips as widely could also affect hip development. In contrast, the incidence of developmental dysplasia of the hip is lower in African countries where babies are carried on parents' hips, which flexes the legs and abducts the hips, allowing the babies' hips to become more stable.

Clinical hip instability was first reported in 1879, with the clinical test for assessment of hip instability – a test of hip reduction – being described in 1910 and brought to prominence by Ortolani in 1937. Barlow's test to provoke subluxation was developed in 1962. Both tests are used in conjunction with one another to identify unstable hips today.

Prior to performing the Ortolani and Barlow manoeuvre it is usual to look for other signs that may indicate a hip problem. With the baby undressed, the midwife should look to see if there is limited abduction of the hip with the baby lying in a relaxed position on a flat surface. Inspecting for asymmetrical groin creases, asymmetrical gluteal creases and a widened perineum will add to the overall examination and as previously mentioned apparent leg shortening with uneven knee heights (Galeazzi sign) is a positive marker that there may be some hip instability.

Ortolani and Barlow manoeuvres

It is usual to examine the hips prior to discharge and the procedure needs to be repeated again at six weeks of age. A midwife or advanced neonatal nurse practitioner who has been specially trained in the use of these techniques should perform the manoeuvres.

It is common practice to perform the Ortolani manoeuvre followed by the Barlow test (Figure 4.3). Both should be performed in sequence and not as separate tests, although they are usually described indi-

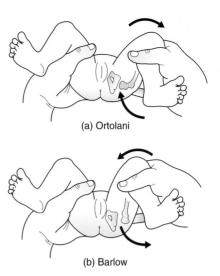

Figure 4.3 Clinical diagnosis of developmental dysplasia of the hip. (Reproduced with permission from Patel K (2006) *Complete Revision Notes for Medical Finals*. London: Hodder Arnold)

vidually. Some examiners prefer to examine both hips simultaneously whereas others find supporting the pelvis with one hand and examining each hip separately preferable. This is a matter of personal choice and either way is acceptable practice. It should also be remembered that this aspect of the physical examination will be last, the baby may be upset or fractious by this time and the midwife should attempt to calm the baby down before an attempt to assess the hips is made.

In the Ortolani test the midwife applies forward pressure to the femoral head, attempting to move a posterior dislocated femoral head towards the acetabulum. Any palpable movement suggests that the hip is dislocated or subluxatable, but is reducible. The test should aim to put a dislocated hip back in place. In the Barlow test the midwife applies backward pressure to the femoral head and a subluxatable hip is suspected if there is complete or partial displacement. If a clunk is felt, often described as feeling like putting the car in gear, it indicates instability of the hip(s). The amount of force required to push the femoral head in or out of the acetabulum is minimal. If a 'click' is felt it is usually insignificant and due to lax ligaments or tendons and does not require any follow-up.

Babies with positive Ortolani or Barlow manoeuvres will require an orthopaedic referral. An ultrasound scan will be performed to determine the shape of the acetabulum and the degree of instability in the hip joint. Once a diagnosis of developmental dysplasia of the hips has been made, the treatment will depend upon the degree of instability. It is usually sufficient to splint the hips into a position of flexion and abduction for up to three months. This enables the femoral head to stay in the correct position and allows for the bones to grow normally and for the ligaments to tighten. The Pavlik harness is successful in splinting the hips, however in smaller babies double or triple nappies can be used until they have grown enough for the Pavlik harness to fit properly.

Treatment using the Pavlik harness will be monitored frequently. If there is no significant improvement the harness will be removed and a closed reduction may be needed. The success of treatment depends upon prompt and correct diagnosis.

Spine

The spine should be examined for any abnormalities by turning the baby over and inspecting for any obvious lesions. Neural tube defects (NTDs) are detected in pregnancy through the antenatal screening programme. The parents and midwives would be well prepared for the delivery of such an infant. However, some women refuse antenatal screening and occasionally women do not have any antenatal care and an undiagnosed NTD may present at birth or on postnatal examination. A sacral dimple is usually insignificant but if the midwife cannot see the base a second opinion should be sought. This also applies if there is any leakage or discharge from the dimple.

A haemangioma or tuft of hair along the spine should be investigated to rule out spina bifida occulta, which is a mild form of spina bifida that is very common. It can affect between 5 and 10 per cent of babies but is of no consequence and there may not be any visible signs that spina bifida occulta is present. The central nervous system and spine develops between days 14 and 23 of pregnancy. Spina bifida occurs when the neural tube fails to close accurately, the vertebrae will also fail to close and this will leave a space connecting one or more of the vertebrae. The visible signs will be a sac or cyst on the back, covered by a layer of skin.

There are two types of spina bifida cystica:

- *Meningocele*: This form of spina bifida is the least common and is where a cystic sac containing the meninges and cerebrospinal fluid overlies the open vertebral arches.

- *Myelomenigocele*: This is more common and more serious and is where the cyst not only contains tissue and cerebrospinal fluid but also nerves and part of the spinal cord. The spinal cord will not be fully developed and will also be damaged. This will result in some paralysis and loss of feeling below the defect.

The cause of spina bifida is unknown, however it is now known that by taking folic acid preconceptually and for the first 12 weeks of pregnancy, women can reduce their incidence of having a baby with spina bifida.

Scoliosis is a curvature of the spine and is not easily detected at birth. Infantile scoliosis may be a result of malposition and will rectify itself as the baby grows, but the baby should be examined again at a later stage to confirm a diagnosis. However, severe curvature of the spine is a result of vertebral defects, either failure of formation or failure of segmentation. The treatment will be based purely on the extent of the defect.

Torticollis is a contraction of the neck muscles and is usually unilateral. It is thought to be due to birth trauma or ischaemia from *in utero* position. Torticollis may not be detected in the newborn period; formation of a swelling or haematoma may be palpated in the soft tissue over the sternomastoid muscle. At two weeks of age torticollis will appear as a hard fibrous mass and will be immobile. Babies with this condition will tilt their head to one shoulder with the chin pointing away from the affected side. An orthopaedic referral will be required for babies where torticollis is suspected.

Chest

Intrapartum history is an important indicator of the baby's condition on examination and the following should be noted:

- significant maternal history
- method of delivery
- assessment at birth (colour, tone, breathing, heart rate)
- prolonged rupture of membranes
- fetal distress
- meconium-stained liquor
- gestation
- maternal sedation (narcotics) in labour
- maternal drug abuse.

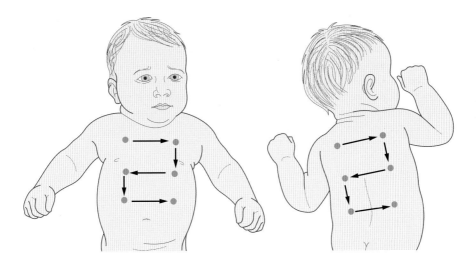

Figure 4.4   Areas of auscultation of the chest. (Reproduced from Tappero EP, Honeyfield ME (2003) *Physical Assessment of the Newborn*. Santa Rosa: Neonatal Network, NICU Ink Book Publishers. © Elizabeth Weadon Massari)

At rest the newborn baby's respiratory rate should be around 30–40 breaths per minute. The assessment of the chest and lungs should begin with a thorough inspection including colour and tone. Acrocyanosis is common after birth and may still be present up to 48 hours following delivery. Central cyanosis is described as a bluish colour of the lips, skin, tongue and nail beds. The breathing should be easy, with no nasal flaring, expiratory grunting or recession. There should be symmetrical chest movement with each breath, with the diaphragm being the major muscle of respiration. If there is any difficulty with the breathing, such as tachypnoea or apnoeic episodes, they will normally be accompanied by cyanosis, mottling or pallor. Tachypnoea, apnoea, grunting and recession are all indicators that there is an underlying cause.

Asymmetrical chest movement is associated with diaphragmatic hernia, pneumothorax and nerve damage. Babies who are experiencing any of these difficulties should be transferred to the neonatal unit for further investigation and treatment.

On auscultation the lungs in a healthy baby should sound clear, with inspiratory and expiratory breaths sounds being similar in pitch and duration (Figure 4.4).

The newly born infant will clear around 100 mL of lung fluid at birth with the onset of regular respirations. Oral or nasal secretions may be noted in the early neonatal period and are usually white in colour. Secretions that are thicker in consistency, cream, yel-

Signs of respiratory distress

- Tachypnoea
- Apnoea
- Grunting
- Nasal flaring
- Intercostal recession
- Retractions
- Cyanosis
- Head bobbing.

Causes of respiratory distress

- Transient tachypnoea of the newborn
- Diaphragmatic hernia
- Congenital pneumonia
- Surfactant deficiency disease
- Pneumothorax
- Meconium aspiration syndrome
- Upper airway obstruction.

low or green in colour are associated with infection and a sample will need to be sent to the laboratory for culture and sensitivity.

Auscultation of the chest should be performed using the bell of the stethoscope. The midwife should listen systematically to the front and the back of the chest, commencing at the top, working from side to side until all four quadrants of the chest have been auscultated, including under each axilla. Localizing breath sounds in the neonate can be difficult because of the small size of the chest compared with that of an older child or adult. Abnormal breath sounds are a sign of underlying disease and can be described as follows:

- Crackles are bubbly sounds, similar to the sound of a fizzy drink, usually intermittent. Can be fine or coarse.
- Wheezes are usually louder on expiration, not often heard in the newborn.
- Rub is associated with inflammation, sounding similar to a dry rub.
- Stridor is a high-pitched, coarse sound usually caused by partial obstruction of the airway and sometimes heard in babies who have been ventilated.

It is not essential for the midwife to be able to identify these individual sounds but she should be able to distinguish the abnormal from the normal, taking into consideration the other signs that may be apparent.

Heart

Midwives have concerns about 'missing' abnormal heart sounds (Lumsden, 2005). However, it must be emphasized that the midwife may not have 'missed' a problem at the time of examination, it could be that the abnormal sound was not there when the examination took place. The timing of this aspect of the examination is significant because of the circulatory adjustments that are taking place in the early neonatal period. Changes in ductal flow, with decreasing pulmonary resistance and increasing vascular resistance, mean that there is turbulent blood flow in the first few hours of life. If women are going home 6 hours after delivery, it could mean that this early assessment may not identify potential congenital heart defects and all babies should be given the opportunity to be examined again at 48 hours.

A recent study (The PulseOx study, 2009) has been looking at whether measuring the level of oxygen in newborn babies could help in the early detection of potential heart problems. Preliminary, as yet unpublished results from this study have been positive in early identification of congenital heart defects.

As with assessment of the lungs, the midwife should establish a whole picture of the baby, looking at the colour, tone, posture, respirations and feeding history. These parameters give a clear indication of the overall condition of the infant before auscultation of the heart takes place, since auscultation should never be performed in isolation. Capillary refill is performed by pressing with the thumb on the sternum until blanching has occurred. The midwife should count the time it takes for the skin to return to its normal colour. Normal capillary refill time is 3 seconds. Anything greater than this is abnormal.

The examination of the heart should commence with inspection of the precordium, which is the area on the anterior chest wall under which the heart lies. There should not be any noticeable pulsation of the apex at the 48-hour assessment although visible pulsation may be seen intermittently during the first few hours of life. Additional palpation of the precordium will elicit further information such as heaves and thrills. The medial side of the hand should be placed on the sternum where any vibratory sensations can be felt if they are present and are defined as follows:

- *Heave*: the hand will be felt to 'lift' if a heave is present.
- *Thrill*: a murmur that is loud enough (grade IV) can be felt through the chest wall. The cause is usually a defective valve or stenotic vessel.

The normal heart rate in the newborn period is between 100 and 160 beats per minute. There are four main heart sounds to be heard. The first heart sound (S1) is created by the closure of the tricuspid and mitral valves. The second heart sound (S2) is created by the closure of the pulmonary and aortic valves. However S3 and S4 are very rarely heard in the neonatal period. The first and second heart sounds are usually expressed as 'lub' (S1) and 'dub' (S2). When first starting to listen to heart sounds it is sometimes difficult to differentiate between heart and lung sounds. By watching the breathing pattern during auscultation, the midwife should be able to tell whether she or he is hearing heart or lung sounds, but this takes practice to perfect (Table 4.3).

The heart should be listened to when the baby is quiet and still which allows for a thorough assess-

Table 4.3 Heart sounds

Heart sound	Expressed as	Physiology	Auscultated area
S1	Lub	Closure of tricuspid and mitral valves	Apex or lower sternal edge
S2	Dub	Closure of pulmonary and aortic valves	Second intercostal space

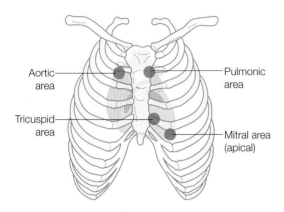

Figure 4.5 Main areas of the heart. (Reproduced from Tappero EP, Honeyfield ME (2003) *Physical Assessment of the Newborn*. Santa Rosa: Neonatal Network, NICU Ink Book Publishers © Elizabeth Weadon Massari)

Table 4.4 Stethoscope placement for assessment of the heart

Stethoscope placement	Area of heart
Second intercostal space, right sternal edge	Aortic
Second intercostal space, left sternal edge	Pulmonary
Fourth intercostal space, lower left sternal edge	Tricuspid
Fourth intercostal space, midclavicular line	Mitral

ment. The four main areas of the heart need to be assessed (Figure 4.5, Table 4.4).

Murmurs are described as prolonged heart sounds or as an additional sound during the cardiac sequence. It is important that the midwife listens to all five areas to identify any deviations from normal. It is not within the midwife's remit to diagnose congenital heart defects but it is well within her or his role to identify normality. Any variations of normal heart sounds therefore will need to be referred for a second opinion.

When a murmur is identified the midwife must establish whether the murmur occurs in systole or diastole. A systolic murmur will occur in between the 'lub' and 'dub,' whereas a diastolic murmur occurs between the 'dub' and 'lub'. In order to confirm whether the murmur is systolic or diastolic the midwife should palpate the brachial pulse at the same time as auscultating the heart sounds.

Heart murmurs are graded in terms of loudness:

- Grade I: very soft, barely audible
- Grade II: Soft but immediately audible
- Grade III: Moderately loud
- Grade IV: Loud and may be associated with a thrill
- Grade V: Very loud again associated with a thrill
- Grade VI: Audible with the stethoscope away from the chest.

Location of maximum intensity is an important factor and the midwife should listen to all areas of the chest to exclude radiation of the heard sound. The heart rate should be counted during auscultation and it should be noted that it is more likely for babies with congenital heart disease to be tachycardic rather than bradycardic.

Palpation of the femoral pulses is the final step in assessing the neonatal cardiovascular system. The femoral pulses are found in the groin, just below the inguinal ligament. Both pulses should be palpated simultaneously using the index or middle fingers and using only light pressure. This skill takes a little practice and quite often with novice examiners a pulse will be found on one side and not the other. This should not cause too much concern, but absent femoral pulses should be investigated further. If the femoral pulses feel weak or bounding, it is useful to palpate the brachial pulse to compare the intensity of the pulsation. Absent pulses could be an early sign of coarctation of the aorta and reliance on the ductus arteriosus will be maintaining the circulation. Medical assessment is always required if a murmur is discovered. It would be useful to perform a standard pulse oximetry test prior to medical assessment.

Congenital heart disease affects 8 per 1000 live births. The causes can be chromosomal, genetic, maternal or environmental. Common congenital heart defects seen in the first two weeks of life are:

- ventricular septal defect (VSD)
- atrial septal defect (ASD)
- patent ductus arteriosus (PDA)
- transposition of the great arteries
- tetralogy of Fallot
- pulmonary atresia
- hypoplastic left heart syndrome
- coarctation of the aorta
- pulmonary and aortic stenosis.

Congenital heart defects can be either acyanotic or cyanotic. With an acyanotic heart defect there will be left-to-right shunt and the baby will not be cyanosed because blood flows from the systemic to the pulmonary system, which causes increased blood flow to the lungs. With right-to-left shunts, blood flows from the pulmonary system to the systemic circulation, where deoxygenated blood mixes with oxygenated blood, thus causing the baby to be cyanosed. Babies will require further investigation, including ultrasound scan of the heart and referral to a neonatal cardiologist.

Neurological assessment

The final aspect of the physical examination is for the midwife to assess the neurological reflexes of the baby. Although a complete assessment in its own right, the midwife will have been able to gain much information about the baby's neurological status throughout the preceding physical examination. For example posture, cry and tone all give clues to the neurological wellbeing, as does the baby's response to handling. A loud, strong cry is usual in the term baby. A weak or feeble cry may be a sign of a premature or sick infant, whereas a high-pitched cry is associated with cerebral irritation, metabolic abnormalities and drug withdrawal.

Babies will lie in the flexed position with the head to one side following birth. Any alteration in neurological status will affect the baby's position and tone; more rarely neuromuscular disorders will also affect the tone. A hypotonic baby will not adopt the flexed position, will be floppy on handling, with head lag and weak extremities. Conversely, hypertonia will result in the baby adopting an extended position. Jitteriness in the early neonatal period is associated with hypoglycaemia or hypocalcaemia and is otherwise benign. If jitteriness is accompanied by hypotonia and irritability then the cause could be a sign of infection or drug withdrawal.

Jitteriness should be differentiated from seizures by observing the baby closely. Seizures are usually much more subtle in neonates than in older babies/children and can present as apnoea, cycling movements, eye-rolling as well as the more obvious clonic and tonic movements. Tonic movements are characterized by extension and stiffness of all limbs, whereas clonic movements are rapid contraction and relaxation of the muscles that can result in violent shaking.

When assessing the neurological reflexes the midwife should ensure that all the baby's movements are symmetrical. Some of this information will have been gained by undressing and examining the baby and should not be discounted. Discussion with the mother will elicit how well the baby is sleeping, how well they wake for feeding, how much they cry and if breastfeeding, how well they latch and suck at the breast. These are all excellent indicators of the baby's behaviour.

Referral pathways

Whether the midwife is working in a midwifery-led unit, obstetric unit or in the community there should be clear routes of referral. Unfortunately these are not always in place and this puts the midwife in a position whereby she or he has to refer to a junior doctor or GP who has less experience of examining babies. Dunn (2001) was adamant that midwives should refer neonatal problems to the junior doctor rather than a registrar as it formed part of the senior house officer's (SHO) training and learning experience and maintained a hierarchy within the medical profession. Attitudes have changed slightly now and midwives can refer directly to the consultant or registrar, bypassing the SHO as this can lead to delay in diagnosis and

Reflexes

- *Grasp reflex*: Placing the little finger into a baby's palm will elicit a grasp reflex. This is a strong response in the term infant, present from 12 weeks' gestation. Stroking the back of the baby's hand will allow the fingers to uncurl and release the grasp.

- *Plantar reflex*: Touching the sole of the foot with a finger will obtain a plantar response. Similar to the palmer grasp reflex.

- *Traction reflex*: Pulling the baby up by the hands will cause the elbows to flex and the baby to assume a sitting position. This reflex is usually seen from 37 weeks' gestation.

- *Rooting reflex*: Stroking the baby's cheek with a finger causes the head to turn towards the finger and the mouth will open.

- *Sucking reflex*: By placing a clean finger in the baby's mouth, the midwife will be able to assess the strength and coordination of the sucking reflex. Sucking is present even in the preterm infant but will be weaker and will lack coordination.

- *Stepping reflex*: Holding the baby under the arms with both hands the baby's feet are allowed to touch a flat surface. A primitive stepping reflex will be seen. This is present from about 34 weeks' gestation.

- *Moro reflex*: Supporting the baby's head in one hand a few centimetres from the cot, the midwife allows the head to fall into her other waiting hand. This should elicit the classic Moro response in which both of the baby's arms are thrown outwards and then brought back into the midline.

anxious waiting for parents. Nevertheless, it is pertinent for anyone undertaking this expansion of role to have agreed criteria and guidelines by which they practice to avoid confusion, embarrassment and delay when identifying a problem in the neonate.

Explanation and documentation

It is usual for the midwife to talk through the steps of the examination as she is performing them. This allows the parents to ask questions and for points to be clarified and explained. It is also a very good opportunity for the midwife to confirm normal features of the baby to the parents, offering reassurance to any worries they may have. The EMREN study

(Townsend *et al.*, 2004) found that maternal satisfaction was higher when midwives examined their babies because of the comprehensive explanations. The study also found that the midwives gave health education at the same time.

Midwives can use this opportunity to talk to the parents about feeding, car safety, smoking, diet, exercise, as well as many other pertinent topics.

Findings from the examination need to be documented in the child health record as well as in the relevant section in the maternal and neonatal notes. The Nursing and Midwifery Council (2008) are clear that nurses and midwives have a responsibility to ensure that all records are contemporaneous, detailed and accurate as well as being completed as soon as possible after an event has occurred.

Conclusion

There is no doubt that by expanding their role to include examination of the newborn, midwives have increased their workload. However, it completes the whole package of care to the family, making midwifery care truly holistic. Time constraints in hospital add to the pressure that midwives are under to free beds by discharging women home early. Six hours post delivery may not be the optimum time to carry out the newborn examination but it is better that babies are given a thorough assessment before they go home rather than not having an examination at all. Midwives are in a key position to perform the examination and will already possess some of the maternal and delivery history before the assessment commences.

It needs to be reiterated here that the midwifery role is to confirm normality and to identify anything that falls outside normal boundaries. Referral for prompt diagnosis is also a key role, knowing who to refer to and when. Advanced neonatal nurse practitioners have a slightly different role in that they can order investigations such as blood tests, X-rays and scans. It would be an advantage if midwives were given the same autonomy with the baby as they have with the mother.

A systematic approach to the examination is crucial so that nothing is missed. Assessing heart sounds and the reflexes while the baby is quiet is essential and leaving hip assessment and neurological assessment until the baby is more awake makes sense so that a comprehensive picture of the baby is elicited.

CASE HISTORY

A community midwife visited a mother and baby on the fifth postnatal day. The midwife was covering for a colleague who was on holiday and had not met this family before. On reading the notes there was nothing of any significance that would cause the midwife to be concerned. The grandmother of the baby was present while the midwife was assessing the baby; she stated that the baby's right arm did not move very much and that there was a lump on the 'collar-bone'.

The grandmother also complained that she had mentioned this to the midwife who had been visiting but that she had not taken any notice. On examination the midwife confirmed that there was a lump on the clavicle and there was reduced movement in the affected arm. The mother was short in stature and the baby weighed 4.2 kg at birth. On questioning the mother about her

labour the midwife was able to elicit that there had been some difficulty delivering the shoulders.

The midwife suspected a fractured clavicle and following referral to the GP an X-ray confirmed the diagnosis and physiotherapy was commenced. The overall outcome was good, but the family were distressed and very angry that this diagnosis had been missed in the first instance.

- What qualities do you think the midwife needed to alleviate the anger and worry from the family?
- Where had there been a breakdown in communication?
- Why do you think that the fractured clavicle had not been recognized before?
- What are the main clues to this diagnosis?

Key Points

- The midwife's role is to confirm normality to the parents and identify deviations from normal.
- It is not the midwife's responsibility to diagnose conditions although she or he may have the experience to do so.
- The midwife should refer for specialist or a second opinion.
- The physical examination forms part of the parent education process and should be seen as a learning opportunity.
- The midwife should be prepared to initiate emergency treatment as and when it is needed.

References

Bannister P (2008) Management of infants born with a cleft lip and palate. Part 1. *Infant* **4**: 5–8.

Campion JC and Benson MKD (2007) Clinical diagnosis of developmental dysplasia of the hip. *Surgery* **25**: 177.

Dunn P (2001) Examination of the newborn infant in the UK: a personal viewpoint. *Journal of Neonatal Nursing* **7**: 55–57.

Fletcher MA (1997) *Physical Diagnosis in Neonatology.* Philadelphia: Lippincott-Raven.

Hall DMB and Elliman D (eds) (2006) *Health for all Children,* 4th edn. Oxford: Oxford University Press.

Hogan M, Westcott C and Griffiths M (2005) Randomized, controlled trial of division of tongue-tie in infants with feeding problems. *Journal of Paediatric and Child Health* **41**: 246–250.

Lumsden H (2005) Midwives' experience of examination of the newborn as an additional aspect of their role: a qualitative study. *MIDIRS Midwifery Digest* **15**: 450–457.

National Screening Committee (2008) Newborn and infant physical examination. Standards and competencies. www.screening.nhs.uk/

Nursing and Midwifery Council (2008) *The Code. Standards of conduct, performance and ethics for nurses and midwives.* London: NMC.

PulseOx (2009) Birmingham Clinical Trials Unit, Birmingham University, Harborne, Birmingham. www.pulseox.bham.ac.uk

Resuscitation Council (UK) (2006) *Newborn Life Support. Resuscitation at birth,* 2nd edn. London: Resuscitation Council (UK).

Townsend J, Wolke, D, Hayes J, Davé S, Rogers C, Bloomfield L, Quist-Therson E, Tomlin M and Messer D (2004) Routine examination of the newborn: the EMREN study. Evaluation of an extension of the midwife role including a randomized controlled trial of appropriately trained midwives and paediatric house officers. *Health Technology Assessment* **8**: 14.

HEREDITARY PROBLEMS AND GENETICS

Debbie Holmes

OVERVIEW

This chapter provides an overview of genetic inheritance patterns. The aim is to present simplified explanations of patterns of inheritance and information on some disorders. Each disorder will look at the incidence, features and effect on lifespan. Contact details for the corresponding association/help for parents and professionals will be listed. The role of the health professional in relation to information-giving and women's choice is also explored.

Introduction

The human body is made up of millions of cells that have evolved from two cells – the product of conception. This miraculous feat is achieved through a complex process of cell division and we may wonder how the majority of human babies are born healthy and normal. These two words, 'normal' and 'healthy', are used to try to show an appreciation of the complexity of human development and not meant to define the parameters of normal or healthy, both of which have expansive and diverse definitions. For 'normal' fetal development to occur cell division must take place at particular critical times and the process is reliant on this division occurring without any errors. We therefore must have some knowledge of cells and cell division to enhance our understanding of how genetic differences may occur.

Cells

The cell is a fundamental unit of the human body. Most cells in the body are somatic; these are cells that contain two copies of each chromosome and are categorized as diploid. Diploid cells contain 23 pairs of chromosomes (46 chromosomes in all) carrying genetic information. When they divide they produce two identical cells through a process of mitosis (Figure 5.1). Although all somatic cells are genetically identical, they are capable of differentiation to enable them to become specialist cells for different tissues and different functions within the body during fetal

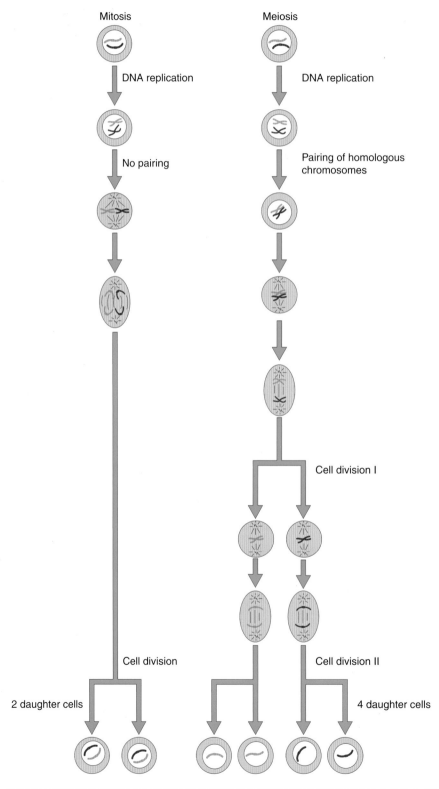

Figure 5.1   Comparison between mitosis and meiosis. To simplify, only chromosome pair number 1 is shown. (Reproduced with permission from Holmes D and Baker P (2006) *Ten Teachers in Midwifery*. London: Hodder Arnold)

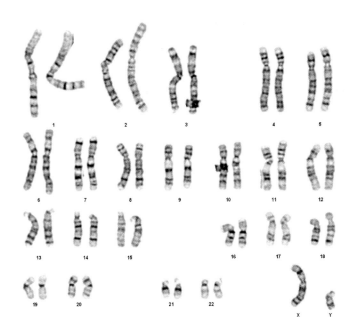

Figure 5.2 Normal karyotype. (Reproduced with permission from Levison D, Reid R and Burt A *et al.* (2008) *Muir's Textbook of Pathology*, 14th edn. London: Hodder Arnold)

development and during cell renewal and growth after birth.

The nucleus of each cell contains DNA (deoxyribonucleic acid). This is the genetic blueprint or information to be passed from cell to cell during division. The DNA is arranged on the chromosomes. DNA must be precisely replicated during cell division and the chromosomes separated successfully so that each new cell produced contains information that makes them genetically identical.

Ova and sperm

Ova (female eggs) and spermatozoa differ from other cells in the human body in that they are required to undergo a process of reduction division (meiosis) (Figure 5.1) to produce a haploid cell containing only one set of chromosomes, 23 in number. If this process did not occur the embryo would have 92 chromosomes (or 46 pairs) and would not develop. After the sperm and the ovum meet and fertilization occurs, the new cell becomes diploid, taking one of each pair of chromosomes, one from the mother and one from the father. The cell is now called the zygote and will go on to divide into the cells that develop into the fetus.

The haploid cells of the sperm and ova will contain 22 chromosomes and one sex chromosome each.

The ova will contain 22 chromosomes plus one X chromosome. The sperm will contain 22 chromosomes plus an X or a Y chromosome. The embryo will have 46 chromosomes in all, two of which are the sex chromosomes, one from the mother and one from the father (Figure 5.2). A female embryo will inherit an X from the mother and an X from the father; a male embryo will inherit an X from the mother and a Y from the father. Thus female = XX; male = XY.

Significance

Despite a decrease in perinatal mortality figures (CEMACH, 2008) in the UK in recent years, the incidence of genetic anomalies is harder to measure. It is estimated that in the general population the risk of having a baby with a serious condition is around 2–3 per cent (Genetic Interest Group, 2008). A high percentage of women will choose to terminate a pregnancy if they discover the fetus they carry has Down's syndrome. Sixty per cent of fetuses who have Down's syndrome are diagnosed antenatally and 45 per cent of women will opt for a termination of pregnancy. Forty per cent are diagnosed in the postnatal period (Morris, 2009). There are obviously many genetic anomalies other than Down's syndrome, but statistics for this condition are good due to the national screening programme in the UK.

Children with genetic anomalies may require specialist support and possible paediatric hospital admission. Their anomaly may contribute to paediatric morbidity and mortality figures.

Already we can see that the ovum and the sperm both have to be in optimum condition when they arrive at the moment of conception. One parent may already have an abnormality in their chromosomes that they may or may not be aware of. If the chromosomes already carry an abnormality when they 'meet' this may manifest as an expressed genetic abnormality in the baby or a chromosomal defect not expressed but carried in the cells of the baby. This genetic information may then be expressed in a future generation. The term 'genotype' applies to the genetic makeup of the individual and may or may not affect appearance, behaviour or lifestyle. The term 'phenotype' refers to the way that the genotype is expressed in the individual through their physical makeup, physiological functioning or behaviour.

There may be other factors involved with the development of a genetic abnormality.

It has been known for some time that women beyond the age of 35 carry a higher risk of conceiving a fetus with Down's syndrome; they have a percentage risk of 0.37 per cent compared with a woman aged 20 who carries a very low percentage risk of 0.066 per cent. The age of the woman around the time of conception can be a factor as it is possible that the chromosomes will not divide correctly (Cuckle *et al.*, 1987).

It is not only the ovum that can be problematic with increasing age, there is current research to suggest that the male sperm may also carry a higher risk of chromosomal abnormalities beyond the age of 35. DNA has been seen to be damaged in the sperm examined in samples from men over the age of 35, suggesting a 'biological clock' for men that entails an optimum time for 'normal' sperm production (Singh *et al.*, 2003).

Environmental damage can also affect the chromosomes in the ova or sperm before they arrive at the point of conception. Radiation, for example, is known to damage the DNA in cells (see Mutations below).

It is thought that around 6 per cent of all zygotes have a chromosomal problem and many will never implant (Stables and Rankin, 2005). Around 50 per cent of conceptions that result in spontaneous miscarriages (abortions) are a result of a chromosomal abnormality (Holmes and Baker, 2006).

Too many or too few chromosomes at conception

It is possible for the chromosomes of the parents to be normal, but for some reason when the meiotic division occurs the chromosomes do not distribute themselves properly between the cells. The result is an ovum or sperm going forward for fertilization with the wrong number of chromosomes in the nucleus, usually 24 instead of 23 chromosomes. Down's syndrome occurs, for example, where there are too many chromosomes as a result of a problem with cell division.

Too few chromosomes will in most cases be incompatible with pregnancy survival as vital data are missing. However, when one of the sex chromosomes is missing (the embryo has 45 instead of 46) survival is possible. An example of this type of inheritance is Turner's syndrome in females, where there is only one X chromosome.

Sometimes there is partial loss of a chromosome, as in cri du chat syndrome (see below), in which the terminal part of chromosome 5 is missing. When there is loss of any genetic material the disorders are often more problematic.

Damaged chromosomes (structural chromosomal defects)

Translocation

Sometimes a chromosome can become damaged, resulting in a small part being lost and attaching itself to another chromosome. If an exchange is made and the detached part swaps places with part of the chromosome to which it attaches, all the genetic material is still there and there will not be a genetic abnormality. This is called a balanced translocation. If, however, the final complement of genetic material is extra there may be an abnormality. An example is another type of Down's syndrome inheritance in which the third chromosome 21 attaches to another chromosome. Parents are often unaware that a balanced translocation has occurred unless the genetic makeup of the fetus has been analysed in an antenatal test (e.g. amniocentesis).

Mutations

Mutation can occur in the DNA during DNA replication. These are common and may have no effect. They will, however, be inherited in the DNA of any offspring. A mutation may be caused by environmental factors, such as radiation exposure.

Inheritance patterns

The fetus will inherit 23 pairs of chromosomes by taking one half of each pair from the mother and one from the father. These pairs provide the genetic instructions, which may or may not be the same on both chromosomes of the pair. For example:

- mother provides a gene for blue eyes only
- father provides a gene for blue eyes only
- the baby inherits blue eyes.

In this case the genes are called *homozygous*. But if:

- mother provides gene for blue eyes only
- father provides gene for green eyes only
- the baby may have a blend of both or if one colour is more dominant they may inherit that colour.

This pattern is called *heterozygous* for the pair.

Recessive genes and inheritance

Where there is a weaker gene it is called the recessive gene. In this case both parents must have the same defective gene for their offspring to be affected. There will be a one in four chance that any pregnancy may be affected (see Phenylketonuria on page 61).

Dominant genes and inheritance

Where there is a dominant gene, as with achondroplasia, if the gene is inherited by the baby the baby will have the disorder (see Achondroplasia on page 62).

What is a genetic abnormality/disorder/ condition/difference?

A genetic 'abnormality' is caused by a chromosomal abnormality that arises from the parents or is caused during cell division around the time of conception.

Support groups

Down's syndrome
- Down's Syndrome Association www.downs-syndrome.org.uk/

Trisomy 13 and 18
- S.O.F.T www.soft.org.uk

Klinefelter's syndrome
- Klinefelter's Syndrome Association www.ksa-uk.co.uk

Cri du chat syndrome
- Cri du Chat Syndrome Support Group www.criduchat.co.uk/researchintocriduchat.html

Muscular dystrophy
- www.nhs.uk/Conditions/Muscular-dystrophy

Phenylketonuria
- National Society for Phenylketonuria www.nspku.org/

Achondroplasia
- Achondroplasia UK www.achondroplasia.co.uk

An environmental factor may be responsible for a problem during cell division.

Some examples of genetic conditions are listed below. As many people live with many of these conditions they are not necessarily considered 'abnormalities/disorders'. Down's syndrome is a good example; many people may have the syndrome but it is not a disease. Down's syndrome is discussed in detail below, identifying some of the screening and diagnostic testing available. Some of the diagnostic testing discussed may also be offered for other disorders discussed later in the chapter.

Conditions where chromosome numbers are duplicated

Down's syndrome (trisomy 21)

Incidence

The incidence of Down's syndrome is 1 in approximately 800 births overall (Stables and Rankin, 2007), although there is an increased risk related to maternal age (Cuckle *et al.*, 1987). Both boys and girls can be affected.

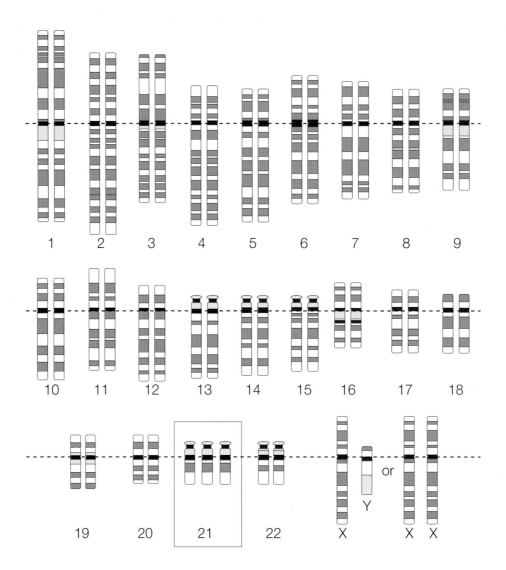

Figure 5.3   Trisomy. (Courtesy: National Human Genome Research Institute)

Genetic explanation

A baby with Down's syndrome will have three copies of chromosome 21 (Figure 5.3) – this is the most common type – meaning that there are 47 chromosomes in all. The reason for this happening is currently unknown although it is linked to maternal age (Cuckle *et al.*, 1987).

In translocation Down's syndrome the third chromosome 21 attaches to another chromosome, keeping the total at 46 chromosomes. This form accounts for around 4 per cent of Down's syndrome cases.

Two per cent of babies with Down's syndrome will have a mosaic form, where only some of the cells have the extra chromosome. There are also other rarer forms of chromosomal disorders that can lead to a baby with Down's syndrome.

Features at birth

The eyes have an upward slant and epicanthic folds, a fold of skin at the inner corner of the eye. A small head is common, flatter at the back with a thickened nuchal fold (fold of skin at the back of the neck). The

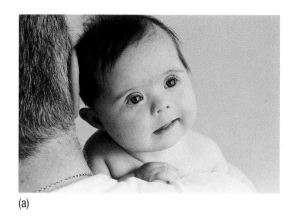

(a)

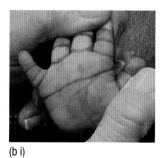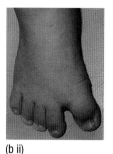

(b i)   (b ii)

Figure 5.4   (a) Baby with Down's syndrome. (b) Single palmer crease and sandal gap. (Courtesy of Down's Syndrome Association, www.downs-syndrome.org.uk)

ears are small. A small mouth makes the tongue appear large and there is often a flattened nasal bridge (Figure 5.4a). Brushfield's spots (white flecks on the iris) are present in most children with Down's syndrome and do not affect vision. Some have cataracts, squint and nystagmus. The limbs and fingers can be short. A single palmer crease can be found in most cases. There is also a wide gap between the big toe and the rest of the toes (sandal toe) (Figure 5.4b). Muscle tone can be poor and the baby may present as 'floppy' and may have difficulty establishing oral feeding. The baby may be small for gestational age. Some babies present with congenital heart conditions or these may have been identified by ultrasound scan in pregnancy.

Life

Lifespan can be up to 60 years of age (Gilbert, 2001). Life experience for people with Down's syndrome is variable, with some children attaining developmental milestones, albeit delayed and attending mainstream school. Other children may have significant delays in developmental and physical milestones and will require specialist input to achieve their full potential. All children with Down's syndrome will have some degree of learning disability. There will be congenital heart defects for approximately 40 per cent of children, some of whom may require surgery. Five per cent of children will have gastrointestinal problems such as duodenal atresia or Hirschsprung disease.

Upper respiratory infections are more likely as the airways are narrowed due to flattened nasal bridge or an impaired immune system. Ear infections and deafness are common.

Thyroid disease is common and there is also a higher risk of developing Alzheimer's disease by the age of 40.

Screening before birth

Some congenital heart defects and some physical markers such as the amount of fluid at the nape of the neck (nuchal fold scanning) may be picked up by ultrasound scan. Blood tests to provide a risk result can be performed and the accuracy of predicting that a problem may be present increases with the advancement of technology and the refining of the tests offered.

Currently the National Institute for Health and Clinical Excellence (NICE, 2008) in the UK are recommending that all pregnant women are offered screening for Down's syndrome. This is a choice and as such women need accurate information about the testing and any subsequent diagnostics that may be offered, such as amniocentesis. Prior to embarking on the screening tests women should be aware of the choices they may be offered if a fetus with Down's syndrome is identified (i.e. counselling about continuing with the pregnancy and preparing to bring up a baby who will need extra support to live a full and rewarding life). For some women the choices may include termination of the pregnancy.

It is suggested that screening for Down's syndrome should take place by the end of the first trimester (between 11 and 13 weeks 6 days). This is the 'combined test' incorporating measuring the fluid around the nuchal fold by scan and performing a blood test. A triple or quadruple blood test is still available for those women who decide to test later or miss this first opportunity. This can be done up to 20 weeks of pregnancy.

If the test returns a result considered to be high risk the pregnant woman requires further information as to what the risk means in terms she can understand before being offered a diagnostic test such as amniocentesis. Amniocentesis is a test where amniotic fluid is taken from around the fetus and the sample analysed, examining the DNA of the fetus. A needle is inserted into the uterus under ultrasound guidance and a sample of amniotic fluid is drawn off and sent to the laboratory. This procedure carries a 1 per cent risk of miscarriage (CEMAT, 1998). If the diagnosis is positive for a fetus with Down's syndrome the woman and her family will require immediate counselling regarding the implications of the diagnosis for them.

Genetic counselling

Future pregnancies will carry an increased risk whatever the inheritance pattern and parents may opt for diagnostic tests earlier without the blood testing for risk. A sample of the chorionic villi can be taken at between 11 and 13 weeks of pregnancy and can provide an early genetic profile of the fetus, as the amniocentesis does. Chorionic villus sampling carries a 2 per cent risk of miscarriage (CEMAT, 1998).

Patau syndrome and Edwards' syndrome will now be discussed briefly as they share similarities with Down's syndrome inheritance and may be seen more commonly than some of the later conditions discussed.

Patau's syndrome (trisomy 13)

Incidence

The incidence of Patau's syndrome is 1 in 6000–8000 births (Gilbert, 2001). This condition is more severe than Down's syndrome and many pregnancies end in miscarriage or stillbirth, and some of the babies born alive will die within the first months of life. Only 10 per cent of babies survive and they suffer severe learning disabilities and often have other congenital anomalies (Gilbert, 2001). There is some evidence to suggest that, as with Down's syndrome, maternal age may be a factor. Both males and females are affected.

Genetic explanation

There are three chromosomes in the 13th position, hence trisomy 13. A mosaic pattern may present when not all of the cells contain 47 chromosomes. These babies are less severely affected and may account for most of those that survive.

Features

Small for gestational age and low birth weight will present, but the clinical features will aid recognition. The head is often microcephalic and may be detected on ultrsound scan. Cleft palate and/or lip are often present along with extra digits. The eyes and jaw are small. Defects in the bony skull may be present, as may heart and renal defects. Chromosomal studies will provide a diagnosis.

Edwards' syndrome (trisomy 18)

Incidence

The incidence of Edwards' syndrome is approximately 1 in every 6000 live births (Gilbert, 2001), or as high as 1 in 3000 (Genetics Education, 2009). The effects can be severe or mild depending upon the form of inheritance.

Genetic pattern

As with Down's syndrome and Patau's syndrome there are three chromosomes, this time in the 18th position. When most cells in the body are affected, the condition is most severe and life expectancy short. A mosaic form where some of the cells are affected will present less severely with a longer life expectancy.

Features

The babies are often hypotonic at birth and may have feeding difficulties. As the baby grows the muscles become hypertonic. Microcephaly is common, as is a short neck and a small, receding jaw exacerbating feeding problems. Up to 95 per cent of children may have a cardiac defect. There is often a single palmar crease and the feet are also often convex on the soles: 'rockerbottom' feet. Renal abnormalities are also common.

Conditions where sex chromosomes are duplicated or lost

Klinefelter's syndrome and Turner's syndrome are two conditions in this category.

Klinefelter's syndrome

Incidence

Klinefelter's syndrome (47-XXY, 48-XXXY, 49-XXXXY, 48-XXYY) is quite common: it is suggested that 1 in 1000 boys could have this type of chromosomal pattern (Gilbert, 2001; Klinefelter's Association, 2009). Unlike people with Down's syndrome, males with Klinefelter's syndrome do not have characteristic physical features and may not be diagnosed until later in life during fertility investigations.

Genetic explanation

Klinefelter's syndrome is caused by an extra X chromosome derived from the sex chromosomes. During the cell division of the parent's sex chromosomes an extra X arrives at conception. The meiotic division has not occurred correctly, resulting in either two XX from the ovum or an XY from the sperm arriving for fertilization, resulting in XXY. There is also a mosaic form where not all the cells have XXY and there are even more complex forms such as XXXY and XXXXY.

Features

These vary greatly and may not present until the child reaches puberty. The only sign at birth may be unusually small testicles. As puberty advances the testes and penis remain smaller than those of other boys, there will be a lowered level of testosterone and a raised level of gonadotrophins, resulting in infertility. Breast development may be seen in some boys.

Life

Life expectancy is normal. Mainstream education and job opportunities are possible unless behaviour is affected badly due to psychological difficulties. Infertility is usual, although men with the mosaic form can sometimes father children. There is an increased risk of osteoporosis.

Genetic counselling

As the syndrome is a result of cell division around the time of conception there is always the same chance of the occurrence for any individual. Kleinfelter's syndrome is not screened for but may be identified if chromosomal studies are performed by amniocentesis or chorionic villus sampling.

Conditions where genetic material on chromosomes is deleted

Examples are cri du chat syndrome and Prader–Willi syndrome.

Cri du chat syndrome

Incidence

The incidence of cri du chat syndrome is approximately 1 in 20 000 births (Gilbert, 2001), although some sources quote incidences of between 1 in 37 000 and 1 in 50 000 (Cornish et al., 2003).

Genetic explanation

This is a deletion of some of the material on chromosome number 5. It often appears as a mutation although one of the parents may have a balanced translocation. If this is the case there remains a risk for future pregnancies. If the loss of genetic material is not in the critical region of chromosome 5 then the child will only be mildly affected, however if it is within the critical region then physical and cognitive development will be affected.

Features

The baby will have a high-pitched cry like a kitten because of a small larynx. There may be intrauterine growth restriction. Microcephaly is present and the baby can have epicanthic folds and a flattened nasal bridge. There may be congenital heart defects present. The baby is often floppy and has difficulty feeding.

Life

Life expectancy can be up to 60 years but life potential will vary with the severity of the symptoms. Children can have respiratory or heart conditions.

Genetic counselling

This would be of value because of the translocation inheritance. It may be picked up via genetic testing, via amniocentesis or chorionic villus sampling but is not screened for routinely.

Examples of sex-linked chromosomal inheritance

Fragile X syndrome, Duchenne muscular dystrophy and haemophilia are three conditions caused by sex-linked chromosomal abnormalities.

Duchenne muscular dystrophy

Incidence

Duchenne muscular dystrophy affects males only and has an incidence of around 1 in 3300 liveborn boys (Gilbert, 2001).

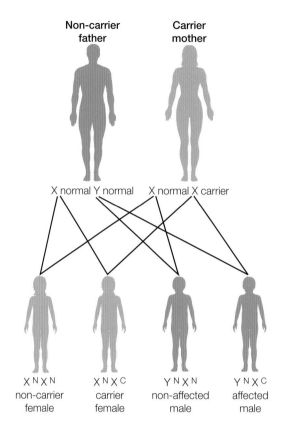

Figure 5.5   Recessive inheritance of an X-linked disorder (e.g. Duchenne's muscular dystrophy): N, normal gene; C, carrier gene

Genetic explanation

This condition is inherited by an X-linked pattern and affects the 23rd pair of genes. The mother is the carrier of the anomaly and as the male fetus must take one of her X chromosomes he has a 50 per cent chance of taking the affected one. Daughters have a 50 per cent chance of being carriers (Figure 5.5). For a female to be affected her father would have to also have an affected X chromosome. If he had an affected X, however, and the mother did not the daughter would not inherit the disease. Mutations can sometimes cause the disease.

Features

Boys often develop normally until they delay walking. Around the age of three years is a common time for diagnosis. The muscles of the body are affected and it

is a progressive disorder. The muscles of organs such as the lungs and the heart may become affected.

Life

Lifespan is shortened, with death usually occurring prior to the mid twenties. Specialist care and support is required to improve the quality of life.

Screening

Determining the sex of the fetus as male in pregnancy can enable genetic studies which would identify an affected male. Sex selection by assisted conception methods could be useful for some couples.

Genetic counselling

This is important for families with a history.

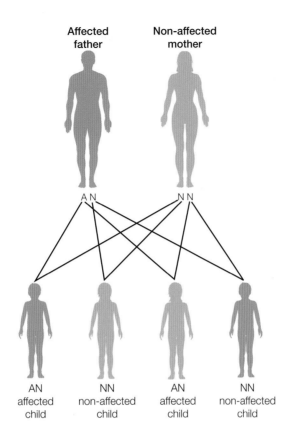

Figure 5.6   Dominant inheritance pattern: N, normal gene; A, affected gene

Recessive inheritance

Phenylketonuria (see also Chapter 3)

Incidence

The incidence is around 1 in 10 000 births (Gilbert, 2001).

Genetic explanation

Phenylketonuria is inherited in a recessive manner. Both parents need to have the affected gene for the fetus to inherit the condition (see Chapter 3 pp 24–25 for inheritance pattern). There is a 1 in 4 chance that a pregnancy can be affected if both parents carry the anomaly.

Features

It is rarely seen in the UK as most babies undergo a screening test at around one week of age and their diet is adjusted to enable normal development and growth. The enzyme to convert phenylalanine is deficient in this metabolic disorder and phenylalanine can build up over time, causing learning disability. Vomiting can occur and the baby's skin becomes dry with a rash. Life expectancy can be shortened if the disorder is not diagnosed.

Life

If diagnosed the child will have to follow a diet that has a monitored restricted intake of phenylalanine. Frequent blood tests will be required. If treatment is put in place normal schooling and lifestyle can be expected.

Screening

The neonatal bloodspot test tests for phenylketonuria among other disorders. Genetic testing in pregnancy can be done but many parents would choose to adjust lifestyle and would not necessarily terminate a pregnancy.

Genetic counselling

If someone with phenylketonuria is embarking on a pregnancy genetic counselling can be helpful as a mother with phenylketonuria may have to look more closely at her diet so that the developing baby is not subjected to high levels of phenylalanine in the uterus. If a family member has the disorder testing of the parents to be before conception can be useful.

Dominant inheritance

Achondroplasia

Incidence

Achondroplasia has an incidence of approximately 1 in 25 000 births (Gilbert, 2001).

Genetic explanation

Achondroplasia is an example of dominant gene inheritance but can also be the result of a mutation. This anomaly means that the fetus (of either sex) has to only inherit one affected gene from one parent to be affected by the condition (Figure 5.6).

Features

Short limbs are a feature but normal body trunk length and obvious short stature are also common. The head is of normal size but may appear bigger due to a pronounced forehead and a flattened bridge to the nose. Hands are broad and short. Spinal and pelvic abnormalities may be present; spinal curvature can cause back problems.

Life

Lifespan can be normal and individuals can lead full lives providing there are no major spinal abnormalities. Slipped discs are not uncommon and spinal cord compression can occur. Emotional problems can affect the individual and some families may need specialist support. The condition will not affect conception or the ability to carry a pregnancy, but birth may be assisted by caesarean section as pelvic abnormalities may be present.

Screening

Normal genetic diagnostics in pregnancy can be utilized or ultraound scan may pick up an unknown familial genetic pattern or mutation

Genetic counselling

If one parent has the disorder then there is a 50 per cent chance for each pregnancy. If both parents have it there is a 75 per cent chance for each pregnancy. Genetic counselling would be helpful.

Consanguinity

Consanguinity for the purpose of this chapter refers to couples who are blood relations that are second cousins or closer. In the UK it is suggested that 50–60 per cent of the British Pakistani community are in consanguineous marriages and it is prevalent in many communities from North Africa and the Middle East (Genepool, 2006). With no history of genetic disease in a family the general population risk for an anomaly is around 2 per cent and that for a consanguineous couple 3 per cent, so the risk is not much higher. There will, however, be a much higher risk for some genetic anomalies, especially recessive inheritance patterns. Genetic counselling may be sought by couples or their families or they may be reassured by a deep cultural belief that this is not required.

Indications for genetic counselling

Genetic counselling may be requested by parents where a family history of genetic anomalies is thought to exist. It may also be offered for future pregnancies when a particular pregnancy has been affected or a baby has been born with a genetic difference. Each case is individual due to the complexity of genetic inheritance differences. Options available need to be discussed and embryo selection may be an option following assisted conception techniques for some couples. For example, it may be advisable to only select a female embryo or an unaffected male embryo where the mother is a carrier for Duchenne's muscular dystrophy.

Screening choices

When they opt for the screening test for their Down's risk, many couples do not realise that the result could mean they are faced with numerous other difficult decisions along the way. The midwife providing the antenatal care must be sure the woman has all the information required to make the right choice for her and her family (Nursing and Midwifery Council, 2004). The possible outcomes should be explained clearly and further choices that may present. Ultimately the choice of terminating a pregnancy should be mentioned, as this may influence the decision of some women whether or not to have the screening in the first place.

Some women will still choose to have the screening done in the hope that they will receive a reassuring low-risk result. They should be informed, however, that even if they receive a result of 1 in 12 000, considered low risk, they could still be the 1 in 12 000. If a woman has had a low-risk result like this and then has gone on to have a baby with Down's syndrome she is unlikely to have confidence in the screening testing for a subsequent pregnancy and she may opt for no testing at all or she may consider a diagnostic test in the first instance.

There are obvious dilemmas for women with the screening testing, and for some women the anxieties around screening can affect their adaptation to pregnancy. Some women will choose to have the screening as they would wish to terminate a pregnancy, other women will choose because they wish to be prepared if their baby is going to require special support because of a genetic disorder.

CASE HISTORY

Claire aged 27 and Michael aged 30 were delighted to inform the midwife of their second pregnancy. The midwife had been involved in their care when their three-year-old daughter Mia was born. At the 'booking' appointment the midwife went over the screening available to identify their risk of having a baby with Down's syndrome. At the time a blood test was offered around 16 weeks of pregnancy, the results of which would be available around a week after testing. Claire and Michael decided that because they had the test with Mia and it was a reassuring low-risk result they would also have the test for this pregnancy.

A week after having the blood test the midwife had to inform them that the result had returned a high-risk chance of them having a baby with Down's syndrome. It was explained that although the risk was 1 in 140 there was a 1 in 139 chance that it was not a problem and that the fetus had a normal genetic makeup. It was also reiterated that the blood test was only a risk-identifying tool and that only a diagnostic test could tell them for sure whether their baby had Down's syndrome or not.

An appointment was made for the following day with the consultant obstetrician and the opportunity for an amniocentesis at the same time if that is what they decided to do. The midwife explained that there was a small risk of miscarriage with the procedure and that if they required longer to consider their decision that this was also fine.

Claire and Michael chose to opt for the amniocentesis the following day. At this point they were unsure of their final decisions if their baby were to have Down's syndrome. They had begun to ask questions about the syndrome and had spent a great deal of time on the Internet doing their own research. The amniocentesis went well and despite a worrying 48 hours no signs of the pregnancy being threatened occurred.

The results of the amniocentesis can take a while to be processed and this was a worrying time for Claire and Michael. Unfortunately the midwife received the news that although the fetus did not have Down's syndrome it had been diagnosed with another genetic disorder, Klinefelter's syndrome, which meant they would also know their baby was a boy.

On relaying this information to the couple the midwife knew that they would require more information than she could possibly provide and an immediate appointment was made with the obstetrician. The results of the genetic testing were presented to the couple and after much soul-searching they decided to terminate the pregnancy.

The midwife continued to support the family during this sad time. The decision to terminate a pregnancy is never an easy one and requires specialist care.

Key Points

- DNA is the genetic blueprint carried in our cells.
- Cell division is a complex process.
- Genetic advances and counselling can assist some couples planning pregnancies.
- Pregnancy screening can present couples with difficult decisions.

References

CEMACH (Confidential Enquiry into Maternal and Child Health) (2008) Perinatal Mortality 2006: England, Wales and N Ireland. London: CEMACH.

CEMAT (Canadian and Mid Trimester Amniocentesis Trial) (1998) The Canadian and mid trimester amniocentesis trial (CEMAT). Randomised trial to assess safety and fetal outcome of early and mid trimester amniocentesis. *Lancet* **351**: 242–247.

Cornish K, Oliver C, Standen P, Bramble D and Collins M (2003) *Cri du Chat Syndrome: Handbook for parents and professionals*, 2nd edn. Cri du Chat Support Group. http://www.criduchat.co.uk/researchintocriduchat.html [accessed 25 March 2009].

Cuckle H, Wald NJ and Thompson SG (1987) Estimating a woman's risk of having a pregnancy associated with Down's syndrome using her age and serum alphfetoprotein level. *British Journal of Obstetrics and Gynaecology* **94**: 387–402.

Genepool (2006) Consangunuity briefing. http://www.library.nhs.uk/geneticconditions [accessed 25 March 2009].

Genetic Interest Group (2008) Genetics information and education, updated 2008. http://www.gig.org.uk/education.htm [accessed 24 April 2009].

Genetics Education (2009) Edwards syndrome. http://www.geneticseducation.nhs.uk/learning/conditions.asp?id=21 [accessed 25 March 2009].

Gilbert P (2001) *A–Z of Syndromes and Inherited Disorders*, 3rd edn. Cheltenham: Nelson Thornes.

Holmes D and Baker P (eds) (2006) *Ten Teachers in Midwifery*. London: Hodder Arnold.

Klinfelter's Syndrome Association (2009) About the Klinefelter's Syndrome Association and the condition. http://www.ksa-uk.co.uk [accessed 25 March 2009].

Morris JK (2009) The National Down Syndrome Cytogenetic Register 2007/8 Annual Report. Barts and The London School of Medicine and Dentistry. Queen Mary University of London.

NICE (National Institute for Health and Clinical Excellence) (2008) *Antenatal Care: Routine care for the healthy pregnant woman*. London: Royal College of Obstetricians and Gynaecologists.

Nursing and Midwifery Council (2004) *Midwives' Rules & Standards*. London: NMC.

Singh NP, Muller CH and Berger RE (2003) Effects of age on DNA double-strand breaks and apoptosis in human sperm. *Fertility and Sterility* **80**: 1420–1430.

Stables D and Rankin J (2005) *Physiology in Childbearing with Anatomy and Related Biosciences*, 2nd edn. Edinburgh: Elsevier.

INFANT FEEDING

Debbie Holmes

OVERVIEW

This chapter will explore infant feeding, discussing both breast and artificial feeding and will include national guidelines and current advice for health professionals and parents. In relation to breastfeeding, anatomy and physiology will be applied and evidence-based advice that midwives and health professionals should provide to encourage successful breastfeeding. Guidance on artificial feeding, sterilization and storage of both breast and formula milk will be provided.

Introduction

In the following text it will be assumed from the outset that human breast milk is the best food for a newborn infant and that it is the only food a healthy newborn infant requires for the first months of life. It will be acknowledged, however, that not all new mothers will be able to or wish to breastfeed their baby. A baby who is born prematurely or who is ill will benefit greatly from breast milk and some mothers will choose to supply breast milk for these babies even if they have an intention to feed formula when their baby is well.

Whatever the choice of feeding method a mother must be given information to allow her to make informed decisions in relation to her infant. Support for mothers who choose to feed formula milk to their baby is just as important as that provided for breastfeeding mothers.

Breastfeeding

To support a mother to successfully breastfeed, the healthcare professional, midwife, doctor, nurse or support worker must have knowledge of the anatomy of the breast and the physiology of breastfeeding. This may be part of initial training but must also be part of updated practice annually. The National Institute for Health and Clinical Excellence (NICE) has issued postnatal care guidance (NICE, 2006) that advises all maternity care providers to implement an externally evaluated structured programme that encourages breastfeeding, using the Baby Friendly initiative (www.babyfriendly.org.uk) as a minimum standard. Many UK hospital trusts and primary care trusts have achieved, or are working towards, these standards. This requires a dedicated lead professional who can manage the implementation, apply for accreditation and then provide continual support and education to maintain the accreditation as a facility. It is also possible to attain this accreditation as an educational institution, allowing universities to educate student midwives and other healthcare professionals to these standards.

Benefits of breastfeeding for the baby

Breast milk is nutritionally balanced and easily digested by newborn babies and because babies regulate the amount they eat they are unlikely to overstretch their stomachs. Breastfed babies are less likely to overfeed and less likely to be obese or develop diabetes when older. The average size of the stomach is shown in Figure 6.1. Babies utilize their jaw muscles to breastfeed and this can enhance speech development. As they feed the eustachian tube (the tube between the

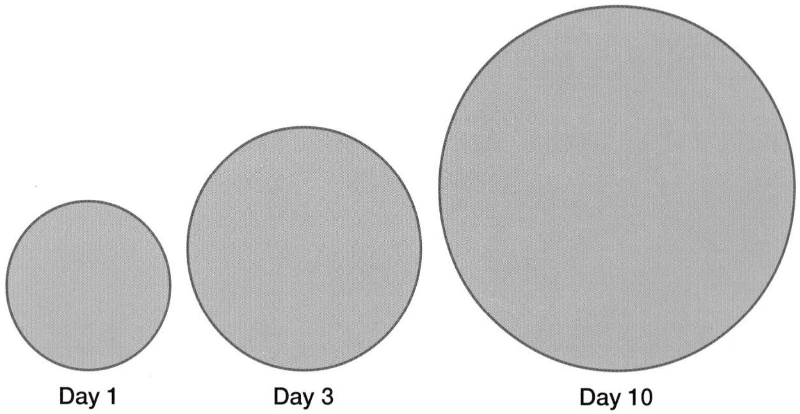

Figure 6.1   Sizes of a newborn's stomach on days 1, 3 and 10

Day 1   Day 3   Day 10

throat and the middle ear) is kept open and this can reduce the chances of middle ear infections (otitis media). A breastfed baby is also less likely to develop allergies as breast milk contains anti-allergenic agents. There is also a decreased chance of other infections of the respiratory, gastric and urinary systems.

Babies who are breastfed are more likely to have higher IQ due to enhanced neural system development

Benefits of breastfeeding for the mother

Breastfeeding is convenient for mothers and is economical, requiring no special purchases. Transportation is easy and sterility is assured; things that come at a cost for the mother who feeds her baby formula.

While breastfeeding a mother releases a hormone called oxytocin that assists the uterus to contract following the birth. Breastfeeding also utilizes energy and helps the woman regain pre-pregnancy weight levels. Fat is laid down in pregnancy to act as an energy store and when breastfeeding this is converted into usable energy, ultimately assisting in weight loss.

Breastfeeding women have fewer incidences of breast and ovarian cancers. There is a reduced risk of osteoporosis and it may be some help in preventing postnatal depression. There is often a delay in ovulation and although this cannot be a substitute for effective contraception, for some women this is the only way they can reduce the chances of another conception.

Anatomy of the breast

The breasts or mammary glands are situated on the anterior chest wall as two hemispherical swellings, either side of the midline. Breast tissue is mainly composed of glandular and adipose (fat) tissue and varies from woman to woman. Until recently the conventional view of the anatomy of the breast has gone unchallenged, but new technology has enabled a different insight into some of the structures. Originally the work of Sir Astley Cooper in 1840 suggested that there were many openings onto the nipple and that the glandular breast tissue was mostly towards the back of the breast, with reservoir-type sinuses behind the nipple. New evidence has come to light, however, following work by Ramsay *et al.* (2005) using ultrasound images of the lactating breast. The new information suggests that there are no reservoirs or ampullae as once thought, and the ducts are uniform in width. Breast tissue can be found directly behind the nipple, instead of being towards the back of the breast, and an average of nine ducts open onto the nipple instead of the textbook 15–20. This is important new information that needs to be considered as we learn more about how the baby feeds at the breast and how we can best support women to be successful at breastfeeding (Figure 6.2).

The breasts develop at puberty under the influence of oestrogen. During pregnancy further development occurs under the influence of oestrogen and progesterone. New glandular tissue is seen and the

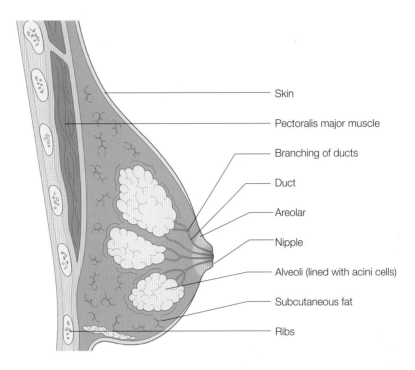

Skin

Pectoralis major muscle

Branching of ducts

Duct

Areolar

Nipple

Alveoli (lined with acini cells)

Subcutaneous fat

Ribs

Figure 6.2 Anatomical drawing of the breast

areolar increases in size and may become more pigmented. Montgomery's tubercles develop (sebaceous glands) and secrete lubrication to keep the nipple moist. Colostrum is present in the breasts from around 16 weeks of pregnancy. Body fat increases in anticipation of increased energy needs for lactation.

Physiology

Although the breasts will produce small amounts of colostrum during pregnancy, following the birth a miraculous process occurs to produce the only food a baby will need for the coming months. Changes occur rapidly in the woman's body, increasing amounts of blood are supplied to the breasts, enabling the glandular tissue to act under the influence of hormones to produce a supply of milk to meet the baby's needs.

Four hormones are involved with the initiation of milk production: oestrogen, progesterone, prolactin and oxytocin. Just prior to birth the blood levels of oestrogen rise and progesterone falls and it is thought that this may be responsible for releasing the acini cells in the alveoli from their inhibitory state, enabling

them to respond to prolactin and begin the production of milk (galactopoiesis). Prolactin is produced by the anterior pituitary under the influence of the hypothalamus. Following the birth of the baby and the expulsion of the placenta, prolactin levels decrease, but remain much higher than those of a non-pregnant woman. Prolactin levels peak in the woman's blood around 30 minutes after a feed; they are lower in the morning and highest in the night. The main stimulus for release of prolactin is the baby suckling at the breast.

Oxytocin is produced in the hypothalamus and stored in the posterior pituitary gland. It is required to cause contraction of the myoepithelial cells (small muscles surrounding the alveoli) and the smooth muscle surrounding the ducts. By contracting the muscle tissues the milk is propelled through the duct system to be available for the baby (the 'let down' reflex). Oxytocin levels rise before a feed and can be stimulated by the baby suckling or the cry of the baby. The stimulus directs a message to the brain that allows oxytocin to be released. Efficient emptying of the milk from the breast will result in the release of prolactin to produce more milk. The sensory stimulus from suckling is the main reason that oxytocin is released: the nipple hypothalamic pathway. This pathway can be overridden by messages from other parts of the brain related to emotion. This emotive–hypothalamic pathway can override the nipple–hypothalmic pathway, especially if the mother is stressed or embarrassed.

The feedback inhibitor of lactation

As well as the endocrine control of milk production and ejection there is also an autocrine control that works individually in each breast. If the milk is not removed from the breast the feedback inhibitor of lactation (FIL), an active whey protein, will inhibit milk production if the alveoli become distended. FIL concentration increases if milk is not removed. When milk is removed from the breast the concentration declines and milk production recommences. This is a protective process within each breast.

Constituents of breast milk

Colostrum

Colostrum is low in volume but higher in protein, minerals and fat than mature milk and is present in the breasts during pregnancy and the first few days after birth. It also contains more anti-infective agents than mature milk and is invaluable to the newborn infant.

Mature milk

Mature breast milk is produced from around three days following the birth. Breast milk changes during a single feed, between feeds and also over time so that it constantly meets the needs of the growing baby.

Protein

In the early days the protein is mostly in the form of whey and some casein. This is easily digestible and contains valuable substances, such as:

- lactoferrin, which binds with iron to prevent bacteria growing;
- lysozomes to help kill bacteria and viruses; and
- immunoglobulins – antibodies passed from mother to baby improving immunity.

As the baby grows, the casein content increases and as this is more difficult to digest it keeps the hungrier baby fuller.

Carbohydrates (sugars)

Lactose is the main carbohydrate and is important for the growth of the brain and gives the milk a sweet taste. Lactose helps the absorption of calcium, important for bone and teeth strength. *Lactobacillus bifidus* grows in the presence of lactose and increases the acidity in the gut, reducing the risk of infection and increasing the absorption of calcium.

Fats

Fats are a major source of energy for the baby and vary depending upon the stage of pregnancy, ensuring a premature baby receives the most suitable milk. The amount is also affected by the time of day (more in the late afternoon), by the time of year (more in the winter) and is depends on the mother's diet. A healthy diet will produce milk richer in fat content. There is also an enzyme present to help digest the fat. Although there is cholesterol present this is necessary and aids cardiovascular development.

The fat content also varies throughout a feed, allowing the baby to receive the more fat the longer the feed (hindmilk). The milk at the beginning of a feed or the milk of a very short feed has less fat and is commonly known as foremilk.

Vitamins

- Vitamin A – responsible for eye development.
- Vitamin D – for bone strength.
- Vitamin K – the levels in colostrum and hindmilk are higher and it is needed to assist blood to clot. Eventually babies produce adequate amounts of this themselves but women are usually offered the choice to supplement their baby with administration of vitamin K via an injection or an oral preparation to reduce the risk of haemorrhagic disease of the newborn.
- Vitamin B complex – needed for development of the nervous system and blood cells.
- Vitamin C – assists iron absorption.

Minerals

Iron is present in small amounts and helps in the formation of blood. its absorption is enhanced because of the vitamin C present in breast milk. As babies do not store iron until the latter weeks of pregnancy some premature babies will be offered supplements of iron until their own bodies are efficient at production.

This does not mean that breast milk is inferior to formula milk, which already has extra additives.

Antenatal preparation for breastfeeding

During the antenatal period a woman may make a decision about how she is going to feed her baby. To enhance the chances of her choosing to breastfeed it is advisable that the midwife does not ask the woman how she will feed but just gives information about the benefits of breastfeeding. At this time some women will be certain they wish to give formula to their baby but it is still important that they are informed of the benefits of breastfeeding based on current evidence. There is no physical preparation required for breastfeeding but some women may wish to express colostrum from 37 weeks. This can be of great benefit to the diabetic mother as the small amounts of colostrum can be frozen and then used in the early neonatal period if the baby has difficulties maintaining its own glycaemic status (see Hypoglycaemia on page 76).

Women may wish to buy a supporting bra for day wear and to sleep in as the breasts become heavier. They may also wish to invest in disposable or washable breastpads if they find they leak colostrum. Not all women will see colostrum in pregnancy. This has no effect on the ability to breastfeed successfully.

It is useful to advise women to educate themselves about how to succeed with breastfeeding; learning about the anatomy and physiology would be beneficial. There may be local classes run by midwives, health visitors, peer support workers, the National Childbirth Trust (NCT) or the La Leche League (LLL). Otherwise books, leaflets and Department of Health guidance are all available in the UK. These contacts can also provide useful support after the birth of the baby.

The first breastfeed

Skin-to-skin contact should be offered to all mothers irrespective of feeding choice. Immediately following birth the baby can be placed on the mother's abdomen or chest taking care to be observant about heat loss for the baby. Some babies will 'crawl' or root towards the nipple from this position. If not the baby can be brought towards the nipple.

The first feed should take place as soon after birth as possible as this has a priming effect on the acini cells and can influence their potential milk-producing

---

Breastfeeding support

- Baby Friendly Initiative www.babyfriendly.org.uk
- La Leche League www.laleche.org.uk
- National Childbirth Trust www.nct.org.uk
- Breastfeeding Network www.breastfeedingnetwork.org.uk

Benefits of skin-to-skin contact

- Helps prevent heat loss
- Can help initiate first breastfeed
- Helps regulate the baby's heartbeat and breathing
- Is calming for mother and baby
- Can help in building a relationship with between mother and baby.

---

properties, enhancing the chance of successful breastfeeding. If for some reason this is not possible but milk can be expressed, then this should be offered and the milk given via cup or nasogastric tube. This will assist in priming the receptors in the acini cells and will mean the baby receives early colostrum. Women should be offered help to initiate the first feed and it is useful if the midwife observes the feed to ensure good positioning and attachment are achieved.

Early days of breastfeeding

Some women will require more support than others in the early days. If in hospital the midwife should make the woman aware that she can call for support or assistance. If at home the woman may benefit from other support as the midwife may not visit daily. If there is an identified need for breastfeeding support that need could be met with a visit from the midwife, a maternity support worker or a peer supporter.

The most important aspect in the early days is achieving correct positioning and attachment of the baby to the breast. If this is not correct it can result in sore nipples or poor emptying of the milk from the breast. Sore nipples will be painful and will interfere with successful feeding as the woman may be reluctant to feed. If the baby is not correctly positioned and attached and the breast milk is not effectively removed this can result in a reduced supply, a hungry, unsettled baby or engorgement which makes it difficult for the baby to attach for the next feed.

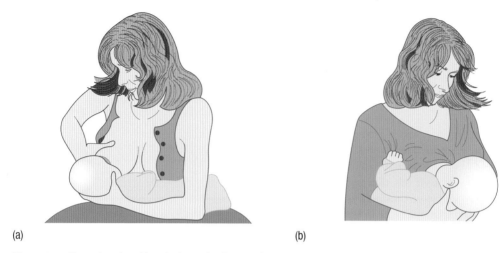

(a)   (b)

Figure 6.3   Examples of positions for breastfeeding. (a) 'Cross-cradle' hold; (b) 'rugby football' hold. (From Lim, 2008)

The midwife must take into account and educate the mother about some of the following factors.

Comfort

It is important for the mother to be comfortable not only physically but also emotionally. Oxytocin release is required for the 'let down' reflex to function and allow the baby to suckle and receive the milk. Oxytocin can be inhibited by stress, therefore it is important that privacy is assured in hospital and any inhibiting factors controlled for. This may mean educating the family and visitors if the woman is not comfortable feeding with them present. Some hospitals provide a special quiet area for breastfeeding mothers; in others the curtain can afford some privacy. This also applies if the woman is expressing her milk when separated from her baby. In this case a photograph or video clip of her baby may help the let down reflex.

Positioning and attachment

Bringing the baby towards the breast and not taking the breast to the baby is important. The midwife should teach the mother to do this without the midwife handling the woman's breasts. Encouragement and direction should be all that is required. The midwife may wish to demonstrate with a model breast and doll. The baby should be brought towards the breast with the baby's nose in line with the nipple. The front of the baby's body should be facing the mother's abdomen so that no twisting of the head is needed. Although the back of the neck needs to be supported, the head should

not be held into the breast as this prevents the baby from adjusting his or her own position (Figure 6.3).

The baby's mouth needs to be open wide; sometimes the mother will need to tease the baby's nose or lips with the nipple to stimulate this (Figure 6.4). As the baby's mouth opens bring the baby towards the nipple, with the lower lip meeting the breast first.

There is a lot for women to think about as they learn to feed their baby, so support and consistent advice is crucial to success. The mother whose baby has been receiving expressed milk until able to be offered the breast will also require this level of support in the early days. It is important that staff on neonatal special

---

Signs of good attachment

- No pain
- Baby's body facing mother
- Head and spine in a straight line not twisted
- Baby held close to mother
- Head not restricted from moving
- Baby's lips rolled outwards and tongue down
- No dimpling of cheeks
- Jaw muscles moving around the ears
- Less areolar seen underneath the baby's mouth than above
- Baby's chin and nose close to breast
- Mother not distorting the shape of the breast with her hands.

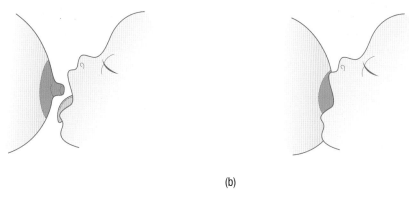

(a)   (b)

Figure 6.4   (a) Baby with a wide gape about to go to the breast. (b) Well-attached baby with a wide gape. (From Lim, 2008)

and intensive care units are also trained and updated about factors that influence successful breastfeeding.

Supply and demand

Breastfed babies should be fed on demand to allow the supply and demand system to meet their daily needs. They require nothing else other than breast milk, so if a baby is thirsty the breast milk will meet that need too – water is not required. The more a baby empties milk from the breast the more prolactin is released and more milk is produced. Night feeds are important as the amount of prolactin produced is greater at night. Mothers who are expressing milk for their baby should be encouraged to express during the night as well as throughout the day.

Mothers need to be made aware of feeding cues so that they can respond to their baby and offer the breast on demand. In hospital it is common practice for the baby to be kept with the mother at all times, allowing her to learn about her baby and her baby to get to know her. Where mothers and babies are separated, the staff in hospital will facilitate and allow contact even if the baby is sick. If the baby is ill on a special or intensive care unit, assisting a mother to feed her baby her breast milk will allow her to feel some control in a frightening situation. She will also be providing her baby with one of the best medicines: human breast milk.

Engorgement of the breasts

If the milk is not removed, the breasts will feel full and engorged. They may also become red and quite painful. Around the third day following the birth the breasts are adjusting to an increased vascular supply and there is often some oedema present. This differs from milk engorgement and expression will not ease the problem. A good supporting bra is required and if the mother is not breastfeeding the fluid will reabsorb and the breasts will settle. Expressing the milk if not intending to feed will only encourage the breasts to produce more milk and will not ease the situation. Mild analgesics may be useful.

If the engorgement is there because the baby is not removing as much milk as is being produced the following recommendations may help:

- encourage demand feeding;
- ensure correct positioning;
- allow the baby to finish the feed before offering the second breast;
- use warm flannels.

It may be that the mother needs to express a small amount of milk to enable the baby to attach to the breast correctly as the nipple area may be stretched flat by the engorgement. Remember the feedback inhibitor of lactation: if the milk is not removed by effective feeding or expression from the breast the milk production will reduce in that breast. Do not encourage the mother to stop feeding.

Sore/cracked nipples

Correct positioning and attachment are essential to avoid the development of sore or cracked nipples. Pain is abnormal while breastfeeding and so if the mother experiences pain encourage her to break the baby's attachment by inserting her finger into the corner of the mouth and begin the process again. Check the positioning and attachment for the mother and suggest another way of holding the baby. A 'rugby ball hold' might take pressure from the sore area. Encourage the mother to express a small amount of colostrum or breast milk and smear it around the nipple. If possible expose the nipples to the air. Creams and lotions are not particularly helpful.

Suckling

Babies are born with several reflexes to enable them to suckle as soon as they are born. Some of these reflexes are only fully developed in the full-term baby (see Chapter 4). The rooting reflex causes babies to turn towards a stimulus such as a nipple and open their mouths. The suckling reflex stimulates babies to take breast tissue into their mouths and compress it into the roof of the mouth.

Some of the new evidence from Geddes *et al.* (2008) is making us think about the rest of this process. It was commonly believed that the baby stripped the milk from the ampullae just behind the nipple, but it is now suggested that a vacuum is also formed by the baby as well as compression to enhance milk ejection.

The swallowing reflex and the baby's ability to breath through the nose are also contributory.

Use of bottles and teats

To feed from a teat and bottle breastfed babies will need to use a completely different action and this may confuse them when they return to the nipple. It is not advisable to use a teat and bottle while establishing breastfeeding. Cup feeding can be used to give a baby expressed milk if a mother is unable to put the baby to the breast. It is also not advisable to give breastfed babies any formula, no matter how small the amount, as this can sensitize them to allergies.

Use of a dummy or pacifier

The decision whether to use a dummy or not can be confusing for parents and health professionals, as a dummy has been identified as possible protective factor against sudden infant death syndrome and yet traditionally it is frowned upon. In general it is not advisable to use a dummy while establishing breast-

feeding as it may mean the feeding cues are missed and the breasts will not have been able to respond to the demand to make more milk (see Chapter 16, p180).

Expressing breast milk

There will be times when a mother is unable to actually put her baby to the breast to feed; for example if mother and baby are separated for any reason, perhaps due to illness in the baby. It is vital in these circumstances that midwives are able to teach mothers how to successfully express breast milk, which will ensure the milk supply is not hindered.

Breast milk can be expressed by hand or by using a breast pump. Breast massage prior to hand expression has been associated with an increased prolactin release, as has hand expression, which will obviously influence the amount of milk produced.

Hand-expressed breast milk has been shown to have a higher fat content than pumped breast milk (Stutte *et al.*, 1988) so it is worth considering this as the first option. In addition there are other advantages, such as convenience, as it requires no specialist equipment, except containers, to collect the milk and there is less risk of contamination.

Oxytocin release, which influences the let down reflex, can also be enhanced by stimulating other senses while expressing breast milk. These can include visual stimulus (looking at the baby or the baby's picture) and smell (holding a blanket or piece of clothing that baby has worn). It has also been shown by Raimboult *et al.* (2007) that exposing preterm infants to the odour of their mother's expressed breast milk can have a positive influence on their sucking behaviour.

Breast massage

Teaching mothers to massage their breasts prior to expression can assist in the let down reflex and has been linked with effective ejection (Jones *et al.*, 2001). There are a number of techniques that can be implemented as part of the massage.

The mother should be advised on hand washing prior to commencing massage or hand expression. Make sure she is sitting somewhere comfortably with some privacy, otherwise any anxiety she feels may be counter-productive to the let down reflex. If possible, she should sit near her baby or have any photographs or blankets close.

The use of warm flannels placed around the breast tissue may help to stimulate the milk flow before starting. Advise the mother to use first two fingers and gently rotate them, starting from the outer part of the breast, moving down towards the nipple. This movement should be repeated all round the breast. This method is particularly useful for blocked ducts.

Some mothers may also find it effective to use their knuckles, with the hand formed in a fist, in a gentle rolling/kneading movement, again from the upper part of the breast towards the nipple. This is sometimes more useful if still clothed.

It may be necessary to perform this for around 5 minutes prior to expression, although it may also be useful to repeat it half-way through if the milk supply seems to be slowing.

Hand expression

Best practice standards identified by the Baby Friendly Initiative, a worldwide programme of the World Health Organization and UNICEF, recommend that all breastfeeding mothers and all mothers with a baby on the neonatal unit should be taught hand expression. Mothers should be advised to express 6–8 times in each 24 hours, including the night period. Early, frequent and effective expression is important in establishing lactation and is linked to greater milk production.

After a period of breast massage, encourage the mother to form her hand into a 'C' shape using the thumb and first two fingers. She should place her fingers around the breast about 2–3 cm from the base of the nipple, although this will obviously vary with each individual. It may be possible for the mother to differentiate a difference in the tissue (it may feel more lumpy or fibrous) around this area and this would be the best area to start.

The fingers (in the 'C' shape) should be pushed inwards toward the chest wall and then the fingers/thumb allowed to 'roll' towards the nipple, in a press and release motion. The fingers should not drag or slide along the breast tissue as this may lead to damage. Encourage this 'press and release' movement until milk flow slows. The mother should then move the hand around the breast in order to express all ducts in the breast. Suggest she changes to express the other breast as the milk flow slows and continue to do this throughout. It may be necessary to alternate between the breasts around 5 or 6 times during an expression.

During the first few days there may be only small amounts of colostrum expressed, which tends to be thick and 'drip'. It may be useful to collect this dripping colostrum using a syringe. As the milk supply comes in, the milk will flow steadily or even 'spurt'. Milk may also drip from the other breast at the same time.

The milk should be collected in a wide-necked container. Although this will need to be sterile for the newborn, as the baby grows it will simply need a very hot soapy wash, ensuring all milk debris is removed.

This whole process of expression would normally take 15–20 minutes, but as the mother becomes more adept, it may become shorter.

Breast pumps

Breast pumps can be manually or battery operated or electric. A manual or handheld pump can assist in helping to relieve full breasts. Some of these are difficult pieces of equipment to sterilize effectively, and they may be less useful when the breast milk needs to be saved and fed to the baby.

A battery-operated pump creates a vacuum, as does a manual pump, but is less tiring to use. They are generally more portable than an electric pump which can be quite heavy and cumbersome. However, for long-term use, many women may prefer an electric pump. Using an electric pump can allow for double pumping; that is, simultaneous pumping of both breasts. This has been linked with an increase in prolactin levels and may therefore assist the milk supply (Jones *et al.*, 2001), while reducing the time taken to express, although some women find it difficult to manage (Lang, 2002).

Care must be taken not to press the collecting funnel into the breast tissue too deeply as this can restrict the ducts and impede the milk flow (Jones *et al.*, 2001). Hill *et al.* (1996) discuss the problem of ensuring that the vacuum pressures used are not too great as this can affect milk flow. However recent work by Kent *et al.* (2008) suggests that using the maximum comfortable pressure tolerated by the mother improves both milk flow and milk yield.

Storage of expressed breast milk

It is recommended to use wide-necked containers, but at least an inch of space should be left to allow for the milk to expand as it freezes. It is possible to add freshly expressed milk (layering) onto previously frozen breast milk (Biaglioli, 2003) although it should not be warm as it may partially thaw the frozen milk. The containers can be either glass or plastic if the milk is to be frozen. White blood cells within breast milk can adhere to a glass container if stored for less than 23 hours but seem to detach after this time (Hopkinson *et al.*, 1990). This may be less vital if the milk is being frozen but it should be remembered that fat also adheres to the sides of plastic bottles so potentially affecting the amount of available calories. Glass bottles are less likely than plastic to absorb any nutrients. Plastic storage bags may also be used providing the milk is being not being stored longer than 72 hours (Williams-Arnold, 2002); however it has been noticed that lipids and secretory immunoglobulin A can stick to plastic storage bags (Hopkinson *et al.*, 1990).

Hanna *et al.* (2004) highlight the effect of storing breast milk. Both refrigerating and freezing breast milk will lower its antioxidant activity, with freezing having the greatest effect. However, despite this, the researchers claim that frozen breast milk still has more antioxidants than formula milk. Antioxidants, including vitamins C and E, selenium and carotenoids, play an important part in protecting cell membranes and improving the immune system.

- Ideally, expressed breast milk should not be stored at room temperature (up to 25°C) for longer than 6–8 hours; it is recommended that it is refrigerated as soon as possible.
- Milk can be stored in a cooler bag, with ice packs for up to 24 hours.
- Expressed breast milk can be stored in the fridge (below 4°C) for up to five days, ideally at the back of the body of the fridge, not in the door where it will be subject to alterations in temperature every time the door is opened.
- If freezing, the milk should also be stored towards the back of the freezer.
- If it is in a freezer compartment inside the fridge (with temperature of –15°C) it can be stored for up to two weeks; in a separate fridge/freezer (–18°C) between 3 and 6 months; and in a deep freezer (–20°C) for between 6 and 12 months.
- Milk that has been frozen and thawed can be stored in the fridge for up to 24 hours but should not be refrozen.

These guidelines apply to healthy term infants, not ill, or preterm infants.

Bottle feeding

Making up formula milk feeds

There have been changes to the advice given regarding making up formula feeds over recent years. This followed information issued by the milk companies regarding the non-sterile nature of their product and potential contaminants of *Enterobacter sakazakii* and *Salmonella*. It was then recommended that parents adopt strict hygiene practices and ensure all formula feeds are made up as needed, not in advance, as had been previous practice. Current guidelines are identified in the box below.

Preparing a feed using powdered infant formula

Each bottle should be made up *fresh for each feed*.

1. Clean any surface thoroughly where the feed is prepared
2. Wash hands with soap and water and then dry
3. Boil fresh tap water in a kettle. Alternatively bottled water that is suitable for infants can be used for making up feeds and should be boiled in the same way as tap water
4. Allow the boiled water to cool to *no less than 70°C*. This means in practice using water that has been left covered, for less than 30 minutes after boiling
5. Pour the amount of boiled water required into the sterilized bottle
6. Add the exact amount of formula as instructed on the label always using the scoop provided with the powdered formula by the manufacturer. Do not add any extra powder than instructed as this could make the baby ill
7. Re-assemble the bottle following manufacturer's instructions
8. Shake the bottle well to mix the contents
9. Cool quickly to feeding temperature by holding under a running tap, or placing in a container of cold water
10. Check the temperature by shaking a few drops onto the inside of the wrist – it should feel lukewarm, not hot
11. Any feed that has not been used within 2 hours should be discarded.

Nasogastric tube feeding

Some babies will need nasogastric tube (NGT) feeding because breast or artificial feeding is inappropriate for some reason. This is usually a short-term measure until full oral feeding is established. The most common reasons that babies require NGT feeding are that they are premature, ill or small for gestational age (transitional care). Midwives can pass NGTs and care for babies who are being tube-fed on the postnatal ward and although this is not a common occurrence there are some wards where transitional care babies are being cared for alongside other postnatal babies. Where mothers wish to breastfeed, they should be encouraged to express and store their milk so that it can be used to tube-feed their baby.

Please note: Trust guidelines should always be followed and full training should be given prior to passing a NGT on a baby. The following is for information only and is not intended to replace clinical instruction. A size 6 or 8 FG NGT should be used and will need to be measured before insertion. Careful measurement of the NGT should be made before it is inserted. Keeping the tube in its plastic cover, measure the tube from the baby's nose to the tragus of the ear and then to the xiphisternum, noting the mark on the tube (Figure 6.5).

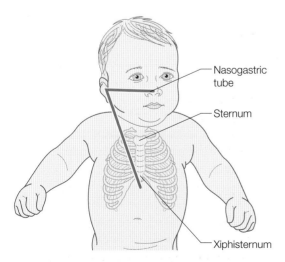

Figure 6.5 Measuring for nasogastric tube

Equipment list:

- NGT
- Gloves
- pH testing paper
- Adhesive tape
- Hydroactive or hydrocolloid dressing
- 10 mL syringe.

With clean, gloved hands pass the tube into one nostril with a backward and downward movement. Inserting the tube too quickly can stimulate a vagal response, therefore a tube passed more slowly will have an improved outcome. The baby should be observed throughout the process for gagging, vomiting and cyanosis. If any distress is noticed, the procedure should be stopped immediately. Once the tube has been inserted, the position should be checked. Aspirate a small amount of gastric contents and test it using pH paper. The National Patient Safety Agency (NPSA, 2005) recommends the use of pH paper to reduce harm caused by misplaced tubes in neonates. A pH of 5.5 and below should indicate correct placement. The tube can be secured with tape applied to the hydroactive or hydrocolloid dressing already in place on the baby's face.

The importance of checking the placement of the NGT cannot be overemphasized and it should always be checked following insertion, before giving medication and before each feed, or if the tube appears misplaced or the baby has been vomiting, coughing or retching.

There are several factors that will affect the pH, such as the gestational age of the baby, small amount of aspirate, medication, postnatal age and if the baby is being continuously fed. In addition to these causes, if the baby has amniotic fluid or milk in the stomach the pH could be falsely alkalotic. The NPSA (2005) advise that if the pH is 6 or above, the baby should not be fed and the tube should be checked for placement by waiting 15–30 minutes, replacing the tube or seeking senior advice. While it may not be practical to wait if the baby is on hourly feeds and re-passing the tube may be traumatic for the baby, it is essential that the feed does not take place until correct tube placement is confirmed. If the baby is due for an X-ray the placement of the tube can be checked using this method. However, the X-ray should not be performed solely to confirm the tube's placement.

Interestingly an audit by Chambers *et al.* (2008) found that on X-ray 30 per cent of babies where the tube was thought to be in the correct position were in fact misplaced, either being in the lower end of the oesophagus or through the pylorus into the duodenum.

Only an appropriate oral feeding syringe should be used when feeding a baby or administering medications via an NGT. The NPSA (2007) issued guidance to be followed and state that healthcare professionals should only use labelled oral/enteral syringes that cannot be connected to intravenous catheters or other ports and should not use intravenous syringes to measure and administer oral liquid medicines.

NGT feeding is essentially a safe and simple procedure provided correct guidelines and procedures have been followed. The current practice in most hospitals is to feed by gravity rather than plunge feed. This allows for a slower feed and will create less turbulence in the stomach, which in turn will cause less vomiting and regurgitation.

Hypoglycaemia (low blood sugar)

Hypoglycaemia is defined according to a blood glucose level that conforms with World Health Organization guidelines (<2.6 mmol/L) or an evidence-based, local protocol at the hospital where the baby is born.

When glucose is used for energy more quickly than it is made, the baby can develop hypoglycaemia. Healthy term babies are very adept at managing their energy requirements and should not routinely have their blood glucose levels monitored. There are some babies, however, who are more at risk of developing hypoglycaemia and they will require closer surveillence. These include intrauterine growth-restricted newborns, newborns whose mothers are diabetic, preterm newborns and those newborns who have experienced fetal distress.

Babies who are 'at risk' need to be correctly identified and managed appropriately. For all babies, the aim should be to ensure that needs are met as far as possible by breastfeeding, or by the use of expressed colostrum/breast milk, as breast milk may enhance the baby's ability to counter-regulate, whereas large volumes of infant formula can suppress this ability. If the baby is unable to breastfeed effectively, the mother should be encouraged to express her milk in order to maximize her future lactation (Baby Friendly Initiative, 2008)

A lack of feeding may be a sign of illness and close observations of the baby in the early period following birth are vital to assess that there is a normal level of arousal. The baby should be woken and lifted from the cot to enable effective assessment; sometimes changing the nappy is useful in a reluctant feeder. Blood glucose measurements taken in the first 3 hours of age are not particularly useful; blood tests immediately after birth are a reflection of the mother's blood levels. The baby's blood glucose levels may then drop sharply while counter-regulation is initiated. If blood glucose levels remain lower than the agreed minimum despite breastfeeding or giving expressed breast milk, the baby should be reviewed by a paediatrician with a view to further investigation and appropriate management. Should any baby develop clinical signs of hypoglycaemia, such as altered level of consciousness, abnormal tone or seizures, blood glucose measurements will be taken and this can indicate underlying illness. If blood glucose levels remain low despite frequent breastfeeding, supplementary expressed breast milk should be provided by NGT or cup. Frequent small volumes of colostrum will be easily digested and absorbed by the baby.

When blood glucose remains below accepted levels and breastfeeding/giving expressed breast milk is not successful or has been insufficient to raise the blood glucose level, formula milk may be required. Should infant formula be required, an appropriate volume (e.g. 8–10 mL/kg) is offered by cup to the breastfed baby to optimize the chances of continuing to breastfeed.

It is recommended the first blood glucose to be measured is after 2 hours of age in the at-risk baby and prior to the second feed unless the baby is symptomatic when the baby's needs will be monitored and managed individually.

Key Points

- Human breast milk is the best food for newborn babies.
- Knowledge of anatomy and physiology is needed to support women to successfully feed.
- Mothers need support whatever the choice of feeding method.
- All mothers should be taught about hand expression.
- Guidance for safe 'making up' of artificial feeds and correct storage is important for infant health.

References

Baby Friendly Initiative (2008) Hypoglycaemia policy guideline. http://www.babyfriendly.org.uk/pdfs/hypo_policy.pdf [accessed 9 September 2009].

Biagioli F (2003) Returning to work while breastfeeding. *American Family Physician* **68**: 2199–2222.

Chambers F, Mahadevan S, Mohite A, Roy K and Pillay T (2008) Utility of chest radiography to assess nasogastric tube position in neonates. *Journal of Neonatal Nursing* **14**: 124–125.

Geddes DT, Kent JC, Mitoulas LR and Hartmann PE (2008) Tongue movement and intra-oral vacuum in breastfeeding infants. *Early Human Development* **84**: 471–477.

Hanna N, Ahmed K, Anwar M, Petrova A, Hiatt M and Hegyi T (2004) Effect of storage on breast milk antioxidant activity. *Archives of Disease in Childhood. Fetal and Neonatal Edition* **89**: F518–F520.

Hill PO, Aldag JC and Chatterton RT (1996) The effect of sequential and simultaneous breast pumping on milk volume and prolactin levels: a pilot study. *Journal of Human Lactation* **12**: 193–199.

Hopkinson J, Garza C and Asquith MT (1990) Human milk storage in glass containers. *Journal of Human Lactation* **6**: 104–105.

Jones E. Dimmock PW and Spencer SA (2001) A randomised controlled trial to compare methods of milk expression after preterm delivery. *Archives of Disease in Childhood. Fetal and Neonatal Edition* **85**: F91–F95.

Kent JC, Mitoulas LR, Creegan MD, Geddes DT, Larssaan M, Doherty DA and Hatmann Pl (2008) Importance of vacuum for breastmilk expression, *Breastfeeding Medicine* **3**: 11–19.

Lang S (2002) *Breastfeeding Special Care Babies*. Edinburgh: Ballière Tindall.

Lim P (2008) *Successful Breastfeeding*. London: Hodder Education.

NICE (National Institute for Health and Clinical Excellence) (2006) Routine postnatal care of women and their babies. http://www.nice.org.uk/Guidance/CG37 [accessed 9 September 2009].

NPSA (National Patient Safety Agency) (2005) How to confirm the correct position of naso and orogastric tubes in babies under the care of neonatal units. Interim advice for healthcare staff. http://www.npsa.nhs.uk/nrls/alerts-and-directives/alerts/feedingtubes/ [accessed 9 September 2009].

NPSA (2007) Patient Safety Alert 19. Promoting safer measurement and administration of liquid medicines via oral and other enteral routes. http://www.npsa.nhs.uk/nrls/alerts-and-directives/alerts/liquid-medicines/ [accessed 9 September 2009].

Raimboult C, Saliba E and Porter RH (2007) The effect of the odour of mother's milk on breastfeeding behaviour of premature neonates. *Acta Paediatrica* **96**: 368–371.

Ramsay DT, Kent JC, Hartmann RL and Hartmann PE (2005) Anatomy of the lactating human breast redefined with ultrasound imaging. *Journal of Anatomy* **206**: 525–534.

Stutte P, Bowles B and Morman G (1988) The effect of breast massage on volume and fat content of human milk. *Genesis* **10**: 22–25.

Williams-Arnold LD (2002) *Human Milk Storage for Healthy Infants and Children*. Sandwich, MA: Health Education Association.

CHAPTER 7

NEONATAL SKINCARE

Sharon Trotter

OVERVIEW

Current thinking on skincare is discussed in this chapter with recommendations on the correct advice the midwife can give parents. Common skin problems, their causes, prevention and treatments will be examined. Implications for practice will be discussed in the light of the latest evidence surrounding neonatal skincare and cord care. Advice for parents will be recommended in line with up-to-date guidelines from the National Institute for Health and Clinical Excellence. Before reading this chapter, refer to the Reflective practice box on page 87.

Introduction

Fashions in healthcare dictate how women will birth their babies and the same is true regarding the introduction of baby skincare products from birth. While no evidence exists to support their use, parents and professionals continue to regard baby skincare products as safe and even beneficial. Parents retain the misguided belief that these products are a necessity to newborn skincare, actively buying up cupboards-full ready for the baby's arrival. It could almost be seen as rites of passage. Comments like 'We used it on all our babies' and 'They smell nice' are hard to challenge, and it takes courage and conviction to question what has become the socially accepted norm.

Many parents buy into an 'ideal' of family life, as portrayed through advertising that has somehow become ubiquitous in modern life. This process can be so subtle that parents and professionals alike are unaware of its effect. In turn, habits and practices which lack credibility may be adopted and can prove hard to break. Midwives and health visitors are autonomous practitioners, responsible for their own actions. It is vital that their practice is based on best practice at the time of providing care. It is no longer appropriate for hospitals and maternity units to supply free baby products when there is no evidence to support their use. Although predominantly involving skincare and cord care, it is important to remember that anything placed on in or around the neonate has the capacity to harm (Trotter, 2004).

Neonatal skin environment

Before considering new guidelines for neonatal skincare or cord care, it is important to explain the physiological role of the skin as a protective organ and describe the natural process of cord separation in the neonate (Figure 7.1).

The epidermis, or outer layer of the skin, is divided into four layers, the stratum corneum (inert) and three living layers: stratum granulosum, stratum spinosum and stratum basale.

The stratum corneum itself is made up of 10–20 microscopic layers in the term infant, similar to that seen in an adult. In premature infants, this number drops to between two and three layers. In extremely premature infants, of less than 23 gestational weeks, the stratum corneum may be virtually non-existent

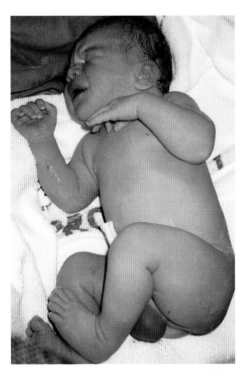

Figure 7.1   Newborn skin – the perfect start. (© TIPS Ltd)

(Holbrook, 1982; Nonato, 1998). Consequently, the risk of damaging these babies' skin is even higher.

Babies are born with an alkaline skin surface, with an average pH of 6.34 (Peck and Botwinick 1964). However, within days the pH falls to about 4.95 (acid), forming what is known as the 'acid mantle' – a very fine film that rests on the surface of the skin and acts as a protector. The development of this 'acid mantle' happens within days of birth, irrespective of gestational age, and probably occurs as a direct result of the skin's exposure to air (Harpin and Rutter, 1983; Evans and Rutter, 1986).

The stratum basale is at the junction of the epidermis and dermis and is where the renewal of the basal cells is carried out. Basal cells, called keratinocytes, constantly divide. The granules in the keratinocytes of the stratum granulosum are bags full of newly synthesized and stored lipids. These will be released before the cell dies and are processed enzymatically to form the lipid barrier. These lipids surround lifeless keratin discs that are formed from keratinocytes after their death and are now called 'corneocytes'. These can be thought of as the bricks in a wall, with the mortar between made up of lipids or fat molecules. This whole structure forms the skin barrier and is situated in the stratum corneum, the most superficial layer of skin. When intact, this 'wall' regulates temperature, acts as a barrier to infection, balances water and electrolytes, stores fat and insulates against the cold. The skin is also a large tactile area used for the interpretation of stimuli.

The structure and function of this delicate layer is easily damaged, leading to a wide spectrum of inflammatory symptoms. The two main causes of such symptoms are the destruction of the skin's barrier (delipidization) within the stratum corneum by the overuse of detergent-based products (sulfates) and also the stimulation of an inflammatory immune response which in turn compromises the skin's barrier (Kownatzki, 2003).

Vernix caseosa

At birth a baby's skin is covered with vernix caseosa (VC) which gives added protection over the first few days of life. The thickness of this layer varies according to the gestational age of the infant. The vernix caseosa is a highly sophisticated bio-film consisting of antimicrobial peptides/proteins and fatty acids. These combine to form a barrier that is not only antibacterial but also antifungal. A study by Tollin *et al.* (2005) goes further by stating that: 'Studies confirm that maintaining an intact epidermal barrier by minimizing exposure to soap and by not removing VC are simple measures to improve skin barrier function.'

Meanwhile the skin becomes colonized with microorganisms and develops its own stable microbiota (Tierno, 2006). This transitional environment, from alkaline to acid (known as the 'acid mantle' and described above) further adds to the protective barrier. Its delicate balance must be maintained if the skin is to achieve an optimum level of protection. There is no evidence to prove that the acid mantle exists beyond this point, so acidic pH detergents are not thought to provide any protection (Kownatzki, 2003).

'Epidermal lipids play a key role in maintaining the skin's barrier, integrity and health' (Ertel, 2003). This is backed up by evidence of reduced levels of epidermal lipids seen in individuals suffering from atopic eczema (Di Nardo *et al.*, 1996). As the epidermis continually sheds, it is vital for the lipid seal around each skin cell (keratinocyte) to be left undisturbed. This protective layer ensures that the skin does not dry out, but can only be achieved in the presence of certain enzymes and the right lipid precursors (Kownatzki, 2003). This barrier cannot be reproduced by artificial means. Great care must therefore be employed to avoid its destruction by delipidization caused by chemicals used in manufactured personal care products.

Once damaged, the epidermis is more prone to transepidermal water loss, which leads to dry skin. This in turn increases the likelihood of sensitization by foreign materials such as microorganisms and allergens, and aggravates the damaging effects of chemical irritants.

Interaction with keratinocyte surface molecules or membrane lipids leads to cell activation. Once released, cytokines send signals requesting assistance to blood vessels and white blood cells. Activation of Langerhans cells initiates an immune response which is particularly effective when a foreign substance is encountered repeatedly. Once a certain level of response has been exceeded, inflammatory symptoms (for example skin irritation and eczema) become evident.

Delipidization

Delipidization just means the selective removal of lipid (fat molecules) components from the stratum corneum. There have been many studies carried out on the damaging effects of surfactants (detergents) to the skin, subsequent changes to the skin's pH, drying effects of hand cleaners and the associated swelling of stratum corneum (Rhein *et al.*, 1986; Ertel, 2003; Kownatzki, 2003). All are agreed that any method used to clean the skin affects the surface fat content thereby reducing the effectiveness of the skin barrier against the introduction of irritants, allergens and microorganisms. Natural antibacterials are removed by washing, alongside the lipid and water-soluble substances. This could lead to increased bacterial growth that jeopardizes the original skin cleansing technique.

It is interesting to note that damage to the skin's lipid barrier caused by overhydration as a result of using latex gloves actually recovers quickly due to evaporation. This is in stark contrast to skin that has a damaged lipid barrier caused by detergent use, which takes many days to recover. The kinetics of damage and its repair and epidemiological evidence suggest that modern synthetic detergents (as used in foaming liquid cleansers) are the major offender (Kownatzki, 2003). If such disturbing findings have been reported on adult skin, the implications for neonatal skin are obvious.

Umbilical cord separation

Physiology

The umbilical cord is a unique tissue consisting of two arteries and one vein covered by a mucoid connective tissue known as Wharton's jelly, which is covered by a thin layer of mucous membrane (a continuation of the amnion). During pregnancy, the placenta provides all the nutrients for fetal growth and removes waste products simultaneously through the umbilical cord.

Following delivery, the cord quickly starts to dry out, harden and turn black (a process called dry gangrene). This is helped by exposure to the air. The umbilical vessels remain patent for several days, so the risk of infection remains high until separation.

Colonization of the area begins within hours of birth (Figure 7.2) as a result of non-pathogenic organisms passing from mother to baby via skin-to-skin contact. Harmful bacteria can be spread by bad hygiene, poor handwashing techniques and especially cross-infection by healthcare workers.

Separation of the umbilical cord continues at the junction of the cord and the skin of the abdomen, with leukocyte infiltration and subsequent digestion of the cord. During this normal process, small amounts of cloudy mucoid material may collect at the junction. This may unwittingly be interpreted as pus. A moist and/or sticky cord may present, but this too is part of the normal physiological process. Separation should be complete within 5–15 days, although it can take longer. The main reasons for prolonged separation include the use of antiseptics and infection.

Antiseptics appear to reduce the number of normal non-pathogenic flora around the umbilicus. This prolongs the healing process and hinders cord separation.

After the cord has separated, a small amount of mucoid material is still present until complete healing

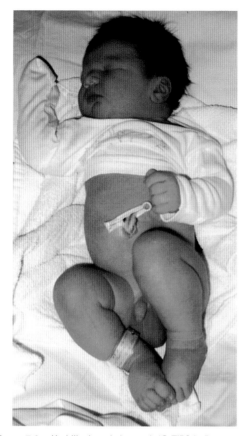

Figure 7.2   Umbilical cord clamped. (© TIPS Ltd)

takes place a few days later. This means that there is still a risk of infection, although not as great as in the first few days.

The evidence

Many studies have been carried out to compare differing treatments and their effect on infection rates, colonization and length of cord separation (Barr, 1984; Mugford *et al.*, 1986; Salariya and Kowbus, 1988; Verber and Pagan, 1992; Bain, 1994; Medves, 1997; Dore *et al.*, 1998; Pezzati *et al.*, 2002). The overall results conclude that the more the cord is treated, the longer it will take to separate. Prolonged cord separation rates are also associated with reduced colonization levels.

This would suggest that a certain level of colonization is actually a healthy sign and not necessarily a precurser to infection. This is why 24 hour rooming-in is such an important factor in the care of the new-born, since it not only avoids cross-infection by healthcare workers, but also encourages early colonization of non-pathogenic organisms, which in turn promotes faster healing (Rush *et al.*, 1987).

Maybe Barr (1984) was right when she postulated that: 'Wharton's Jelly may possess an, as yet, unknown factor, that is essential to the natural healing processes.' It certainly seems to be true that the use of treatments on the umbilical cord appears to interrupt and prolong the natural process of cord separation.

As there is no evidence to recommend the widespread use of topical treatments for cord care, further studies would be helpful, especially in developing countries where neonates are at higher risk of contracting infections. However, for the healthy term infant 'open cord care' using no topical treatments continues to be the safest and most cost-effective practice. These guidelines are based on the World Health Organization (1998) review of the evidence and the recent Cochrane Database Systematic Review (Zupan *et al.*, 2004) on topical umbilical cord care at birth.

Common skin conditions seen in the neonate

Erethema neonatorum

This is a non-infective rash that is commonly seen in the first few weeks of life. There is no treatment and it usually clears within a few days. Great care must be taken to avoid all manufactured skincare products or contact with carers' make-up and perfumes as these can also be a cause of irritation to newborn skin.

Heat spots

This is similar to the erythema rash but the cause is overheating and the rash is more evident around skin folds. Take care to dress a baby in layers so you can add or remove them in order to maintain a stable temperature. A baby's room should be kept at a constant 16–20°C. Do not cover a baby's head, avoid duvets and if possible use lightweight baby sleeping bags to avoid overheating.

Miliaria (milk spots)

This is due to obstruction of the sweat glands and is seen in babies who become overheated. It will resolve once normal temperature control is maintained.

Napkin rash (ammoniacal dermatitis)

This is usually confined to the nappy area and is caused by the skin's reaction to high levels of ammonia from urine and faeces. Frequent nappy changes, gentle but thorough washing (using only water for neonates) plus a thin layer of barrier cream will help to avoid and control this condition.

Conjunctivitis

This is a very common condition affecting neonates which often necessitates treatment with chloramphenicol eye drops or ointment. A simple remedy is the application of a few drops of fresh colostrum. Colostrum and breast milk are known to contain many anti-infective properties. They are commonly used to treat eye infections in developing countries (Singh et al., 1982).

Cradle cap (infantile seborrhoeic dermatitis)

This is a greasy scaly rash usually confined to the scalp of a baby. It is thought to be caused by an overactivity of the sebaceous glands due to increased circulating hormones from the mother or overuse of harsh skincare products in the early weeks of life. It can be treated with an application of vegetable oil (which should be left overnight) followed by gentle combing of the loosened skin flakes. Strong shampoos aimed at the treatment of cradle cap should be avoided.

Infantile eczema

A diagnosis for this condition is not made until three months old. The cause is unknown but reactions to harsh ingredients in skincare products are known to exacerbate the condition. Atopic eczema is the commonest type seen in babies and can also signal an allergic reaction to proteins such as milk, eggs or wheat. Treatment includes avoiding contact with any suspected allergens plus maintenance of the delicate epidermal barrier by way of emollient treatments.

Infective skin conditions affecting the neonate

The development of more serious skin conditions including pemphigus neonatorum (staphylococcal infection), paronychia (infection of the nail bed), omphalitis (infection of the umbilical cord) and, ultimately, septicaemia can be avoided by allowing the skin to maintain its essential protective barrier. Implemented nationally, standardized guidelines for neonatal skincare practice can go a long way to minimize confusion and provide consistency for parents as well as for health professionals.

Baby products and the potential dangers associated with early overuse

Due to the myriad of potentially toxic ingredients used in skincare products today, it would seem sensible for manufacturers of baby products to remove any chemicals that have been shown to cause irritant/sensitizing reactions. The object of washing newborn skin is to clean without removing the lipid barrier that is essential to the surface ecosystem (Gelmetti, 2001). Studies have shown that using mild soap as opposed to water has minimal effects on skin bacterial colonization in the neonatal period, so plain water is sufficient. Bathing should also be avoided until the separation of the umbilical cord is complete so as not to disrupt the flora at the base of the cord and potentially hinder the natural process of cord separation (Trotter, 2003).

All cleansing agents, even tap water, influence the skin's fat content to some degree. However, the dissolution of fat molecules in the upper epidermis by synthetic detergents is not only worrying but avoidable. It should be considered that even short-term effects, when repeated several times a day, can disturb the 'acid mantle' and its protective function, leading to dry and squamous skin in some infants (Fatter et al., 1997).

This is why, once introduced, products should be used sparingly and harsh detergents avoided altogether (see pages 83 and 84).

- It is important to remember that the ratio of skin surface to body weight is highest at birth so the proportion of absorbed product will be greater than in an adult.

- There is no need to bath a baby daily; two or three times a week is adequate.
- Products, however mild, should be used briefly so that potential damage to the skin surface is minimized. For this reason a baby should not be immersed for longer than five minutes.
- Exposure to hard water in the home may further increase the risk of eczema in children of preschool age due to the need for more soap/shampoo to obtain lather (McNally *et al.*, 1998) so extra care must be taken when choosing products.
- Some products have been tested using the Human Repeat Insult Patch Test (HRIPT) and due to the proximity of use to the eyes, many products are tested using the EpiOcular test. A score of 60–90 can claim to be non-irritant on packaging but this is only a guide.
- Statements such as 'dermatologically tested', 'pH balanced', 'natural ingredients' or even 'organic' (just 5 per cent of ingredients originating from organic sources can allow the word 'organic' to be used) do not guarantee safety of ingredients.
- Many ingredients are meant only for discontinuous (short period) use.
- Problems arise when a combination of ingredients are used which have the capacity to exacerbate adverse reactions of individual compounds.
- Ingredients are listed by percentage of total volume. The nearer an ingredient is to the top of the list, the higher its concentration.

Ingredients to avoid

Sodium lauryl sulfate (SLS), also known as sodium dodecyl

SLS is a very harsh industrial degreasant found in 98 per cent of personal care products (Day, 2005). It is known to strip away the lipid barrier and erode the skin leaving it rough and pitted. It can stay in the tissues for days and is known to denature the proteins of eye tissues, impairing eye development permanently. It is also known to strip the skin of moisture, cause cracking and severe inflammation of the epidermis and separate and inflame skin layers. SLS is routinely used in clinical trials as a standard irritant for skin

(Vance, 1999). It is intended for 'discontinuous' use but when added to other chemicals, such as triclosan (which is now common with antibacterial preparations), it can stay next to the skin for many hours which is more likely to damage the skin's natural protective barrier. SLS is used because it is cheap and when added to salt it thickens, making products appear more concentrated.

Sodium laureth sulfate (SLES) and ammonium laureth sulfate (ALES)

When SLS is ethoxylated (a chemical process that increases molecular size which is thought to produce a milder formulation, with potentially less risk of skin irritation) to enhance its foaming properties, it becomes SLES. This is commonly used as a foaming agent in toothpastes, bath gels, bubblebaths and degreasants. It dissolves proteins and can lead to mouth ulcers.

SLES and ALES stay in the tissues for up to five days and can form nitrates and nitrosamines (carcinogens) which go on to make the body absorb nitrates at higher levels. This means that the body is more likely to develop cancers.

During the ethoxylation process the extremely harmful compound 1,4-dioxane is created. This is one of the principal components of the chemical defoliant Agent Orange. Leading toxicologist Dr Samuel Epstein reports: 'The best way to protect yourself is to recognize ingredients most likely to be contaminated with 1,4-dioxane. These include ingredients with the pre-fix word or syllable PEG, polyethelene, polyethelene glycol, polyoxylene, eth (as in sodium laureth sulphate), or oxynol' (Steinman and Epstein, 1995).

Propylene glycol (PG) and polyethylene glycol (PEG)

This is really industrial antifreeze and the major ingredient in brake fluid. It dissolves oil and grease and is widely used in deodorants and toothpastes (as a thickener).

Triclosan

This is registered with the Environmental Protection Agency as a pesticide and suspected to cause cancer in humans. It is used in antibacterial products to kill germs (e.g. the microban range) and is also used in toothpastes to provide 'continued protection' for 12–24 hours!

Alcohol, isopropyl (SD40)

Found in toothpastes, this is very dehydrating and can act as a carrier for harmful chemicals to cross into the oral cavity.

Methylisothiazoline (MIT)

Found in many top brand shampoos, this chemical has been linked with Alzheimer's disease (Adams, 2005), birth defects and neurological disorders. Methylisothiazoline is totally unregulated by the US Food and Drug Administration (FDA) because it is not a prescription drug.

Parabens (methylparaben, propylparaben, ethylparaben and butylparaben)

These synthetic preservatives are used in cosmetics and personal care products, especially baby wipes, baby lotions and shampoo. They are also used as food preservatives.

Parabens have been found to act like the hormone oestrogen in lab experiments, although activity was weak. They may cause dermatitis, rash or allergic skin conditions.

Current guidelines and sensible precautions

The author is a passionate advocate of safe skincare for the neonate and her published work on this subject (Trotter, 2002, 2003, 2004, 2006, 2007, 2008a, 2008c) has led to the promotion of a 'minimal' approach to skincare in the use of products described as cleansers or for skin nourishment. In the UK, this advice is now supported by the latest postnatal care guidelines (NICE, 2006). The guidelines state that: 'Bathing (cleansing agents, lotions and medicated wipes) are not recommended' and 'Parents should be advised how to keep the umbilical cord clean and dry and that antiseptics should not be used routinely.'

The cosmetics industry as a whole has a good safety record considering the number of ingredients and products on offer. However, there is no room for complacency. Ingredients which may seem innocuous on their own have the potential to irritate sensitive skin (specifically in babies and young children) when added to a cocktail of other chemicals. With this in mind, it is sensible to keep exposure to an absolute minimum.

'Babycare – back to basics': a leaflet for parents

This leaflet was first published in 2004 and is regularly updated in line with the latest evidence-based advice (Trotter, 2008b). Extracted from the most recent version of this leaflet, the following information is aimed at new parents and covers the most common topics associated with baby skincare, cord care and related issues.

Introduction

- Recent research suggests that it is safer to bath your baby in plain water for at least the first month of life (Figure 7.3).

- At birth, the top layer of your baby's skin is very thin and absorbent. This means it is more sensitive to damage from germs, chemicals and water loss. Over the first month (longer in premature infants), your baby's skin matures and develops its own natural protective barrier. The maintenance of this barrier is vital and damage can lead to the development of skin conditions.

- It is important to remember that *anything* placed on, in or around your baby has the potential to harm.

- With this in mind, the following guidelines will help to give your baby the best possible start in life.

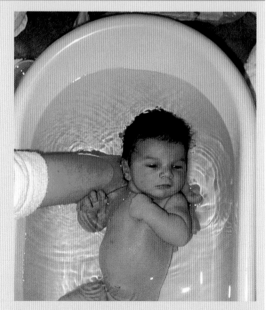

Figure 7.3   Water only for all babycare. (© TIPS Ltd)

'Babycare – back to basics': a leaflet for parents – *continued*

Cord care

Cord care for the healthy term baby

- Keep this area clean and dry. The best way to achieve this is to leave the area alone. After the first bath in plain water, pat dry with a clean towel. Fold the nappy back, at each change, until the cord falls off. In the first few days, it is advisable to only top'n'tail your baby to allow the cord to separate naturally. Wet cotton wool can be used if the area becomes soiled, otherwise leave it alone. There is no need to use antiseptic wipes or powders. The cord clamp may or may not be removed, depending on hospital policy. If the cord or surrounding area becomes red or smelly, notify a member of staff. This advice is based on the World Health Organization (WHO) recommendations published in 1999.

Cord care for the sick or premature baby

- Cord care should be the same as for any other baby. Be guided by staff in the neonatal unit and they will advise you on the best possible care for your baby.

Bath care

- *Before and after carrying out any baby-care it is very important to wash your hands thoroughly.*

- Your baby's first bath will be in plain water. This will help to protect the delicate skin while it is vulnerable to germs, chemicals and water loss. Wash cloths should be avoided as they can be harsh. Handwashing your baby, or using cotton wool (organic is better) or a natural sponge is gentler. A baby comb can be used to gently remove any debris from thick hair after delivery. Please bring a baby comb into hospital with you.

- It is best to leave the delicate area around the eyes untouched. If it does become sticky, please notify a member of staff and they will advise you. The ears and nose should also be left alone and cotton buds should be avoided.

- Vernix (the white sticky substance that covers your baby's skin in the womb) should always be left to absorb naturally. This is nature's own moisturizer and gives added protection against infection in the first few days.

- Premature babies' skin is even more delicate, so it is important to take extra care. Research has shown that massaging premature infants, using pure vegetable oils, can give some protection against skin infections. Be guided by staff in the neonatal unit, who will be happy to advise you.

- If your baby is overdue, his/her skin may well be dry and cracked. This is to be expected, as the protective vernix has all been absorbed. Don't be tempted to use any creams or lotions as this may do more harm than good. The top layer of your baby's skin will peel off over the next few days, leaving perfect skin underneath. Continue with plain water only for at least the first month.

Skin-to-skin contact and baby massage

- The benefits of skin-to-skin contact cannot be overstated and should be positively encouraged from birth. It not only promotes successful breastfeeding but stabilizes your baby's heart rate and temperature. Baby massage follows on naturally from this and is now widely practised. It is advisable to avoid nut oils, petroleum-based oils or oils with perfumes if there is any history of allergies in your family. Choose a properly qualified massage therapist for your baby and ask for their advice on suitable oils.

- Remember not to use any products on broken skin.

Handy tips

- Continue bathing your baby with plain water for at least the first month before *gradually* introducing baby products. By this time the skin's natural barrier will have developed. These products should be free from sulfates (SLS and SLES), colours and strong perfumes.

- Baby wipes should also be avoided for the first month. Once introduced, try to use ones which are mild and free from alcohol and strong perfumes.

- It is safer to file nails with a soft nail file rather than use scissors, which can leave sharp edges. Baby nails that have started to come away can be peeled off gently.

- Shampoo is not necessary when your baby is under a year old. Once you have introduced baby bath products, simply rinse your baby's hair in the bath water solution. If used, shampoo should also be sulfate free (SLS and SLES).

- It is advisable to use a thin layer of barrier cream on the nappy area. The ideal preparation should be free from preservatives, colours, perfumes and antiseptics, and clinically proven to be effective treatment for nappy rash.

- If after a few weeks you wish to use a moisturizer, choose products that are emollient based. These will not dry out the skin, but they will give it some protection.

- When washing your baby's clothes and bedding remember not to overload the machine to ensure thorough rinsing. Fabric conditioners, if used, should be mild and free from colours and strong perfumes.

- Cloth nappies are as efficient as disposable ones and do not present a higher risk of nappy rash.

continued ➤

Diet tips

- Breastfeeding is obviously the best choice for your baby as it is known to strengthen the immune system, giving some protection against allergies developing. Skin-to-skin contact in the period immediately after birth, as well as during breastfeeding, is an excellent way of helping to colonize your baby's skin with friendly and protective bacteria, which in turn will reduce the risk of skin infections developing.

- Whether you breastfeed or bottle-feed, remember that weaning should be done very carefully. The World Health Organization advises that weaning should not start before your baby is six months old.

- Your health visitor or dietician will be happy to advise you on what foods to introduce and when. This is especially important if there is a history of allergies in your family. Like breastfeeding, weaning should always be 'baby-led'.

- From the age of six months babies should also start to drink from cups without teats or spouts, these are often called 'open top cups'. The UK Committee on Medical Aspects recommends that babies over one year old should not drink from bottles.

- You may still receive free samples while in the maternity unit or shortly afterwards. However, we recommend you do not introduce the baby skincare products until your baby is at least one month old.

Conclusion

'It is the responsibility of midwives to deliver care based on current evidence, best practice and where applicable, validated research where it is available' (Nursing and Midwifery Council, 2008). Midwives therefore have a 'duty of care' to advise parents of the potential dangers associated with the early overuse of manufactured baby products and inform them of the safe alternatives that are available.

Manufacturers must play their part by re-evaluating formulations in light of the growing evidence against the use of synthetic detergents. These chemicals are likely to be a contributory factor in the huge rise in skin-related conditions observed over the past 30 years. The widespread use of baby products is coincident with this statistic.

CASE HISTORY

The following testimonial was written by a mother of six who had experienced ongoing skin conditions in all of her first five children. She followed the 'Babycare – back to basics'™ leaflet guidelines, and the outcome for her new baby was life changing.

'As a 40-year-old mother of five children aged between 18 and 3 I thought I knew just about all there was to know about care of the newborn and wouldn't have taken kindly to just anyone trying to tell me otherwise! However, Sharon approached me with her views on skincare and I have to admit she seemed to make sense. I had always been someone who liked their baby to smell nice as well as clean which is why I used manufactured baby products. However all my babies had all been plagued with rashes, cradle cap and dry skin. I knew that using strongly perfumed lotions and wipes was not good for delicate skin and always used what I thought were reliable brands, designed especially for babies but this did not seem to lessen the reactions my baby's developed.

When pregnant with my sixth child I decided to try Sharon's advice. From the day Harry (Figure 7.4) was born I used nothing but water on him, from his hair to his bottom. I had been used to using the small antiseptic wipes on the babies cord but here too I just used water and kept it dry. I went from having babies whose cord would take up to a week to dry and fall off, often being quite wet and horrible, to a baby whose cord dried and fell off after two days. His skin had no rashes or redness and no dryness round his wrists and ankles. At nearly three years of age he is my only child not to have had cradle cap and he still only gets his hair washed when he really needs it not as a matter of course each bath time. If I had known 20 years ago what I know now I would have done things very differently. I must have spent a fortune over the years on different creams and shampoos (probably made by the same manufacturers that made the perfumed lotions!) to remedy the problems caused by using perfumes and lotions on my babies in the first place. All of this had the added bonus of allowing me to smell my baby's own true smell which often disappears soon after birth, for much longer.'

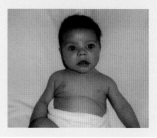

Figure 7.4   Baby Harry. (© TIPS Ltd)

Reflective practice

The following questions can be used to evaluate your under-standing of neonatal skincare as a result of reading this chapter. Answer the following questions honestly (try not to guess):

Part 1 – to be completed *before* reading the chapter on neonatal skincare

1 How does neonatal skin differ from that of older babies?

2 Have you heard of a 'water only' regime for bathing babies?

3 Do you recommend parents use baby products on newborns?

4 Do you recommend parents shampoo their baby's hair?

5 If you have answered no to question 3, at what age do you recommend they introduce products?

6 What advice do you give parents regarding vernix?

7 Do you recommend the use of massage oils or moisturizers?

8 Do you understand the term 'open cord care'?

9 Do you remove the cord clamps in your maternity unit and if so when?

10 Do you continue to bath babies until the cord separates?

11 Do you use any products on the cord area? If so what and why?

12 What advice do you give parents about skin-to-skin contact and natural colonization of the skin?

13 Has your unit got a baby skincare policy?

14 Does your maternity unit have supplies of free products in postnatal areas for use by parents?

Part 2 – to be completed *after* reading the chapter on neonatal skincare

1 Have your opinions changed on the subject of neonatal skincare as a result of the reading this chapter? If so why?

2 Will you change practice as a result of this?

3 Would you like your maternity unit to implement a policy on baby skincare?

4 Will you be spreading the word about best practice in baby skincare?

5 Have your views changed on vernix?

6 Have your views changed on cord care?

7 Will you seek to change practice on cordcare in your unit?

8 Do you feel better able to advise parents on baby skin/cord care issues?

9 Would you use baby skincare products on your baby?

10 Do you now identify this as a clinical risk?

11 Can you think of other practices that may be a clinical risk?

12 Have you any questions or queries?

Key Points

- Avoid using any manufactured baby skincare products for at least the first month of life. Instead, use plain water and cotton wool (preferably organic and unbleached).

- Once introduced, opt for baby products that are free from sulfates (SLS and SLES) as such products are less likely to irritate.

- Read the label of any skin product and if in doubt contact the manufacturer.

- Stick to a few tried and tested products, preferably within one range as this will reduce exposure to ingredients.

- Never mix different preparations.

- Use products before the 'best before date'.

- Shop around for simple preparations that are ecologically sound and contain as few preservatives as possible.

- When washing baby clothes and bedding, do not overload the washing machine. This will ensure thorough rinsing.

- Opt for diluted essential oils rather than synthetic fragrances.

References

Adams, M (2005) Popular shampoos contain toxic chemicals linked to nerve damage. http://www.newstarget.com/003210.html [accessed 7 October 2008].

Bain J (1994) Umbilical cord care in preterm babies. *Nursing Standard* **8**(15): 32–36.

Barr J (1984) The umbilical cord: to treat or not to treat? *Midwives Chronicle and Nursing Notes* **97**(1159): 224–226.

Day P (2005) *Cancer – Why we're still dying to know the truth.* Marden, TN: Credence Publications.

Di Nardo A, Sugino K, Wertz P *et al.* (1996) Sodium lauryl sulphate (SLS) induced irritant contact dermatitis: a correlation study between ceramides and in vivo parameters of irritation. *Contact Dermatitis* **35**: 86–91.

Dore S, Buchan D, Coulas S, Hamber L, Stewart M, Cowan D *et al.* (1998) Alcohol versus natural drying for newborn cord care. *Journal of Obstetrics, Gynaecology and Neonatal Nursing* **27**: 621–627.

Ertel K (2003) Bathing the term newborn: personal cleanser considerations. In: Maibach HI and Boisits EK (eds) *Neonatal Skin: Structure and function.* New York, Marcel Dekker, Chapter 11, pp. 211–238.

Evans NJ and Rutter N (1986) Development of the epidermis in the newborn. *Biology of the Neonate* **49**: 74–80.

Fatter G, Hackl P and Braun F (1997) Effects of soap and detergents on skin surface pH, stratum corneum hydration and fat contents in infants. *Dermatology* **195**: 258–262.

Gelmetti C (2001) Skin cleansing in children. *Journal of European Academy of Dermatology and Venereology* **15**(suppl 1): 12–15.

Harpin VA and Rutter N (1983) Barrier properties of the newborn infant's skin. *Journal of Pediatrics* **102**: 419–425.

Holbrook KA (1982) A histological comparison of infant and adult skin. In: Maibach HI and Boisits EK (eds) *Neonatal Skin: Structure and function.* New York, Marcel Dekker, pp. 3–31.

Kownatzki E (2003) Hand hygiene and skin health. *Journal of Hospital Infection* **55**: 239–245.

McNally N, Williams H, Philips D, Smallman-Raynor M, Lewis S, Venn A and Britton J (1998) Atopic eczema and domestic water hardness. *Lancet* **352**(9127): 527–531.

Medves J (1997) Cleaning solutions and bacterial colonization in promoting healing and early separation of the umbilical cord in healthy newborns. *Canadian Journal of Public Health* **88**: 380–382.

Mugford M, Somchwong M and Waterhouse IL (1986) Treatment of umbilical cords: a randomised trial to assess the effect of treatment methods on the work of midwives. *Midwifery* **2**: 177–186.

NICE (National Institute for Health and Clinical Excellence) (2006) *Routine Postnatal Care of Women and their Babies. Quick reference guide.* London: NICE.

Nursing and Midwifery Council (2008) *The Code – Standards of Conduct, Performance and Ethics for Nurses and Midwives.* London: NMC, p. 7.

Nonato L B (1998) Evolution of skin barrier function in neo-nates. Unpublished doctoral dissertation, University of California, Berkley. UMI Publication number AAT9827176.

Peck S and Botwinick J (1964) The buffering capacity of infants skin against an alkaline soap and neutral detergent. *Journal of Mt. Sinai Hospital* **31**: 134.

Pezzati M, Biagotti EC, Martelli E, Gambi B, Biagotti R and Rubaltelli FF (2002) Umbilical cord care: the effect of eight different cord care regimens on cord separation time and other outcomes. *Biology of the Neonate* **81**: 38–44.

Rhein L, Robbins C, Fernee K *et al.* (1986) Surfactant structure effects on swelling of isolated human stratum corneum. *Journal of Society of Cosmetic Chemists* **37**: 125–139.

Rush JP, Hempal V and Dotzert L (1987) Rooming-in and visiting on the ward: effects on newborn colonization rates. *Infection Control* **2**(suppl 3): 10–15.

Salariya EM and Kowbus NM (1988) Variable umbilical cord care. *Midwifery* **4**: 70–76.

Singh N, Sugathan PS and Bhujwala RA (1982) Human colostrum for the prophylaxis against sticky eye and conjunctivitis in the newborn. *Journal of Tropical Pediatrics* **28**: 35–37.

Steinman D and Epstein S (1995) *The Safe Shoppers Bible: Guide to non toxic household products, cosmetics and food.* New Jersey: Wiley.

Tierno Jr, PM (2006) How to protect your baby against harmful germs. In: Ettus S. *The Experts' Guide to the Baby Years.* New York: Clarkson Potter.

Tollin M, Bergsson G, Kai-Larsen Y *et al.* (2005) Vernix caseosa as a multi-component defence system based on polypeptides, lipids and their interactions. *Cell Molecular Life Sciences* **62**: 2390–2399.

Trotter S (2002) Skincare for the newborn: exploring the potential harm of manufactured products. *RCM Midwives Journal* **5**: 376–378.

Trotter S (2003) Management of the umbilical cord – a guide to best care. *RCM Midwives Journal* **6**: 308–311.

Trotter S (2004) Care of the newborn: proposed new guidelines. *British Journal of Midwifery* **12**: 152–157.

Trotter S (2006) Neonatal skincare: why change is vital. *RCM Midwives Journal* **9**: 134–138.

Trotter S (2007) Baby products – it's all in the labelling. *MIDIRS Midwifery Digest* **17**: 263–266.

Trotter S (2008a) Neonatal skin and cordcare – the way forward. *Nursing in Practice* (January/February) Number 40 (Dermatology): 40–45.

Trotter S (2008b) *Baby Care – Back to basics™.* Troon: TIPS Limited.

Trotter S (2008c) Neonatal skincare and cordcare – implications for practice. In: Davies L and McDonald S (eds) *Examination of the Newborn and Neonatal health – a multidimentional approach.* Edinburgh: Churchill Livingstone, Elsevier Worldwide, Chapter 14.

Vance J (1999) *Beauty to Die For: The cosmetic consequence.* USA: iuniverse.com.

Verber IG and Pagan FS (1992) What cord care – if any? *Archives of Disease in Childhood* **68**: 594–596.

World Health Organization (1998) Care of the umbilical cord: a review of the evidence. Reproductive Health (technical support) Maternal and newborn Health/safe motherhood. WHO document WHO/RHT/MSM/98.4.

Zupan J, Garner P and Omari AAA (2004) Topical umbilical cord care at birth. *Cochrane Database of Systematic Reviews* (3): CD001057. DOI: 10.1002/14651858.CD001057.pub2.

CHAPTER 8

THERMAL CARE OF THE NEWBORN

Hilary Lumsden

OVERVIEW

The care of the baby's temperature is a fundamental role for the midwife and, when managed well, can prevent unnecessary admission to the neonatal unit for hypothermia. Effective care of the neonatal temperature on the delivery suite and postnatal ward can also accelerate discharge into the care of the community midwife. Term newborn babies are able to maintain their own body temperature from birth although they will not be as efficient as older children or adults, with the neonate's temperature being maintained over a narrow range of ambient conditions. Newborns therefore require some support in stabilizing their temperature in the first few days of life.

Thermoregulation is the balance between heat loss and heat production and the mechanisms of maintaining temperature equilibrium. A sound understanding of the physiology of thermoregulation is essential to enable the midwife to care for the baby appropriately and to also be able to advise parents correctly about temperature control. There are four ways in which babies lose heat and there are several ways in which to prevent heat loss as well as encouraging heat production.

Temperature control of preterm babies presents more of a challenge to midwives and neonatal nurses. The aim of this chapter is to discuss the physiological aspects of temperature control along with practical methods of maintaining skin temperature within normal limits for the term and preterm infant.

Fetal temperature

During pregnancy the woman will generate approximately 35 per cent more heat than in her non-pregnant state. This will result in an increased tolerance to cold weather and an increase in the activity of sweat glands and leads to warmer skin temperature. It is normal for the maternal temperature to increase by around 0.5°C. Therefore the fetal environmental temperature is linked to the maternal temperature with the fetus not being able to maintain its own temperature independently during pregnancy. Fetal temperature is 0.5°C higher than that of the mother, making the fetal core temperature in the region of 37.6° to 37.8°C (Tucker Blackburn, 2007). If there are changes to the maternal temperature because of fever or exercise, there may be a rise in fetal temperature at the same time. This naturally warm environment ceases however, when the baby is delivered.

At birth

The importance of keeping babies warm cannot be over-emphasized. Silverman *et al.* (1958) recognized the clear link between temperature control and neonatal mortality. In their study Silverman and colleagues found that keeping babies warm in incubators resulted in an unqualified reduction in mortality by 25 per cent. According to Lyon (2007) no single change in practice has had such a remarkable effect on reducing the mortality of newborn babies. And while Silverman *et al.*'s (1958) study examined the effects of hypothermia on preterm babies, the principles of maintaining the temperature in the term baby still applies today. Interestingly, the CESDI 27/28 project (CEMACH, 2003) showed that for babies born at 27 and 28 weeks' gestation a temperature below 36°C was found in 73 per cent of those who died compared with 59 per cent of those who survived.

The neonate has to establish and maintain its own temperature at birth. Heat loss is rapid due to the baby's large surface area and can exceed heat production if the baby is left exposed in an ambient room temperature that is too cool or draughty. Term and preterm babies have a large surface area-to-weight ratio, they lack subcutaneous fat and the skin is permeable to water, all of which makes the conservation of heat difficult. Most babies will have a fairly well-developed thermoregulatory capability; however, it is the narrow range of normality that makes them vulnerable when there is poor temperature control.

Although skin vasoconstriction in response to cold in babies is similar to that of adults, even in the term baby the insulation provided by subcutaneous tissue is less than half that of the adult (Rennie and Roberton, 2002). At birth the fetus moves from the warm interuterine environment to the colder extrauterine environment. Term babies have a limited ability to maintain their temperature by shivering, they will also have some ability to change their position in order to reduce their surface area to conserve heat, but they lack subcutaneous fat and are born wet into a cooler environment.

Non-shivering thermogenesis is the process that occurs in babies during the first few weeks of life in order to maintain their temperature and is activated immediately after the separation of the placenta. An increase in oxygenation plays an important role in initiating this system. The sympathetic nervous system is stimulated by cutaneous cold receptors. This activates the release of noradrenaline which in turn stimulates brown adipose tissue (BAT) metabolism. Thyroid-stimulating hormone (TSH) is also released from the anterior pituitary with the thyroid hormones playing

Brown adipose tissue (BAT)

The main role of BAT or brown fat is heat production. It is found around the neck, between the scapulae, along the sternum and clavicles. It also covers all the major thoracic vessels, with the largest amount of BAT padding the kidneys. Brown fat is excellent at producing heat energy. Within the brown fat cell there are several mitochondria and it is these that provide energy for metabolic conversion. BAT is found in the preterm infant in small amounts; in the term infant, however, it can account for up to one-tenth by volume of the total adipose tissue.

The unique structure of BAT gives it the ability to generate more energy than any other tissue in the body. These features include:

- many mitochondria – produce energy for heat production;
- glycogen stores – a source of glucose for the production of adenosine triphosphate (ATP) and energy;
- a prolific blood supply – brings nutrients to the cell and transports the heat that is produced to other parts of the body;
- an abundant sympathetic nerve supply – mobilizes the metabolism of BAT by noradrenaline.

Rennie and Roberton (2002) suggest that the exothermic pathways release approximately 2.5 kcal/g of brown fat/min and warm the blood passing through the tissues. Oxygen is consumed during brown fat metabolism and in the hypoxic baby the reaction to cold will be put at risk.

a part in mobilizing the enzymes that accelerate glucose oxidation.

In order for non-shivering thermogenesis to take place there needs to be energy in the form of glucose. If glucose levels are low, for example, in the baby affected by intrauterine growth restriction following fetal distress or resuscitation, the baby will need to convert protein and lipids into glucose. This process is called gluconeogenesis. It may be inhibited in preterm or small for gestational age infants (Figure 8.1).

Heat loss

Heat is lost from the baby to the environment in four different ways: evaporation, radiation, convection and conduction (Figure 8.2). These are described in Table 8.1.

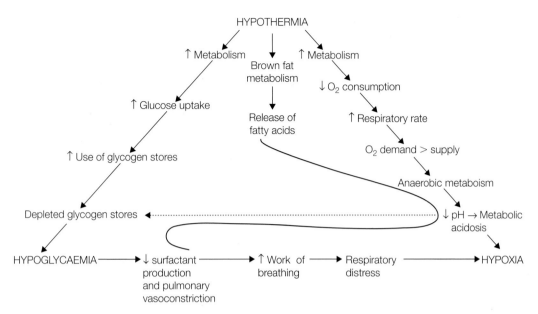

Figure 8.1   Integrated physiology underpinning the neonatal energy triangle. (Adapted with permission from Aylott M (2006) The neonatal energy triangle. Pt 2: Thermoregulatory and respiratory adaptation, *Paediatric Nursing* **18**:7. © RCN Publishing)

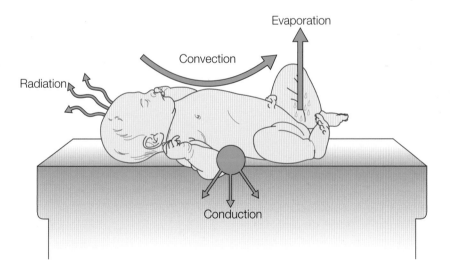

Temperature measurement

The World Health Organization (1997) recommend that the normal body temperature for a neonate in the first few days should be between 36.5 and 37.5°C. It has long been argued that the rectal temperature is the 'gold standard' of temperature measurement (Rennie and Roberton, 2002), but there is a risk of perforation of the rectum as well as a risk of vagal stimulation leading to bradycardia when the temperature is taken via the rectal route. For these reasons axillary temperature measurement is accepted practice in the UK. Axilla and skin temperature measurements tend to be slightly lower than the core rectal temperature but

Table 8.1   Four mechanisms of heat loss

Mechanism	Description	Prevention
Evaporation	The wet baby is exposed to the environmental air, and with the conversion of water to vapour there is a subsequent loss of heat	Dry the baby well at delivery paying attention to the head. Once the wet towel has been removed, wrap the baby in warm dry towels
Radiation	The transfer of heat from the exposed area of the baby to the surrounding surfaces	Make sure that the baby is not placed near to cooler surfaces such as windows or walls
Convection	Heat is lost due to the movement of air at the surface of the skin	Close windows and doors, switching off any fans prior to birth. Free flowing facial oxygen can also cause convective heat loss
Conduction	Heat is lost from one surface to another, placing the baby on a cold surface	Any surface that the baby is placed onto such as the resuscitaire or scales should be pre-warmed. Cold hands can also cause conductive heat loss

these methods will still reflect the increases and decreases in temperature consistent with differences in core temperature and can be as accurate as the rectal route.

Rosenthal and Leslie (2006) strongly suggest that obtaining an accurate measurement of the baby's temperature is a basic step in providing thermoneutrality. The initial temperature recording of a newborn provides the foundation for the baby's subsequent care and management.

Historically, mercury thermometers were used, but because of the hazards associated with mercury this type of thermometry is no longer used in the developed world. In place of mercury thermometers there are several alternatives now in use.

Suretemp and Lightouch thermometers are currently used in many hospitals. Their accuracy has been studied and they have been found to be more reliable than traditional methods of temperature recording (Rosenthal and Leslie, 2006). It is important that midwives are conversant with current methods of temperature measurement in order for appropriate care to be given.

Hypothermia

Babies who are sick are more susceptible to hypothermia and if the delivery room is not well prepared or if the birth takes place outside the delivery room hypothermia becomes a real risk. Non-shivering thermogenesis requires oxygen to metabolize the BAT and if the baby has respiratory problems this will affect the process. Babies with a high surface area-to-body mass ratio, such as small for gestational age babies, have low levels of subcutaneous fat and glycogen stores and are more vulnerable to a cold environment.

Transepidermal water loss increases with lower gestational age because of the preterm infant's very thin skin. With high levels of water loss the temperature will lower. For preterm babies on the neonatal unit high levels of humidity can reduce water loss and therefore conserve the temperature.

Babies at risk

It is important to identify those babies who might be at risk of hypothermia so that efforts can be made to prevent hypothermia occurring. This will include:

- preterm babies, particularly those under 30 weeks' gestation;
- babies with birthweight below 2.5 kg;
- sick babies;
- small for gestational age;
- babies who have needed resuscitation at birth (Neonatal Bedside Guidelines, 2007).

Cold stress

Since newborn babies are at risk of cooling, it is the role of the midwife in the delivery room to ensure that the baby does not become cold. Cold stress particularly affects babies where there are risk factors such as being preterm, requiring resuscitation or transportation. Other risk factors are hypoglycaemia, nutritional problems, respiratory problems, neurological conditions and congenital anomalies such as gastroschisis, exomphalos, myelomeningocele, where insensible water loss is high which may cause the core temperature to plummet.

Babies who are born by caesarean section are also at risk of hypothermia because they have not undergone the processes associated with vaginal delivery and may be slow to breathe and are more at risk of needing resuscitation.

Cold stress affects oxygenation by increasing the pulmonary artery resistance and as a result affects surfactant production. Anaerobic metabolism is increased because of poor perfusion, which can cause acidosis. This reduces the amount of blood flowing to the lungs and can result in hypoxia. The baby will use extra glucose because of the increased metabolism and this may cause hypoglycaemia, which in turn leads to further acidosis.

The clinical signs of cold stress are non-specific but can include:

- pallor
- grunting
- tachypnoea
- cool skin
- lethargy
- poor feeding
- hypotonia
- apnoea
- irritability
- bradycardia
- mottling.

Since these signs can be attributed to other clinical conditions in the newborn the midwife should make an objective assessment of the baby's condition, which will include taking the temperature, measuring blood glucose and seeking medical assessment.

The consequences of hypothermia are detailed in Table 8.2.

Cold stress can increase postnatal weight loss and decrease subsequent weight gain. Severe cold stress may present with peripheral oedema and sclerema,

Table 8.2 Consequences of hypothermia

Consequences of temperature <36.0°C	Hypoglycaemia Metabolic acidosis Hypoxia with increased oxygen demands
Consequences of temperature <35.5°C	Increased metabolic rate Clotting disorders Shock Apnoea Intraventricular haemorrhage Persistant fetal circulation Decreased surfactant production

Neonatal Bedside Guidelines (2007).

can affect coagulability and increases the incidence of neonatal mortality.

Perinatal asphyxia can cause moderate or severe encephalopathy in approximately 2:1000 births, which can subsequently lead to cerebral palsy. In the TOBY trial research study currently being undertaken in the UK, babies who have experienced moderate or severe asphyxia are randomly allocated to receive either standard intensive care or intensive care with cooling. The aim of the study is to determine whether whole body cooling improves survival and reduces the neurological effects of asphyxia. Those babies who have been cooled have their body temperature reduced to 33–34°C for 72 hours, followed by gradual re-warming (National Perinatal Epidemiology Unit, 2008). Selective cooling may in the future be an acceptable practice in the prevention of neurological problems in babies where there has been perinatal asphyxia.

Overheating

Similar to cold stress, overheating can have a deleterious effect on the neonate. Babies who are too warm will have increased fluid loss by sweating and evaporative heat loss, which can contribute to dehydration. This can, in turn, lead to hypernatraemia and may increase postnatal weight loss. There is also an increased risk of jaundice. It must be pointed out that although the neonate has more sweat glands than the adult they have limited ability to use them for cooling. The sweat glands of babies under 36 weeks' gestation do not function.

Overheating has been linked to apnoea and sudden infant death syndrome (SIDS). The advice for parents from the Foundation for the Study of Infant Deaths (Department of Health, 2009) is 'Do not let your baby get too hot (or too cold)'.

Babies may become too hot by being in a room with a high ambient air temperature, lying in direct sunlight or under phototherapy, or as a result of overdressing or swaddling. Overheating should be differentiated from pyrexia. Babies with pyrexia will usually have other signs of illness such as apnoea, poor feeding/vomiting, tachypnoea, pallor, tachycardia and hypotonia. The pyrexial baby will often have temperature recordings that are unstable, vacillating between high and low. Further observation, screening and investigations will be needed to rule out infection or other causes in the pyrexial baby.

Transport

While it is acknowledged that transportation to other hospitals can affect the baby's temperature, simply transporting the baby to the neonatal unit or postnatal ward in some instances can cause the temperature to drop to worrying levels. In one study an audit of babies' temperatures on admission to the neonatal unit revealed that some were at suboptimal levels. The geography of the maternity unit seemed to add to the risk in cases where babies had to be transported longer distances to the neonatal unit, regardless of how the transfer was conducted (West Midlands Perinatal Register, 2005). A similar finding by Loughead et al. (1997) found that 45 per cent of very low birthweight babies were hypothermic on admission to the neonatal unit.

A pre-warmed transport incubator is the ideal method of transferring vulnerable babies to the neonatal unit, but many maternity units use the resuscitaire as a method of transferring babies.

Efficient management of the baby's temperature both at birth and in the first few hours of life can prevent unnecessary admissions to the neonatal unit/transitional care unit and separation from the mother. Likewise it is common to find babies with lower temperatures on admission to the postnatal ward even though the temperature may have been recorded as within normal limits on the delivery suite. Transferring babies to the postnatal ward with their mothers, providing skin-to-skin contact, may help prevent hypothermia on admission.

Hypothermia is one of the three most common reasons for admission to the neonatal unit. In an attempt to reduce unnecessary admissions for hypothermia, Hubbard (2006) suggests that babies with a temperature of 36.3°C and rising and who are otherwise well do not need to be admitted to the neonatal unit. It means that babies with borderline temperatures do not need to be separated from their mothers and are not subjected to unnecessary interventions and are allowed to recover their temperature on the postnatal ward.

Thermoneutral environment

The thermoneutral environment is the ambient air temperature at which energy expenditure and oxygen consumption are at a minimum to maintain the baby's normal activities. The temperature of a thermoneutral environment will depend on the baby's birthweight, postnatal age and whether they are naked or clothed. Infants who use a great deal of their own energy (calories) to maintain their temperature are sacrificing energy that could be used for growth and development. As previously discussed, babies will utilize oxygen in the process of keeping warm or if they are too hot, so it is essential that the ambient air temperature allows them to maintain their temperature without the need to utilize additional oxygen.

Range of environmental temperature

The temperatures at which newborn babies should be nursed, clothed and in a draught-free environment are listed in Table 8.3.

Table 8.3   Temperatures for newborn babies

Day	Birthweight 2.0 kg	Birthweight 3.0 kg
0–1	25–29°C	22–28°C
5	23–28°C	20–27°C
10	21–27°C	19–26°C

Adapted from Hey (1971) in Rennie and Roberton (2002).

Prevention of hypothermia

The midwife plays a significant part in the prevention of hypothermia. Following a few simple rules the midwife can enable the baby to remain warm, prevent hypoglycaemia and potential longer term problems.

In hospital

- Delivery room, operating theatre and recovery rooms should have an ambient air temperature of 23–28°C and be free from draughts.
- The baby should be dried immediately following delivery, the wet towel should be removed and the baby wrapped in *warm* dry towels.
- The mother should be offered skin-to-skin contact with the baby.
- The baby should be offered a breast or bottle feed in the delivery room.
- The baby should wear a hat for the first few hours.
- Weighing the baby should be deferred.
- Keep the mother and baby together for transfer.
- Pre-warmed bedding should be used. This can be achieved by placing a pre-warmed wheat bag into the cot before delivery.
- If delivering in a birthing pool, the temperature of the water should be 37°C.
- Hands and stethoscope should be warmed before examining the baby.
- Dress the baby in pre-warmed clothes.

In the community

- Keep the room warm, closing all windows and doors.
- Reduce the flow of 'traffic' through the rooms to prevent draughts.
- Set up a 'resuscitation' area for the baby (i.e. a changing mat with prepared, checked equipment).
- Put towels, blankets and the baby's clothing on the radiators to warm.
- Offer skin-to-skin contact, offer breast feed.
- Pre-warm baby's bedding.

Methods of heat gain

Preterm babies

Babies who are 30 weeks' gestation or less should have the following care in the delivery room:

- Keep the delivery room or theatre 23–28°C and free from draughts.
- Put the preterm baby in a plastic bag up to their neck – do not dry the baby beforehand.
- Dry the head well.
- An overhead radiant heater must be switched on in order for the plastic bag method to be effective.
- Put a hat on the baby's head.
- Keep the baby in the plastic bag until it is in a pre-warmed, humidified incubator on the neonatal unit.

The use of plastic bags for preterm babies has been shown to be effective at reducing water loss and heat loss during resuscitation (Lyon and Stenson, 2004). However, to date no studies have concluded whether this method of reducing heat loss has had any effect on perinatal mortality. Preterm babies are particularly vulnerable to heat loss.

The current practice is to place any baby born before 30 weeks' gestation into a food preparation standard plastic bag until the baby has been transferred to the neonatal unit (Resuscitation Council (UK), 2006). The baby should not be dried before putting into the bag, the face and head should be left exposed and most importantly the baby should be placed under a radiant heater. Attention must be paid to the head, which should be dried well and a hat should be put on the baby's head to prevent heat loss through the large surface area of the head.

Term babies will also benefit from wearing a hat, particularly for transfer to the ward or until the temperature is stable on the postnatal ward. Clothes act as a significant thermal barrier to heat loss, and term, well, newly born babies should be able to maintain their temperature in a cot in a warm room. However, it is advisable to pre-warm the baby's clothes by placing them on the resuscitaire with the radiant heater in pre-warm mode. Clothes are very often cold when they are taken out of the mother's case and it will defeat the object if the baby is put into cold clothing.

On admission to the postnatal ward the midwife should check the baby's temperature and ensure that the baby is not still in a wet towel and that the baby has been fed. If, despite these measures, the baby becomes hypothermic there are a few simple measures the midwife can do to increase the baby's temperature. Mild hypothermia can be managed with putting a hat on the baby if one is not already in place and making sure that the baby is fully clothed, including bootees and mittens. Extra blankets can provide additional warmth and should be pre-warmed before use. The ambient air temperature of the room should be increased if possible with the use of a heater if the overall ward temperature cannot be improved. Skin-to-skin care can be provided and will be discussed further later in this chapter.

Cot lids provide a safe, cheap and effective method of minimizing convective heat loss and can if necessary be used in conjunction with a radiant warmer. A clear Perspex cot lid can be put onto the cot when the baby is dressed and has blankets in place; the mother will be able see her baby through the lid from the bedside.

Heated mattresses or gel-filled mattresses are effective in increasing the temperature of the hypothermic baby, as are radiant heaters which can increase the temperature quickly. Care should be taken that babies do not become overheated and as soon as normal levels are achieved the heater can be switched off. Care should be taken, however, as there may be a fall in the baby's temperature once the heater has been turned off and the axilla temperature should be monitored closely.

If none of these methods succeed in raising the baby's temperature, the next stage would be to put the baby into an incubator.

Tog values of baby clothing and bedding

The tog values of various items of clothing and bedding are listed in Table 8.4. Most infants will require a tog value of 6–10 to prevent hypothermia and hyperthermia in a room temperature of 16–20°C (Johnston et al., 2003). It is recommended by Foundation for the Study of Infant Deaths that blankets rather than quilts or duvets are used because it is easier to control the tog level by adding layers to increase the temperature since duvets/quilts can increase the temperature quickly to dangerous levels. The World Health Organization (1997) also recommends that babies are dressed in several layers of loose clothing and bedding, requiring one or two more layers of clothing than an adult.

Babies who are hypothermic are at risk of also becoming hypoglycaemic since they will have used some of their energy in generating heat. A capillary blood glucose test from a baby's heel should be taken

Table 8.4   Tog values of clothing and bedding

Item	Tog value
Vest	0.2
Babygro	1.0
Jumper	2.0
Cardigan	2.0
Trousers	2.0
Disposable nappy	2.0
Sleep suit	4.0
Sheet	0.2
Old blanket	1.5
New blanket	2.0
Quilt	Around 9

Adapted from Johnston et al. (2003).

and tested using a reagent strip because hypothermia and hypoglycaemia are so closely linked.

Jaundiced babies under phototherapy will lose heat if the room is cold or draughty. Some babies could be at risk of transepidermal water loss, which may or may not affect their temperature control. Fluid balance should be monitored and adjusted when necessary. The use of a 'Biliblanket', which is a lightweight, fibreoptic pad that delivers up to 45 μW of therapeutic light for the treatment of jaundice, can be considered. The Biliblanket allows the infant to be swaddled, held and cared for by parents and hospital staff, while allowing jaundice to be treated without the baby becoming cold.

It is usual to record the baby's temperature twice a day, as long as it is stable. If the baby has been hypothermic or hypoglycaemic, the temperature should be taken more frequently until it is stable and recorded in the baby's notes.

Skin-to-skin care

The World Health Organization (1997) recommends skin-to-skin care as one of the ten steps to successful breastfeeding (Baby Friendly Initiative, 2000). It should be offered to all mothers in the delivery room whether they are intending breastfeed or not.

Skin-to-skin or kangaroo care was first recognized as being useful for warming babies in Bogotá in 1978 where small, preterm babies were being cared for in hospitals where the facilities were poor, with a lack of incubators resulting in higher death rates among premature babies. It has been seen to be successful in neonatal units in the UK in recent years. It can encourage bonding, facilitate breastfeeding and helps to maintain the body temperature of the sick, small and premature baby.

Kangaroo care also promotes cardiorespiratory stabilization, improves thermoregulation, increases rate of infant weight gain, has a high incidence of exclusive breastfeeding, shortens hospital stay and reduces maternal stress levels (Hunt, 2008).

Although there have been several studies that support the use of kangaroo care in the neonatal unit, few have been carried out in relation to term, well babies. Nevertheless, skin-to-skin care has to be seen as an effective method of preventing heat loss in newborn babies whether they are preterm or term.

When the baby is placed on the mother's chest or abdomen, the warmth from the mother will ensure that the baby will not have to use any valuable energy stores to generate heat. The technique of skin-to-skin care is simple: the baby is held upright or diagonally and prone against the skin of the mother, between her breasts with the baby's head under the mother's chin. The baby should be naked except for a nappy. The mother should sit in an upright position to allow the head, neck and abdomen to be extended and not in a slumped position so that the baby's airways are not obstructed. The baby should be dried well before putting skin-to-skin, a hat is placed on the head and the mother and baby should be covered in a blanket or shawl.

If the mother is unwell, recovering from surgery or the idea does not appeal to her, skin-to-skin care with the father will be just as effective at increasing the temperature or preventing hypothermia.

Following a caesarean section or complicated delivery some mothers may become cold due to the environment or because of blood/fluid loss as well as the poor quality of hospital gowns. Midwives caring for mothers in the recovery room or on the postnatal ward should bear in mind that, if the mother is cold, she should also be covered with a blanket or dressing-gown and that skin-to-skin care may not be as efficient at warming the baby as where the woman has had a straightforward normal delivery with minimal blood loss.

The warm chain

The World Health Organization (1997) recommend the 'warm chain' as a method of preventing heat loss in the newly born baby. This involves the following:

- warm delivery room
- immediate drying
- skin-to-skin contact
- breastfeeding
- bathing and weighing postponed
- appropriate clothing and bedding
- mother and baby together
- warm transportation
- warm resuscitation
- training and awareness raising.

CASE HISTORY

Baby A was born by normal delivery at 23.30 hours to a primiparous insulin-dependent gestational diabetic woman. The baby weighed 2.95 kg and passed meconium at birth, although passing urine could not be confirmed. The baby was put to the breast in the delivery room and fed reasonably well. The baby's temperature in the delivery room was 36.7°C. The blood glucose was measured with a reagent strip, the result was 3.4 mmol/L. Baby A was transferred to the postnatal ward with Mum. The blood sugar was tested again 3 hours following delivery (as trust policy on management of the infant of an insulin-dependent gestational diabetic patient) and the result was 3.2 mmol/L. The

baby was offered a breastfeed but was asleep and was left alone.

At 08.00 the blood sugar was again checked as per hospital policy. The midwife noticed that baby A's feet were very cold and this made obtaining a capillary blood sample difficult. The axilla temperature was checked and read 36.2°C. It was also noted that the room temperature in the six-bedded bay where the mother and baby were situated was particularly cool. There were no overhead heaters available so extra blankets were given, a

continued ➤

CASE HISTORY *continued*

hat was put on the baby and the temperature was checked again half an hour later. The temperature on this occasion was 36.0°C. The baby was put to the breast, did not latch well, was still sleepy and urine had still not been passed. The mother was given the baby for some skin-to-skin contact. The temperature had increased to 36.6°C in an hour and to 37.1°C an hour after that. The baby was then tried at the breast once again, latched well and fed well. When the nappy was changed it was noted that baby A had now passed urine.

Questions to ask:

- What are the contributing factors to this baby's hypothermia?

- What are the physiological principles underpinning hypothermia?

- Are there any other ways in which this baby's temperature could have been managed?

Key Points

- An understanding of the mechanisms of heat loss means that midwives are in an excellent position to prevent hypothermia in the newborn.

- Identifying and dealing with hypothermia in a practical way can reduce more complex, longer-term complications.

- Managing the temperature in the delivery room is the key component in the 'warm chain'.

References

Aylott M (2006) The neonatal energy triangle part 2: Thermoregulatory and respiratory adaptation. *Paediatric Nursing* **18**: 38–43.

Baby Friendly Initiative (2000) Hypoglycaemia policy guideline. http://www.babyfriendly.org.uk/pdfs/hypo_policy.pdf [accessed 9 September 2009].

CEMACH (Confidential Enquiry into maternal and Child Health) (2003) CESDI 27/28 Project. An enquiry into quality of care and its effect on the survival of babies born at 27/28 weeks. Norwich. The Stationery Office.

Department of Health (2009) Reduce the risk of cot death. http://www.dh.gov.uk/en/Publicationsandstatistics/Publications/PublicationsPolicyAndGuidance/DH_4123625 [accessed 9 September 2009].

Hubbard M (2006) Reducing admissions to the neonatal unit: a report on how one neonatal service has responded to the ever increasing demand on neonatal cots. *Journal of Neonatal Nursing* **12**: 172–176.

Hunt F (2008) The importance of kangaroo care on infant oxygen saturation levels and bonding. *Journal of Neonatal Nursing* **14**: 47–51.

Johnston PGB, Flood K and Spinks K (2003) Essential care of the newborn baby. In: *The Newborn Child*, 9th edn. Edinburgh: Churchill Livingstone.

Loughead MK, Loughead JL and Reinhart MJ (1997) Incidence and physiologic characteristics of hypothermia in the very low birth weight infant. *Pediatric Nursing* **23**: 5–11.

Lyon A (2007) Temperature control in the neonate. *Paediatrics and Child Health* **18**: 155–160.

Lyon AJ and Stenson B (2004) Cold comfort for babies. *Archives of Diseases in Childhood. Fetal and Neonatal Edition* **89**: F93–F94.

National Perinatal Epidemiology Unit (2008) TOBY: Whole body hypothermia for the treatment of perinatal asphyxial encephalopathy. http://www.npeu.ox.ac.uk/toby [accessed July 2009].

Neonatal Bedside Guidelines (2007) Hypothermia. The Bedside Clinical Guidelines Partnership in association with Shropshire, Staffordshire and Black Country Neonatal Networks, Stoke-on-Trent. http://www.newbornnetworks.org.uk/staffs/documents/Hypothermia2007.pdf [accessed July 2009].

Rennie JM and Roberton NRC (2002) *A Manual of Neonatal Intensive Care*, 4th edn. London: Hodder Arnold.

Resuscitation Council (UK) (2006) *Newborn Life Support. Resuscitation at Birth*, 2nd edn. London: Resuscitation Council (UK).

Rosenthal HM and Leslie A (2006) Measuring temperature of NICU patients: a comparison of three devices. *Journal of Neonatal Nursing* **12**: 125–129.

Silverman WA, Fertig JW and Berger AP (1958) The influence of the thermal environment upon survival of newly born preterm infants. *Pediatrics* **22**: 876–885.

Tucker Blackburn S (2007) *Maternal, Fetal and Neonatal Physiology: A clinical perspective*, 3rd edn. Edinburgh: Elsevier Saunders.

West Midlands Perinatal Institute (2005) www.perinatal.nhs.uk/manners/

World Health Organization (1997) *Thermal Protection of the Newborn: A practical guide*. Geneva: WHO.

CHAPTER 9

CARE OF THE JAUNDICED BABY

Carole England

OVERVIEW

Physiological jaundice is common in term and preterm babies. It results from temporary immaturity of the liver's excretory pathway for bilirubin at a time of its heightened production. For most of these babies it is mild and resolves spontaneously. The ability to predict which babies are at greater risk remains imprecise and, with current trends for early transfer home soon after birth, it is important for both hospital and primary care midwives to be able to recognize exaggerated physiological jaundice from truly pathological jaundice that necessitates investigation and possible treatment.

Jaundice is the commonest reason for readmission to hospital in the first week of life. When a baby develops significant hyperbilirubinaemia, concerns arise about the possible long-term effects, which may take the form of bilirubin encephalopathy. This chapter will focus upon the midwife's role in the assessment and differential diagnosis of clinical jaundice including knowledge of bilirubin metabolism and its patterns in the fetus and neonate along with issues of contemporary management to include phototherapy. Referral to and working with the multiprofessional team will be included as essential requisites of the role. The healthy term baby will be the main focus, but given that midwives care for healthy low birthweight babies from 34 weeks' gestation to term, reference will be made to preterm and babies small for their gestational age (SGA) where relevant.

Introduction

Midwives need to have a thorough knowledge of the physiology of why newborn babies develop jaundice so that they can communicate effectively with their clients and the multiprofessional team.

Red blood cells and bilirubin production

Why does the fetus need so many red blood cells?

The placenta is a poor oxygenator of the blood compared with the lungs. The oxygen tension in fetal blood is only 20–30 mmHg (3–4 kPa), which is really low when compared with the healthy newborn value of 90–100 mmHg (12–13 kPa). To compensate, the fetus has to enhance its oxygen-carrying capacity by producing more circulating red blood cells and so has a haemoglobin of 18–22 g/dL compared with a late neonatal level of around 11–12 g/dL. Therefore at birth about 20 per cent of circulating red blood cells need to be removed from the blood.

Bilirubin metabolism in the fetus and newborn

The biggest difference between fetal and neonatal handling of bilirubin is that the fetus uses the placenta and maternal liver rather than its intestines as the major elimination pathway. Most of the bilirubin produced by the fetus is converted to a fat-soluble form that can be readily cleared by the placenta. The mother will excrete it through her liver. Small remnants of water-soluble bilirubin that remain make up the composition of meconium. After birth the liver of the newborn baby must assume full responsibility for bilirubin metabolism. Immaturity of the liver and intestinal processes for metabolism and excretion can result in physiological jaundice. Different degrees of physiological jaundice are seen in 60 per cent of term babies and in 80 per cent of preterm babies.

The production of bilirubin

With clamping of the umbilical cord the ductus venosus gradually constricts and the flow of blood to the liver increases. The liver is a unique organ that houses many different types of cells that perform different functions. The reticulo-endothelial cells are responsible for haemolizing (breaking down) the haemoglobin of red blood cells into globin and haem. Globin is broken down into amino acids, which are reused by the body to make proteins. Iron is stored in the liver to make new red blood cells when needed at a later time. From the haem a pigment called biliverdin and carbon monoxide are produced. Biliverdin is converted into bilirubin by an enzyme called bilirubin reductase. One gram of haemoglobin will produce 600 µmol/L of bilirubin. Bilirubin then becomes virtually insoluble in water. It takes on lipophilic properties, which means it is fat-soluble and able to cross cell membranes, including biological boundaries such as the blood–brain barrier, and diffuse into any cell.

Potential benefits and threats of fat-soluble bilirubin

At low levels fat-soluble bilirubin is thought to act as a potent intracellular antioxidant and helps protect the fetus in moving from the lower oxygenation of the intrauterine environment to the oxygen-rich extrauterine environment. At extremely high levels, fat-soluble bilirubin is thought to be toxic to the brain, which is why the bilirubin is carried around the body buffered against this undesirable effect.

Bilirubin encephalopathy

When serum levels rise excessively, particularly in the first three days of life, it is thought that unconjugated bilirubin becomes toxic and acts like a generalized cellular poison. The blood–brain barrier is derived from the tightness of the junctions between the endothelial cells of cerebral blood vessels and in normal circumstances they do not leak fluid or electrolytes as other blood vessels may. It is thought that if the blood–brain barrier is disrupted, free unbound unconjugated bilirubin will flow into the brain tissues.

Coexisting risk factors such as anoxia, particularly hypercarbia, will increase cerebral blood flow and will open the blood–brain barrier. Preterm infants are more susceptible to this process as their systems and cells are less well developed. Clinical manifestations of bilirubin encephalopathy arise from the susceptibility to damage of the basal ganglia, brainstem, auditory (eighth cranial nerve) pathways and oculomotor nuclei (third cranial nerve) and are related to increased blood flow and metabolic activities in these areas.

Bilirubin encephalopathy is historically known as kernicterus, a term derived from the same root as 'kernel', referring to the way the basal ganglia sits as an island of grey matter in the white fibres of the cerebrum. Kernicterus is technically a pathologic diagnosis and when used in the clinical setting should be used to denote the chronic and permanent sequelae of bilirubin toxicity. Its use is therefore inappropriate for the neonatal period. Instead, the term *acute bilirubin encephalopathy* should be used.

The baby may present with a high-pitched cry, lethargy and hypotonia followed by hypertonia, rigidity (arching of the back called opisthotonus) and convulsions. Should the baby survive, it will be diagnosed with *chronic bilirubin encephalopathy* and may suffer athetosis, partial or complete deafness, limitations of upward gaze, dental dysplasia and intellectual deficits. The clinical problem is that there is no prescribed level of safety from bilirubin encephalopathy in healthy term newborns, but a threshold of serum bilirubin somewhere between 425 and 510 µmol/L is used as a yardstick for guidance.

From liver to blood

Once produced, bilirubin is transported from the reticulo-endothelial cells into the blood attached to serum albumin, which acts as a carrier plasma protein. Fat-soluble bilirubin and serum albumin have a special affinity or bond for each other and while attached to albumin, the fat-soluble bilirubin will not attach to other fat cells in the body. One mole of bilirubin will be carried by one mole of albumin. However, to be excreted from the body, the fat-soluble bilirubin needs to go through a process to make it water-soluble. The process is called conjugation and can only happen in specific liver cells called hepatocytes. Therefore the fat-soluble bilirubin, otherwise known as unconjugated bilirubin or indirect bilirubin, will be carried from the blood back to the liver and into the hepatocyte.

According to Blackburn (2007) the hepatocyte will only accept the bilirubin if bound to albumin. This is why the bilirubin cannot be transferred directly from the reticulo-endothelial system cells to the hepatocytes. The hepatocytes lining the liver sinusoids are able to extract the unconjugated bilirubin from the albumin and, by a process of carrier-mediated diffusion, the unconjugated bilirubin is transported to the hepatocyte which also has an affinity for it. In the hepatocyte, ligandin Y proteins and to a lesser extent Z proteins transport the bilrubin to a specific area called the smooth endoplasmic reticulum. Here the fat-soluble bilirubin is converted to a water-soluble compound in a process called conjugation (Lissauer and Fanaroff, 2006).

The conjugation process in the hepatocyte

There are two requirements for conjugation to take place. The hepatocyte needs to produce glucuronic acid, which is dependent upon a rich supply of oxygen and glucose. Blackburn (2007) argues that if these substances are not available or only in small amounts, the conjugation process will be correspondingly slowed down or even stopped. This fact illustrates that the liver is not working in isolation from other bodily systems which may be compromised. It is not uncommon for initial respiratory problems or cooling of the baby to adversely affect feeding and then glycaemic control. These coexisting problems may render the baby more susceptible to clinical jaundice.

The second requirement is an enzyme called hepatic uridine diphosphate glucuronyl transferase (UDPGT). This converts the unconjugated bilirubin into bilirubin diglucuronide, which is a water-soluble compound then called conjugated bilirubin or direct bilirubin. The bilirubin is then actively transported by carrier-mediated active transport out of the hepatocyte into the biliary canaliculi. The conjugated biliru-

bin becomes a component of bile and ready for excretion via stools and urine. This is a rate-limited process and oversaturation of the carriers will result in accumulation of conjugated bilirubin in the blood and can be measured as direct bilirubin if the blood is sampled (Blackburn, 2007).

UDPGT activity is minimal during the first 24 hours after birth but rises rapidly to reach adult levels by 14 weeks postnatal age. Activity is lower in preterm infants but is more related to postnatal age than gestational age. An increase in bilirubin levels in the newborn may help induce more UDPGT activity and conjugation processes in the liver after birth but hypoxaemia (low levels of oxygen in the blood) may reduce blood flow to the liver (in favour of brain, heart and lungs) and alter hepatocyte function.

Conjugated bilirubin is a golden colour, is mixed with bile and acted upon by bacteria to form stercobilinogen, some of which is reabsorbed into the plasma and excreted via the kidneys to form urobilinogen. The majority of the conjugated bilirubin continues to undergo bacterial degradation by colonic bacteria to become stercobilin. Hence conjugated bilirubin colours both the urine and the stools (Figure 9.1).

Entero-hepatic circulation

In the fetus the bowel and urinary systems are not functional for bilirubin excretion so conjugated bilirubin is converted back to unconjugated bilirubin by an enzyme called beta-glucuronidase which is found in the fetal small intestine, contained within the brushborder mucosa. The unconjugated bilirubin is absorbed across the intestinal wall into the portal circulation and is transported via the placenta into the mother's circulation to be excreted by the mother. This process is referred to as entero-hepatic circulation. In the newborn, the bowel is initially sterile and peristalsis is poor. The longer conjugated bilirubin remains in the small intestine, the greater the likelihood it will be converted back to unconjugated bilirubin via the entero-hepatic circulation.

Levene et al. (2008) assert that this also applies to bilirubin-laden meconium, thus babies with delayed passage of meconium (e.g. with meconium ileus, intestinal atresias or obstruction and Hirschsprung disease) are more likely to develop physiological jaundice. Babies who are fed within the first hour of birth and continue to feed regularly will tend to have earlier

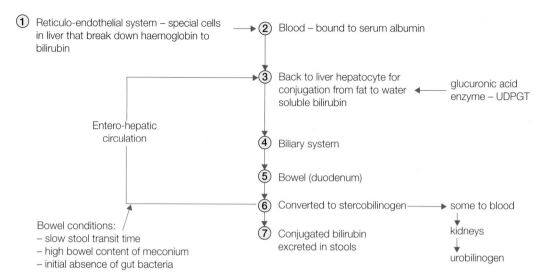

Figure 9.1   The metabolism of bilirubin

passage of meconium and have a lower incidence of physiological jaundice. Among breastfed babies, bilirubin levels tend to be lower in those who defecate more frequently. Formula-fed babies tend to excrete more bilirubin in their meconium during the first three days after birth because their stools are bulkier.

The importance of albumin binding

When there is a clinical sign of jaundice this indicates that there is too much unconjugated bilirubin for the available serum albumin. There is a limit to binding capacity and as soon as that is reached any surplus unconjugated bilirubin is left free in the blood plasma.

Factors affecting bilirubin–albumin binding

When the hydrogen ion levels in the extracellular fluid rise, the potential hydrogen (pH) level falls from normal values of 7.35 and the baby is described as being acidotic as a result of hypoxia (metabolic acidosis) and/or an accumulation of carbon dioxide (hypercapnoea) resulting in a respiratory acidosis. Free fatty acids are produced by the liver to provide energy for the body cells. These normally circulate attached to serum albumin. If free fatty acids reach a molar ratio with albumin in excess of 4:1 they will interfere with bilirubin binding. Levels of free fatty acids increase when the baby is hypoxic, hypoglycaemic, hypothermic and/or infected. In the same way, the affinity of bilirubin increases for the tissues so that fat tissues become very attractive to the bilirubin; thus tissues such as subcutaneous fat become more stained by the fat-soluble bilirubin. When these tissues become saturated, other fatty cells such as brain cells and myelinated nerves may stain too.

Albumin binding and the preterm baby

In the preterm baby the problem is an increased bilirubin load coupled with poor albumin production. Molecular concentrations of serum albumin must be greater than those of bilirubin for binding to occur. Also, in the immature baby albumin and bilirubin do not bind so effectively. There is an increased potential for the preterm baby to suffer the effects of hypoxia, acidosis, hypoglycaemia and sepsis and it may in addition be in receipt of medicines that can also compete for albumin-binding sites.

Jaundice – a clinical sign

At birth, the lungs oxygenate the blood from the first breath, at which point large quantities of red blood cells are surplus to requirements. Unconjugated bilirubin in normal circumstances will be below 80 μmol/L; however if the rate of haemolysis of red blood cells is greater than that at which the transport and excretion systems can process them, the levels will rise and jaundice will result. By definition, jaundice is a sign and is the yellow discoloration of the skin (as a result of staining of the underlying fat) and this staining can extend to the sclera (whites of the eyes).

Jaundice is detected by blanching the skin with finger pressure to observe the colour of the skin and subcutaneous tissues. It progresses in a cephalo-caudal direction (Levene *et al.*, 2008). The highest bilirubin levels are associated with jaundice seen below the knees and in the hands and soles. Visual inspection is not a reliable indicator of serum bilirubin levels but provides a good guide.

Physiological jaundice in the healthy term baby

Ives (2005) asserts that although the word physiological is helpful in an understanding of the common patterns of neonatal jaundice, it may convey the false impression of being something totally safe and benign. Levels of unconjugated bilirubin may be high enough to cause transient auditory derangement and, rarely, permanent neurological damage. When there is no identifiable disease process, the term 'exaggerated physiological jaundice' may be more appropriate. The midwife must be able to recognize when a disease/pathology is contributing to the baby's condition.

Johnston *et al.* (2003) argue that traditionally physiological jaundice appears on the second to third day, peaks by the fourth or fifth day and is resolved by the seventh to tenth day. Jaundice that is present within 24 hours of birth is not considered physiological, and when the total serum bilirubin is <250 µmol/L in the first 48 hours, <275 µmol/L by 72 hours and <300 µmol/L by 96 hours. This implies an exaggerated haemolysis process (Ives, 2005). Thus the timing of when the jaundice first appears is vital in assessing its possible aetiology but it is futile to attempt to assess whether the cause is physiological or pathological by serum bilirubin level ranges alone. The baby needs to be assessed holistically to include patterns of feeding and excretion.

Physiological jaundice in the healthy term breastfed baby

Given that exclusive breastfeeding should be the recognized physiological norm, midwives need to ques-tion what constitutes normality related to physiological jaundice if a mother chooses to exclusively breastfeed her baby. Laurence and Laurence (2003) assert that the term 'exclusively' means that the baby is only fed breast milk and has received no formula milk at all. Over the past 30 years or more, many of the notions associated with the patterns of physiological jaundice have been influenced by the frequent use of formula or mixed feeding. It appears that the exclusively breastfed baby is underrepresented in a population of breastfeeding women but in examining jaundice trends it is becoming more accepted that breastfed babies may have a serum bilirubin that peaks at the end of the first week and may not resolve until the end of the second week.

Ives (2005) argues that bilirubin levels can commonly reach 205 µmol/L and may reach 256 µmol/L. Up to one-third of babies remain clinically jaundiced beyond two weeks of age and these may need screening to exclude pathological causes because their pattern of jaundice is perceived as prolonged.

Breastfeeding jaundice and breast milk jaundice

These are two commonly recognized forms of jaundice.

Breastfeeding jaundice

Breastfeeding jaundice or the early onset form is often referred to as 'breastfeeding-associated jaundice' and is believed to be related to the actual process of feeding. Such babies have higher bilirubin levels after three days of life than formula-fed babies. The lower calorific intake and slower passage of meconium is sometimes referred to as 'lack of breast milk jaundice' or 'breast-non-feeding' jaundice. These descriptions reflect the underlying problem. The importance of a good calorie intake in the first few days of life to prevent or lessen the risk of jaundice is vital.

Babies who exclusively breastfeed and do not suffer significant weight loss are no more likely to develop jaundice than exclusively formula-fed babies. Babies who experience excessive weight loss who are breastfed and in addition receive formula supplementation are more likely to develop jaundice. It is thought that the prolonged form of jaundice in breastfed babies is enhanced by increased entero-hepatic shunting due to lower fluid and calorific intake, less frequent stooling patterns, increased levels of beta-glucuronidase and decreased formation of urobilins (Riordan, 2005).

Breastfeeding-associated jaundice is not thought to be caused by increased bilirubin production or abnormal hepatic uptake or conjugation of bilirubin, and given that human milk contains beta-glucuronidase perhaps breastfeeding physiology is aimed at maintaining a low but constant level of unconjugated bilirubin in the blood for its antioxidant effects. This may account for some of the health benefits conferred by exclusive breastfeeding. However, adequate calorie intake is considered essential and any significant decline results in physiological adaptations that lead to increased fat breakdown for energy and fatty acid production that increases intestinal fat absorption and may indirectly interfere with UDPGT and ligandin activity. When fatty acids reach the liver they may inhibit UDPGT activity or saturate the hepatic protein carrier system. The increased absorption of fat from breast milk may also increase intestinal bilirubin absorption.

It is known that breastfed babies produce lower weight individual stools, have a lower initial stool output and have stools that contain less bilirubin than formula-fed babies. Greater weight loss and less frequent stooling are associated with higher bilirubin production.

These babies also have slower urobilinogen formation, possibly due to different intestinal colonization patterns after birth. It is easy to think that large stools are desirable, but they are as a result of an incomplete digestive process that is not physiologically normal and caution should be exercised when comparisons are made with artificial, factory-made milk consumption.

Breast milk jaundice syndrome

Breast milk jaundice syndrome, or the later onset form, is less common and thought to be due to the milk itself. It is characterized by increasing bilirubin levels from day 4, peaking at 10–15 days, followed by a slow decrease in bilirubin levels over 3–12 weeks. These babies show good weight gain and do not have any signs of haemolysis or abnormal liver function. The cause is unknown but has been attributed to specific factors in breast milk that appear to be minimal in colostrum but appear in transitional and mature milk. However the presence of the steroid pregnane 3 alpha-20 beta-diol has been disproved.

Babies with breast milk jaundice syndrome are more likely to have increased entero-hepatic circulation and reports of encephalopathy in otherwise healthy breastfed term babies do exist, although other coexisting factors contributed to the outcome and the cases are extremely rare. Mothers with babies who have breast milk jaundice syndrome have a recurrence rate of 70 per cent in future pregnancies.

Once a diagnosis of breast milk jaundice is made, and this can only be done after medical assessment and investigation to rule out pathological jaundice, parents should be warned that resolution of jaundice in their breastfed baby may take up to 2–3 months. They should be advised to report to their GP if the nature of the jaundice changes, starts deepening instead of getting lighter, stool colour changes from yellow to pale or there is failure to thrive or the jaundice persists beyond three months.

Although interruption of breast milk feeds with formula feeds for 24 hours may be associated with a marked decline in the serum bilirubin levels, this practice is rarely justified. Supplementing breastfed babies with water, dextrose or formula is also strongly discouraged. It appears that once physiological adaptations have occurred to a specific type of milk, changing from, for example, breast to formula is disruptive to the overall physiological processes of the baby.

Although regarded as physiological jaundice the serum bilirubin may be high enough to warrant serial bilirubin measurement and treatment.

Pathological jaundice

When the cause of jaundice is thought to be as a result of a disease process, it is called pathological. To distinguish physiological from pathological jaundice the midwife needs to know and understand the more likely causes of pathological jaundice and categorize them according to age of onset.

When the baby is under 24 hours of age

In this timeframe jaundice as a result of haemolytic anaemia and congenital infection are more likely to be seen.

Haemolytic jaundice

This is jaundice that occurs within 24 hours of birth that is caused by increased red blood cell haemolysis or destruction secondary to antibodies to red blood cell antigens. The bilirubin is predominantly unconjugated and therefore potentially neurotoxic.

Rhesus disease

Maternal rhesus status and blood group should be sought. Babies of known rhesus-negative mothers are likely to have had cord or postnatal blood sent for a direct antiglobulin test (DAT). The most severe form of haemolytic disease is rhesus disease, which starts *in utero* when maternal rhesus-positive antibodies break down the red blood cells of the fetus. The progressive anaemia results in loss of colloid osmotic pressure in the circulatory system and tissue oedema results. This is called hydrops fetalis and the fetus may die of heart failure if not treated. At birth the combination of a falling red cell count and rising unconjugated levels of bilirubin put the baby at continued risk of heart failure and bilirubin encephalopathy.

ABO incompatibility

This occurs in 10–15 per cent of pregnancies but the proportion that result in significant haemolysis is small. When the mother's blood group type is O and the baby's blood type A or B, maternal IgG anti-haemolysins cross the placenta and cause red blood cell haemolysis in the baby.

The onset of haemolytic jaundice is within the first 24 hours. Haemolysis and destruction of red blood cells may progress during the first few weeks of life and need follow-up to monitor levels of anaemia. The finding of a positive DAT is not predictive of the severity of the jaundice. Assessment of cord blood for haemoglobin and bilirubin can help to identify babies who may benefit from early exchange transfusion. The Kell group of antibodies can cause severe haemolytic anaemia whereas Duffy, Kidd and more rare forms are usually less severe.

Haemolytic jaundice as a result of red blood cell defects

Glucose 6 phosphate dehydrogenase is an enzyme that normally protects the red blood cell and other cells from oxidative injury and haemolysis. Glucose 6 phosphase dehydrogenase deficiency (G6PD) is an X-linked recessive disorder that mostly affects males, although females get a less severe form. It affects over 100 million people worldwide and may cause severe neonatal jaundice in African Americans, Chinese and those with genetic variants from the Mediterranean or Middle or Far East parts of the world.

Parents of affected babies should be advised to avoid certain medications that could be passed through breast milk or if given directly to the baby (some antibiotics, aspirin and paracetamol) when the baby has an infection as these circumstances may trigger haemolysis. Contact with moth balls (naphthalene) can also trigger haemolysis.

Hereditary spherocytosis

This condition is uncommon but can cause jaundice in the first day of life. It is an autosomal dominant genetic disease that renders the red blood cell spherical in shape and not biconcave, which can result in severe haemolysis and jaundice that can occur suddenly as the immune system recognizes the abnormal cells. There is usually a strong positive family history. A blood test will show spherocytes.

Congenital infection

Drowsiness, reluctance to feed and vomiting should always raise the suspicion of infection. Bacterial septicaemia and urinary tract infections can cause early onset jaundice.

When the baby is 24 hours of age to two weeks old

Infections that interfere with liver function, namely transplacental infections such as toxoplasmosis (protozoa), rubella, cytomegalovirus, herpes simplex and the spirochete of syphilis (bacteria), can cause jaundice but the bilirubin tends to be of a conjugated form. Viral hepatitis (B and C), coxsackievirus, *E. coli*, group B haemolytic streptococcus, *Listeria monocytogenes*, tuberculosis and staphylococcus are all known to cause jaundice. There is always a need to consider urinary tract infection although it is an uncommon cause of jaundice. The jaundice is more likely due to a combination of factors that include reduced fluid intake, some haemolysis, impaired liver function and increased entero-hepatic circulation.

Prolonged jaundice when the baby is beyond two weeks old in a term baby and three weeks old in a preterm baby

Congenital hypothyroidism

Unrecognized hypothyroidism is rare, as the blood spot screening test performed at 5–7 days should detect a raised thyroid-stimulating hormone (TSH) level to indicate that the thyroid gland is not producing enough thyroxine, hence the anterior pituitary gland is producing TSH to stimulate it. Classical signs of untreated hypothyroidism are poor feeding, constipation, abdominal distension, umbilical hernia, mottled skin, protruding tongue, hypotonia, hypothermia and persistent jaundice. The jaundice is thought to be caused by delay in UDPGT synthesis and impairment of albumin production. Early recognition and treatment with thyroxine is vital to raise basal metabolic rate and prevent mental deterioration.

Galactosaemia

This rare autosomal recessive condition (1:60 000) is caused by a deficiency of an enzyme called galactose-1-phosphate uridyl transferase, which is needed for carbohydrate metabolism, converting galactose-1-phosphate to glucose-1-phosphate. In the absence of the enzyme galactose-1-phosphate accumulates in the blood and can cause severe illness in the first week of life with vomiting, cataracts, jaundice, coagulation disorders and eventually encephalopathy. The urine is tested for reducing substances. If the urine is positive on Clinitest tablet testing, but negative for glucose on a glucose oxidase stick test, then assay of glucose-1-phosphate uridyl transferase should be performed. The baby will be given galactose-free milk.

Neonatal hepatitis syndrome

According to Mupanemunda and Watkinson (2005) any baby with conjugated hyperbilirubinaemia has neonatal hepatitis syndrome. It is defined as a state in the newborn period where, as a result of decreased bile flow, there is accumulation of substances in the liver, blood and extrahepatic tissues that would normally be excreted in bile. Jaundice may result from obstruction to the flow of bile either within the liver (intrahepatic) or from blocked extrahepatic bile ducts. In both situations, the bilirubin is conjugated normally by the liver cells, but because it cannot pass through the bile ducts to the bowel, it is reabsorbed back into the blood, circulated to the kidneys and excreted, colouring the urine dark yellow/brown. The stools remain a pale, putty colour as little or no bile flows into the bowel. There is no risk of encephalopathy but this uncommon picture of a baby with persistent jaundice, conjugated hyperbilirubinaemia, failure to thrive, pale stools and dark urine is serious and needs specific investigations.

There are many different causative disease processes but it is important to differentiate biliary atresia as this condition requires surgery before the baby is 60 days old.

Causes of neonatal hepatitis syndrome

Neonatal hepatitis syndrome is a non-specific condition with a variety of causes:

- Infections include toxoplasmosis, rubella, cytomegalovirus, herpes simplex virus, cocksackie B virus, varicella and human immunodeficiency virus (HIV), all of which have usually been contracted in the first trimester of pregnancy.

- Metabolic causes include fructosaemia, tyrinosaemia, galactosaemia and cystic fibrosis. An autosomal recessive genetic disorder called alpha 1-antitrypsin deficiency affects only babies who are homozygous for the defect. When affected, only half of these recover, the other half develop cirrhosis and often die from liver failure.

- Genetic disorders include trisomies 13, 18 and 21.

- Structural causes include biliary atresia, gallstones and choledochal cyst.

In biliary atresia all or some of the extrahepatic biliary ducts are obliterated, leading to complete bilary obstruction. It is a rare condition (1:16 000 births) with an unknown aetiology, but an early and a late form are recognized. In the early form (20 per cent) biliary atresia is thought to be part of a syndrome and other abnormalities will be found (e.g. heart defects). In the late form the biliary system is normal but appears to undergo a progressive sclerosis with inflammation and scarring, which appears to progress in the first few weeks of life. Hepatomegaly is present. Jaundice can arise from birth or may be delayed until 2–3 weeks and progressively the baby has a yellow-greenish tinge. A hepato-biliary ultrasound scan helps to identify choledochal cysts, tumours, masses, an absent or small gall bladder. A liver biopsy and endoscopy exploration can confirm the diagnosis. The Kasai portoenterostomy is performed with an intra-operative cholangiogram where the damaged extrahepatic tissue is removed and a loop of jejunum is anastomosed to the hepatic hilum. Even with optimal therapy, many babies develop cirrhosis and require liver transplantation.

Clinical assessment of the jaundiced baby

Whether the baby has been born at home or transferred from hospital/birthing centre (or other) to home, the location may change but the care continues until the midwife considers the mother and baby fit for discharge (Nursing and Midwifery Council, 2008). Early transfer home after birth is becoming increasingly common and consequently many babies who stayed in hospital and had their clinical jaundice managed by the hospital multiprofessional team are now at home long before any signs of physiological jaundice are seen. In effect, the responsibility for recognizing early signs of clinical jaundice is shifting from hospital midwives to parents and primary care midwives. All midwives therefore need to educate their parents about the signs and significance of jaundice and for their part parents should know and understand what they need to do should their baby be affected.

Jaundice is often overlooked by parents who may not notice it at all, especially if the baby is assessed under artificial lights and in the winter (Sellwood and Huertas-Ceballos, 2008). Earlier and more frequent follow-up should be provided for babies who have risk factors and it is argued that the importance of assessing the baby for the development of jaundice is as important as the mother's health requirements and home visits should not be based solely upon routine schedules. In the early days, observing a feed and recording information on the baby's excretion patterns is a crucial part of the midwife's role.

Babies who are transferred home before 48 hours will need at least two follow-up visits by the midwife. It is a given that clinical judgement should be used in determining follow-up but it is suggested that if the baby is 24 hours old on transfer, the first visit should be within 72 hours. For the baby transferred between 24 and 48 hours the baby should not be more than 96 hours of age before being seen and if aged between 48 and 72 hours they should receive a first visit by 120 hours of age. The second visit will be determined by the findings of the first.

Preterm infants tend to develop physiological jaundice on the third day, with a peak level at seven days, fading by 14 days. This presentation is often overlooked and should be considered when planning care.

The hospital/primary care midwife should attempt to ascertain:

- the age of the baby when the jaundice first started to show;
- whether the bilirubin is more likely to be conjugated or unconjugated;
- whether there is any potential risk of neurological damage;
- whether the cause is physiological or pathological;
- what referral pathways/Trust guidelines are in place should this baby's care warrant them;
- what further action is needed.

Severe hyperbilirubinaemia is an emergency, immediate referral is mandatory and the initiation of phototherapy is of the upmost importance. Too often a factor is an avoidable delay in initiating appropriate treatment. A systematic approach needs to be used to examine all the presenting evidence.

First the midwife should look carefully at the history of the baby for risk factors:

- Is there a family history of jaundice, particularly haemolytic anaemia?
- A family history of liver disease may suggest galactosaemia or cystic fibrosis.
- Ethnic or geographical variations (e.g. East Asian, Greek, Japanese, Korean and American Indians) are more prone to jaundice and their skin pigmentation may make detection more difficult.
- A sibling with jaundice or anaemia may suggest blood group incompatibility. Was there breast milk jaundice with a need for phototherapy?
- Maternal history during pregnancy may suggest congenital viral or toxoplasmosis infection.
- The labour and birth history may indicate trauma with extravascular bleeding (e.g. a difficult forceps delivery and sub-aponeurotic bleeding). Did the baby need resuscitation at birth? Delayed cord clamping may be associated with neonatal polycythaemia and increased bilirubin load, especially in preterm babies and the recipient baby of twin-to-twin transfusion. Infants of diabetic mothers who are not macrosomic may develop polycythaemia.
- Vomiting may be due to sepsis, or inborn errors of metabolism (phenylketonuria, galactosaemia).
- Breastfeeding. Increased entero-hepatic circulation may be exacerbated by swallowed blood, small and large bowel obstruction, dehydration, poor calorie intake.

Next, listen to the mother. A general impression of the baby's behaviour can be ascertained from the mother by asking certain key questions:

- How is your baby today?
- How is your baby compared to yesterday?
- How is your baby feeding?
- How many feeds a day?
- How many wet/soiled nappies a day?
- Are the stools changing from yellow to pale?
- Is the jaundice deepening or getting lighter?

The general appearance and handling of the baby should indicate to the midwife whether this is a well baby. The degree of any colour changes and/or lethargy should be noted alongside any reports of decreased eagerness to feed. The midwife should listen attentively to the mother and document any concerns she may express. The midwife should see and include a description of the stools, whether they are yellow or pale. An overall impression of a more sleepy/unstable baby with a possibility of a rising serum bilirubin is always of significance and needs serum screening. The primary care midwife should at this point warn the parents that readmission to hospital may be called for with the acknowledgement that it is anxiety-provoking for them and if the care can continue in the home the midwife will make every effort to facilitate this outcome. However, the midwife needs to skilfully inform the parents of the risks of bilirubin encephalopathy.

Physical examination

Babies who are developing clinical jaundice should be examined physically by the midwife for the presence (or absence) of the following risk factors:

- gestational age – preterm babies are more vulnerable;
- small for gestational age – if asymmetrically grown, there could be polycythaemia; if growth is symmetrical, there may be signs of intrauterine infections;
- microcephaly and/or congenital cataracts – could be a sign of intrauterine infections;
- colour variations of the skin (e.g. plethora) – does the baby appear red, which may imply polycythaemia? Alternatively, if pale, is the baby peripherally shut down due to cooling or other metabolic changes (e.g. hypoglycaemia or sepsis)? Also, could the baby be anaemic due to haemolysis processes or extravascular blood loss?

- extravascular blood in the tissues (e.g. bruising where a ventouse cap has been used or a forcep blade has touched the skin). Purpura and/or petechiae may be seen on the face due to a tight cord around the neck (not to be confused with central cyanosis). After 48 hours a cephalhaematoma may start to be noticed on the scalp;
- enlarged liver known as hepatomegaly associated with liver disease, congenital infections or haemolytic anaemia;
- infection of the umbilicus (omphalitis) or skin? Sepsis is a consideration;
- neurological signs (e.g. hypertonia, opisthotonus (arching of the back), convulsions, abnormal eye movements). Hypotonia – the baby is more floppy than expected for gestational age;
- abdominal distension associated with bowel obstruction or hypothyroidism.

Screening blood tests that may be performed

The midwife will take blood from a heel puncture and ask for a serum bilirubin estimation which will provide a single-figure result. If further investigations are required and the baby is at home, the baby will usually have to be taken to a hospital so that blood can be taken by the paediatrician or advanced neonatal nurse practitioner and the results assessed. The following tests may be performed:

- total serum bilirubin to determine levels and whether the bilirubin is unconjugated (indirect) or conjugated(direct);
- direct antibody test (DAT or Coombs' test) to detect the presence of maternal antibodies on fetal red blood cells;
- indirect Coombs' test to detect the presence of maternal antibodies in serum;
- reticulocyte count (may be elevated if there is excessive haemolysis of red blood cells and new immature ones are being produced);
- ABO blood group and RH type for possible incompatibility;
- haemoglobin/haematocrit estimation to assess anaemia;
- white cell count to detect infection;
- serum sample for specific immunoglobulins for transplacental infection assays;

- glucose-6-phosphate dehydrogerase (G6PD) assay. Be aware that this result may be normal if the reticulocyte count is high. The test needs to be repeated to avoid missing the diagnosis;
- urine for reducing substances;
- blood film for spherocytes;
- check TSH result from blood spot screening for hypothyroidism;
- galactose-1-phosphate uridyl transferase assay for galactosaemia.

Treatment of hyperbilirubinaemia

If the jaundice is mild and the baby is well there is no need for any intervention. However if a more marked jaundice is present phototherapy should be considered if it is suspected that the level of unconjugated bilirubin may compromise the baby if it were to increase. Figure 9.2 shows indications of when to commence phototherapy in different categories of babies. Note the first four days are considered when the baby is more at risk of bilirubin encephalopathy.

Phototherapy

Phototherapy does not conjugate in the same way the hepatocyte does and how it works is not clearly understood, but one fact is clear: bilirubin is photolabile which means it absorbs and is changed by light.

Key points in providing phototherapy

- It is vital that any blood samples should be taken before the commencement of phototherapy and that further samples should not be taken from the baby with the lights on as this will result in bleaching of the blood in the collecting vessel and a lower but false result.

- Informed consent from the parents should be sought so that they understand the rationale for the therapy and can contribute to its efficacy.

- Jaundiced babies should not be separated from their mothers, so phototherapy should, whenever possible, be carried out by the mother's bedside in a draft-free room.

- It is not physiologically possible to give prophylactic phototherapy. Decomposition of bilirubin occurs in the skin and it has to be present to be acted upon.

- Bilirubin catabolism is most rapid at the beginning of each phototherapy period. It takes about 3 hours for the bilirubin to return to the skin after removal of the photo-isomers.

- The baby should be naked except for eye covers (when applicable).

- Once a baby has been exposed to phototherapy, the skin can no longer be used to assess jaundice levels. Serum bilirubin levels need to be monitored 24 hourly or more frequently if necessary.

- When there is a satisfactory decline in bilirubin levels, the baby should be removed from phototherapy as soon as possible.

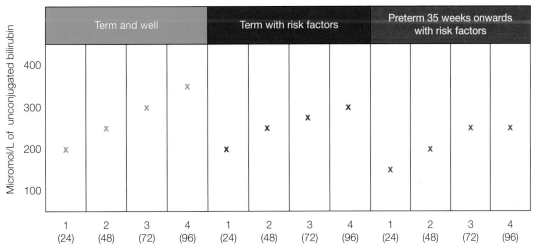

Age in days and hours for each category. The rate of increase in the bilirubin level, the gestational age, generated risk factors and general condition, determine how soon to start phototherapy

Figure 9.2   Indications for phototherapy in three categories of babies.

This means that light can be used to successfully treat mild to moderate hyperbilirubinaemia. Decomposition of unconjugated bilirubin when exposed to phototherapy occurs in the skin in the superficial capillaries and interstitial spaces. Three types of photochemical reactions occur: photo-isomerization, structural isomerization and photo-oxidation.

Photo-isomerization

This takes place in the extravascular spaces of the skin. It is thought that unconjugated bilirubin becomes transformed into a photo-isomer when light energy breaks down the hydrogen bonds around it, causing it to take in water. The substance that is left can then be excreted via bile and bowel without conjugation. However the excretion process is slow and the photo-isomer is readily converted back to unconjugated bilirubin and absorbed from the bowel back into the blood if the baby is not frequently producing stools. Photo-isomerization occurs at low-dose phototherapy in an intensity of 4–10 $\mu W/cm^2$ per nm. It offers no significant benefit from doubling the irradiance.

Structural isomerization

This is the intramolecular conversion of unconjugated bilirubin into lumirubin and is excreted via bile and urine without conjugation. It is an irreversible process and the lubirubin cannot be reabsorbed. The dose of phototherapy is 6–12 $\mu W/cm^2$ per nm and is considered an important pathway for reducing serum bilirubin levels.

Photo-oxidation

This is the slowest and least effective process which converts unconjugated bilirubin to small polar products that are excreted in urine.

Methods of providing phototherapy

Martin and Cloherty (2008) assert that only certain wavelengths are absorbed by bilirubin molecules. Light wavelengths in the blue–green ultraviolet spectrum (425–550 nm) are most effective. Special blue (narrow spectrum) bulbs are the most effective because they provide irradiance at 450 nm, which is the maximum blue wavelength absorbance. Green light favours formation of lumirubin and its longer waves penetrate further into the skin. Thus the use of blue–green light found in a recently introduced light source called a light-emitting diode (LED) device is

thought to be advantageous, especially as it also produces less ultraviolet light, infrared radiation and heat. This means the device can be placed a shorter distance from the baby to deliver high radiances, thus enhancing lumirubin formation.

Some find phototherapy light bank units with alternative blue (narrow spectrum) and daylight fluorescent lights to be effective and they do not make the baby appear centrally cyanosed. If an incubator is used there must be a 5–8 cm space between it and the unit to allow air flow and prevent overheating. The baby's temperature should be carefully monitored on a regular basis. Servo control can be used. The phototherapy unit gives off some heat, as do the photochemical reactions taking place in the skin.

Tungsten halogen or quartz halide spotlights provide white light with output in the blue spectrum, but cover a smaller surface area of the baby and are therefore not as effective in reducing bilirubin levels. They can be used, however, in combination with a fibreoptic blanket in which halogen light beams are transmitted through a cord of fibreoptic filaments to a woven fibreoptic pad. When placed beneath the baby and used in conjunction with overhead phototherapy, this is known as double phototherapy.

When the pad is wrapped around the baby and worn below clothing it is called a biliblanket. These pads remain at room temperature and deliver light within the 425–475 nm wavelength part of the blue–green spectrum. Although they are not thought to be as effective as overhead conventional phototherapy units, they have the advantages that the baby can be cared for in an almost normal way while treatment is given and the baby does not become overheated, although the skin may occasionally become reddened where the sheet is applied. There is also no glare to the eyes. The biliblanket can be used in the home for less severe forms of jaundice.

Side-effects of phototherapy

To give informed consent, parents need to know the side-effects of phototherapy but also the possible risks of not treating their baby. They need to be able to ask questions and this is why the midwife needs to be well informed and be able to provide adequate support and reassurance for them to assume their new role. Whether in the home or hospital, parents should be seen as active partners in care provision.

The baby should be monitored closely when in receipt of phototherapy, given the known side-effects:

Thermal and other metabolic changes may affect the production of glucuronic acid which will directly affect the conjugation process. If the baby is too hot there will be a raised metabolic rate with an increased body temperature and, as a result, increased oxygen consumption, increased respiratory rate and increased skin blood flow. These adaptations may lead to a mild respiratory distress and possible hypoglycaemia. A neutral thermal environment needs to be established whereby the baby is not too hot or cold. Cooling can result in oxygen and glucose consumption to raise metabolic rate. Check for excessive air flow in the room. A Perspex cover can be used over the cot if the room is not warm enough to support a naked baby. The baby's temperature needs to be recorded regularly and if too hot the midwife must check to see that the phototherapy unit is not too close to the baby (see the manufacturer's instructions). Regularly feeding the baby is essential to replace calories and protect against lethargy.

Insensible water loss (water lost through respiration, perspiration, stools, etc.) may be as much as 40 per cent in term babies and 80 per cent in preterm babies. Extra milk should be given to make up these deficits (20–30 mL/kg per day), but not water. The baby needs calories to maintain its metabolic rate and intake should be largely regulated by the baby's thirst.

Watery diarrhoea and increased faecal water loss can be caused by increased amounts of bile in the bowel stimulating gastrointestinal activity.

Temporary altered lactose tolerance can be caused by decreased lactase (enzyme) activity at the epithelial brush border.

Retinal damage has not been reported in humans but eye shields or patches should be closely monitored to ensure they cover the eyes without occluding the nose. The eyes should be checked for any signs of infection.

Skin changes include an erythematous rash (redness) which may occur with an increased release of histamine from the mast cells in the skin as a result of the ultraviolet light. Creams and lotions should not be used. Phototherapy is contraindicated in babies with conjugated hyperbilirubinaemia caused by liver disease or obstructive jaundice as it causes a bronzing of the skin due to deposition of a brown pigment (bilifuscin). This is reversible but takes many months to resolve.

It is beneficial to turn off the lights and remove eye shields (if appropriate) to enable the baby to be held by the mother for feeding and other carers as there are some psycho-behavioural concerns for the baby. It is argued that the baby may lack its usual sensory experiences in skin-to-skin contact such as touch, smell and sight. Lethargy, irritability and altered feeding behaviour can influence parental perceptions of their baby. The midwife should monitor the baby's neurobehavioural status, particularly responses to stress and interactions with the mother and other carers.

Conclusion

The midwife is well placed to support the family who will be providing much of the care for their jaundiced baby. Parents tend to perceive jaundice as an anxiety-provoking occurrence and rely upon a well-informed,

CASE HISTORY

Baby Jade was born at term but was bruised from a forcep delivery. She was being exclusively breastfed but by her third day she was jaundiced and becoming lethargic. She had fewer wet nappies and stools. The midwife checked her serum bilirubin level and the result (280 μmol/L) indicated that she needed phototherapy (see Figure 9.2). The midwife helped Mary to wake Jade with skin-to-skin contact and stayed with Mary throughout the feed to ensure enough milk had been taken. The following day Jade became very sleepy and was not feeding from the breast. Mary expressed her breast milk and attempted to give it via a cup. This also proved to be difficult and eventually a nasogastric tube was passed and remained in situ to ensure each feed was completed. By day 6 the serum bilirubin had fallen to 160 μmol/L and the phototherapy was discontinued. Jade was feeding well at the breast and thriving. Her facial bruising had diminished. The following day, Mary and Jade were transferred home to the care of the midwife.

continued ➤

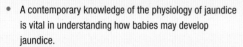

CASE HISTORY *continued*

- The facial bruising put Jade into an at-risk category for a term baby hence the serum bilirubin at 280 µmol/L on her third day was justification for phototherapy.

- An adequate feeding pattern is essential in the management of physiological jaundice.

- Parents need to be prepared for their baby to receive a few days of phototherapy and to stay in hospital a little longer than they hoped.

Key Points

- A contemporary knowledge of the physiology of jaundice is vital in understanding how babies may develop jaundice.

- Physiological jaundice in the healthy term exclusively breastfed baby may last for a longer period compared to traditional patterns of onset, peak and fade times seen in babies that have received formula feeds.

- Early transfer home has placed a greater responsibility onto the primary care midwife to support parents in recognising and managing physiological jaundice.

- Differentiating between physiological and pathological jaundice is at the heart of effective management of neonatal jaundice.

- Phototherapy is a reliable method of reducing serum bilirubin levels, but its use does have recognisable side effects.

- The threat of bilirubin encephalopathy means that in the presence of significant clinical jaundice, an expedient response from the midwife and the multiprofessional team is essential.

- The midwife's support of the parents helps to reduce the considerable anxiety that can surround this area of neonatal care.

confident midwife to guide them through the decision-making process and phototherapy if needed. The trend for early transfer from hospital to the community is set to continue so detection of jaundice and the decision when to refer to the multiprofessional team is a vital component of the hospital midwife's role. For those midwives who work in primary care, extra surveillance, support and education are essential elements of care. Decisions on whether the baby is well enough to stay at home or be readmitted to hospital will ultimately fall to the midwife who will require contemporary knowledge of the physiological and pathological causes of jaundice. Feeding and excretion patterns in the exclusively breastfed baby need close supervision coupled with a view that if jaundice does occur, its pattern of onset, peak level and fade time may be later than many traditional models that are influenced by formula feeding physiology.

References

Blackburn ST (2007) *Maternal Fetal and Neonatal Physiology. A clinical perspective.* Washington: Saunders Elsevier.

Ives NK (2005) Gastroenterology. In: Rennie JM (ed.) *Neonatology.* London: Elsevier.

Johnston P, Flood K and Spinks K (2003) *The Newborn Child.* London. Churchill Livingstone.

Laurence RA and Laurence RM (2003) *Breastfeeding. A Guide for the medical profession.* London: Mosby.

Levene MI, Tudehope DI and Sinha SK (2008) *Essential Neonatal Medicine*, 4th edn. London: Blackwell Publishing.

Lissauer T and Fanaroff AA (2006) *Neonatology at a Glance.* London. Blackwell Publishers.

Martin CM and Cloherty JP (2008) Neonatal hyperbilirubinaemia. In: Cloherty JP, Eichenwald EC and Stark AR (eds) *Manual of Neonatal Care*, 6th edn. London: Lippincott Williams & Wilkins.

Mupanemunda R and Watkinson M (2005) *Key Topics in Neonatology.* London: Taylor and Francis.

Nursing and Midwifery Council (2008) *The Code – Standards of conduct, performance and ethics for nurses and midwives.* London: NMC.

Riordan J (2005) *Breastfeeding and Human Lactation.* Boston: Jones and Bartlett.

Sellwood M and Huertas-Ceballos A (2008) Review of NICE guidelines on routine postnatal infant care. *Archives of Diseases in Children. Fetal Neonatal Edition* **93**: F10–F13.

CHAPTER 10

INFECTION IN THE NEWBORN PERIOD

Lynne Paterson

OVERVIEW

The first month of the neonate's life is a wonderful time for new parents but can be a truly hazardous time for newborns themselves. It is the most dangerous period in their lives since they are more susceptible to infection within the first four weeks than at any other time. The aim of this chapter is to identify why this is the case, outline how this may manifest itself and highlight to midwives how this may be reduced. Management strategies will also be included.

What protection does the newborn have against infection?

Even before it is born, the fetus has some protection from infection afforded by the placenta and surrounding membranes. Few bacteria can penetrate this defence but viruses are able to cross freely and can be particularly vicious to the developing fetus, causing, in some instances, congenital abnormalities.

Some protection from infection in the form of immunoglobulins is passed through the placenta to the developing fetus during pregnancy and from as early as 14 weeks, providing what is called 'passive immunity' (Cant and Gennery, 2005). This passing over of immunoglobulins from mother to baby allows the baby to utilize these immediately after it is born. However, in infants born prematurely before this is complete, their protection from infection is significantly reduced.

Immunoglobulin G (IgG) is the only immunoglobulin that can pass through the placenta during this time. The protection it affords only has a half-life of around 3–6 months and it can only provide immunity to those conditions that the mother has previously been exposed to or vaccinated against. Babies therefore have to develop their own immunity within the first few weeks and months of birth.

Developing fetuses are able to produce B and T lymphocyte cells, which play a role in cell-mediated immunity and in the development of antibodies against antigens. They also have phagocytes and macrophages, which engulf and digest debris, pathogens and bacteria, as well as complement available. Complement is a group of around 20 proteins which, in the presence of infection, is responsible for a biochemical sequence of events in which several processes are coordinated together and the infection is attacked. This cascade includes the release of histamine to cause inflammation and attract phagocytes to a specific area of infection.

Following birth, infants begin to produce their own antibodies and can mobilize immunoglobulin M (IgM) as well as IgG, with immunoglobulin A (IgA) rising very slowly. By two months of age, they are able to produce a good IgG antibody response to protein vaccines. This coincides with the commencement of the routine childhood immunization programme.

Despite these factors, the infant at birth is considered immunologically immature and has the potential to develop an infection given the right set of circumstances (Boxwell, 2000; Cant and Gennery, 2005). It is essential for any carer to know how to prevent infection as well as what to look for postnatally.

The limited immunity that babies do have can be improved if the mother chooses to breastfeed. Breastmilk contains IgA, which acts on the gut, as well as lactoferrin, lysozyme, neutrophils, macrophages and the bifidus factor. Although it is not fully understood how this works, breastmilk appears to have the ability to promote prevention of infection by increasing the infants' capacity to mount a response as well as reducing their incidence of respiratory tract infections, diarrhoea and otitis media (Fewtrell and Lucas, 2005).

When used in preterm babies in the establishment of early nutrition it is thought that breastmilk may be responsible for reducing the incidence of necrotizing enterocolitis by as many as 500 cases a year in the UK, thus reducing a major cause of mortality in the neonatal intensive care unit (Fewtrell and Lucas, 2005).

When born at term, babies are further protected from infection by intact skin and mucous membranes. These act as barriers which prevent bacteria from gaining entry. The protective effect is enhanced by cilia and secretions that are present within the respiratory tract, tears, urine and the acid present in the stomach (Boxwell, 2000; Cant and Gennery, 2005). Each has their own part to play in the prevention of infection. There are, however, some predisposing factors that will result in alterations to this protection and these are listed in Table 10.1.

When can an infection occur?

There are two distinct times in the newborn period when sepsis is more likely. These are described as early onset and late onset infection:

- Early onset infection is defined as that which results in symptoms at birth or within the first 48 hours following birth (Davies *et al.*, 2001). This may have occurred *in utero* due to organisms from the mother so that the baby is born with a congenital infection that may be severe if not immediately treated. Most cases of early onset infection are caused by group B streptococcus (GBS) and infants present with symptoms either immediately or within the first few hours (Dear, 2005).

- Late onset infection is defined as those infections that arise after the initial 48-hour period (Davies *et al.*, 2001). Again, it is possible that these organisms originated from the mother but it is more likely that they came from the environment. The most commonly responsible organism is coagulase negative staphylococci (CONS) (Dear, 2005).

Table 10.1   Factors that affect the risk of infection in the newborn

Before birth	Preterm rupture of the membranes
	Prolonged rupture of the membranes
	Premature labour
	Any sepsis in the mother
	Maternal colonization with group B *Streptococcus* (GBS)
	Previous child affected with GBS
	Chorioamnionitis
	Substance abuse in the mother
	Maternal temperature of >38°C
After birth	Immaturity of the immune system especially if born prematurely
	Loss of intact skin from forcep blade cuts, fetal scalp electrodes and other invasive instruments
	The postnatal ward environment
	Exposure to staff and visitors
	Invasive therapies associated with neonatal intensive care such as line insertion
	Use of broad-spectrum antibiotics
	Any condition affecting the immune system (such as DiGeorge syndrome)

How does an infant become infected?

A newborn can become infected in three main ways: while the fetus is still *in utero* by the transplacental route, during the intrapartum phase via the ascending route or during the postpartum period.

The transplacental route

Several viruses, including rubella, cytomegalovirus, varicella and HIV, are known to cross the placenta relatively easily to infect the developing fetus. This is known as transplacental or vertical transmission. Some of these viruses, namely rubella, cytomegalovirus and varicella, if contracted during early pregnancy may cause severe congenital malformations, including cardiac abnormalities, growth restriction, deafness, eye abnormalities and learning disability.

Toxoplasmosis, a parasitic protozoa usually carried by cats, may also transfer to the fetus using this route and cause similar problems.

Listeria is one of the few bacteria that can cross the placenta. *Listeria monocytogenes* is a bacterium found in soil and water that contaminates fruit and vegetables. It occasionally leads to outbreaks of the disease listeriosis. Two well-publicized examples of this were traced back to coleslaw and maple syrup. *Listeria* is able to penetrate the placental barrier and cross to the growing fetus, which can cause stillbirth or lead to an infection in the fetus. Listeriosis presents as sepsis, pneumonia or meningitis and can be fatal, although the mother may be unaware that she had ever been infected. Infants are treated with intravenous ampicillin and gentamicin.

The ascending and intrapartum route

Ascending infections can occasionally occur before the membranes rupture but this is not common (Dear, 2005). It is more likely that organisms found in the vagina advance towards the fetus once the membranes rupture. Those infants whose membranes have ruptured for 18 hours or more are especially at risk. Once labour starts and the intrapartum phase has begun, the infant is pushed along the birth canal and can become colonized during this active process.

The postpartum route

Once the baby has been born there is risk of contamination via several sources, including not only the mother but also the health personnel and the surroundings. Good handwashing practice is essential to prevent hospital-acquired or nosocomial infection, with overcrowding and sharing of equipment being avoided.

There are also many areas of the neonate that are more easily infiltrated by organisms than others, including the eyes, the fingernails, the umbilicus and any areas of the skin that have been breached, perhaps by fetal scalp electrodes or forcep blades. The umbilical stump, the perineum and the axillae are the areas that become most heavily colonized with organisms within the first few days of life with as many as 65 per cent of infants being colonized with *Staphylococcus aureus* (Dear, 2005). Most term infants will manage to deal with this colonization, however there will be some who develop signs and symptoms of either superficial skin infection or indeed bacteraemia.

Differences in preterm versus term infants

When born early, infants have less immunoglobulin protection because it has not had enough time to pass from the mother. They also have a poor neutrophil and complement response, macrophage ability is not good and the function of their T cells is also impaired. In all, their ability to mount a response to infection is very poor. On top of this, they are admitted to a neonatal intensive care unit where their fragile and thin skin is breached by the insertion of lines and their respiratory system is invaded by the use of ventilators and plastic endotracheal tubes. Lastly, they will also be attended to by many different caregivers, and sadly it is a well-established fact that the longer infants stay in hospital, the more likely they are to develop a hospital-acquired infection.

Signs and symptoms of infection

Infants differ from adults in the signs and symptoms that they present with during an infection. This of course will depend on the type and site of the infection with minor, superficial infections causing fewer problems than bacteraemia.

Initially in the newborn period, the baby may present with subtle signs suggesting that an infection is present. The midwife needs to be alert to these during daily examinations and when the mother complains of any changes in behaviour. Typically, babies who have fed well will suddenly go off their feeds or be disinterested in feeding. They may also have changes in temperature, though these can go undetected. It is generally prudent to take note of the mother who tells you that her baby just 'does not seem right'. Table 10.2 outlines the signs and symptoms that may affect the systems of an infant to which the midwife should be alert.

Table 10.2   Symptoms and signs of infection

System	Symptom/sign
Neurological system	Irritability (may be due to infection or/and pain of the infection)
	Listlessness/lethargy
	Sucks poorly
	Unresponsive
	High-pitched cry
	Jitteriness
	Full or bulging fontanelle
	Hypotonic/hypertonic
	Seizure activity
	Temperature change (up or down)
Cardiovascular system	Tachycardia
	Pale
	Mottled
	Poor cutaneous circulation giving a delayed capillary refill time
Respiratory system	Tachypnoea
	Apnoea
	Recession
	Grunting
Gastrointestinal system	Not interested in feeding
	Vomiting
	Diarrhoea
	Abdominal distension
	Poor weight gain
Hepatic system	Jaundice
	Altered coagulation
Skin	Petechia
	Septic spots
	Heat and redness in an infected area

A high index of suspicion

Since infection can be completely overwhelming in a neonate, the midwife must have a low threshold for intervention. When it is suspected, a full history should be taken from the mother, involving not only the notes but also asking questions around any problems that she had during her pregnancy, including any flu-like symptoms, fevers or rashes. A complete physical examination should be performed on the infant, which involves looking at the naked child in order that every inch of the skin can be observed as well as identifying any other signs and symptoms of sepsis. Typically tachypnoea can be one of the first signs, thus once the chest is exposed, the respirations should be counted for a full minute to establish a true respiratory rate (which is normally less than 60 per minute). Finally, appropriate investigations should be taken such as swabs of infected sites or blood sugars to rule out hypoglycaemia in order that a definitive diagnosis can be made.

In any case of suspected sepsis, the midwife should know who to contact when onward referral is required. This advice should also be sought early and urgently so that the infant can get the appropriate treatment in a timely fashion. It is then likely that once the neonatal team are involved blood cultures as well as other inflammatory markers will be included as part of the overall investigation.

Common newborn infections seen by the midwife

Group B streptococcal infection

Group B streptococcus (GBS) is the scourge of maternity units everywhere since it is the principal cause of early onset neonatal sepsis. The reason that this is an important infection to prevent is because it poses a particular problem to the neonate and can be fatal yet its effects can be preventable. GBS may colonize the genital tract of as many as 15 per cent of pregnant women; 1 per cent of babies born to these women will subsequently develop early onset sepsis (Davies et al., 2001). Research studies are scarce in the UK but infection rates are described as around 0.60–0.86/1000 births (Davies et al., 2001).

Infants can develop bacteraemia, pneumonia or meningitis with a GBS infection, the latter often leaving them with long-term physical problems such as blindness, deafness and learning disability.

GBS is most commonly passed from mother to baby since it may already live harmlessly in the mother's vagina. The risk for transmission of this infection is increased when the membranes have been ruptured for 18 hours or more, so this is considered to be an antenatal risk factor (Royal College of Obstetricians and Gynaecologists, 2003). Thus, the baby may become infected even before labour begins.

Current evidence as well as professional guidance support providing intrapartum antibiotics for any mothers who are colonized during pregnancy, as well as those who have had a previous child with GBS disease (Smaill, 1996; Royal College of Obstetricians and Gynaecologists, 2003). This has been shown to be 80 per cent effective at preventing early onset infections in the neonate. Antibiotics are therefore required during labour and administration is essential at least 2 hours before the baby is delivered in order that protection has been passed over from mother to infant (Royal College of Obstetricians and Gynaecologists, 2003).

Other risk factors include the development of pyrexia in labour, generally considered to be around 38°C or higher, and a known urinary tract infection caused by GBS in the mother.

Preterm labour is also known to be caused in some instances by GBS.

Infants typically present within the first 48 hours with respiratory symptoms, though the vast majority, 90 per cent, will present in the first 12 hours. Symptoms may include grunting, recession and tachypnoea, and as the disease progresses the infant may also exhibit some of those symptoms seen in Table 10.2. These infants should be referred to a member of the neonatal team in order that that they can be investigated and treated and some will end up being admitted to a neonatal unit or special care baby unit during this time. They may even require ventilatory assistance, depending on how severe the presentation is. Blood cultures will be taken and in some cases, a lumbar puncture may be indicated. Prophylactic antibiotics will be commenced intravenously until the exact causative agent is known. Since GBS is such a harmful bacteria to the neonate all will be treated prophylactically for GBS until this is proven otherwise. The first-line drugs of choice for the treatment of GBS are generally penicillin and gentamicin given intravenously.

GBS can also be the causative agent in late presenting sepsis, though the mechanism for this is less clearly understood.

Conjunctivitis

The conjunctiva covers the eye and lines the eyelids. It is common for the infant to present with inflammation of this lining in the first 24–48 hours of life, presenting as conjunctivitis. Many babies will initially have eyes that appear watery or sticky and these will generally settle with regular cleansing using saline drops. Some infants may have a simple blocked nasolacrimal duct, which is not infected. If the exudate persists, however, if the discharge becomes purulent and profuse or if there is redness of the sclera, the likelihood is that the eye is infected and therefore medical opinion should be sought. The prospect of an infection in the eyes needs to be identified quickly as the more severe causative bacteria may lead to permanent damage or other disease if left untreated. The eyes should be swabbed and a scraping taken for chlamydia.

The infection can be caused by a common infection, such as *Staphylococcus aureus*, or it may be caused by a sexually transmitted infection such as gonorrhoea, chlamydia or syphilis.

The Health Protection Agency (HPA) monitors all new sexually transmitted infections. Their results from 1998 to 2007 demonstrate that the overall incidence is increasing in the UK among the younger population (Health Protection Agency, 2007). This has also resulted in an increase in the number of cases of both gonococcal ophthalmia neonatorum and chlamydial ophthalmia neonatorum.

Gonococcal ophthalmia generally presents in the first 24 hours of birth whereas chlamydial ophthalmia usually presents a bit later after five days (Dear, 2005). Both infections are notifiable to the HPA. Gonococcal infection caused by *Neisseria gonorrhoeae* generally presents with bilateral profusely discharging eyes, which fill up quickly when cleansed. Marked oedema of the eyelids may also be seen and this disease can go on to cause permanent scarring of the cornea. While swab cultures are awaited, the infant is usually treated prophylactically with penicillin both intravenously and by instilling eye drops.

Chlamydial conjunctivitis caused by *Chlamydia trachomatis* does not cause permanent damage to the eye but left untreated may lead to a chlamydial pneumonia later in the infant's life. This disease manifests in a similar fashion to gonococcal ophthalmia but may present in one eye initially and can spread to both relatively quickly. They may not respond to typical antibiotic treatment and once the causative organism is known, they are generally treated with a two-week course of erythromycin.

The parents in these scenarios will also need further follow-up and treatment.

While eye infections with syphilis are relatively few, the disease is currently on the increase in the UK and as such, this should also be considered as a causative agent.

Staphylococcus aureus skin infection

Staphylococcal aureus can grow very well on newborn skin and can lead to superficial skin infections. This presents typically as spots or vesicles filled with a yellow fluid found commonly on the neck, the groin or the underarms. The infant remains well and if they are few in number and dry by themselves, they may not require treatment. If they continue to increase or surround the umbilical cord, where there is a direct portal of entry to the bloodstream, then swabs should be taken and treatment with either oral or intravenous flucloxacillin will be indicated.

True omphalitis or umbilical cord infections are most commonly caused by *Staphylococcus aureus* and present with redness around the site or peri-umbilical erythema; this can be further complicated by cellulitis and requires urgent intravenous treatment with flucloxacillin to prevent a bacteraemia.

Infection of the nail beds or paronychia is also generally caused by *Staphylococcus aureus*, though *Candida* can also be the causative agent.

Thrush

Candidiasis or thrush is seen fairly commonly in newborn infants. This is a fungal infection caused by the yeast *Candida albicans*. *Candida* lives in the body with few problems in the normal population and works within the gastrointestinal tract. It can, however, cause problems when its balance is affected, as seen in the presence of antibiotics, it subsequently proliferates and leads to an opportunistic infection. It is commonly seen in newborn infants within the first few weeks of life and this may have come from the mother. The baby can either become infected as it is born through the birth canal or it can acquire it from the infected nipples of the mother during breastfeeding.

Thrush presents in infants as either a nappy rash or a coated mouth or both. The tongue and gums in the mouth become coated in a white, creamy substance often described as looking like cottage cheese. These plaques cannot be removed easily and they occasionally bleed. The buttocks and perineum of an infected infant may also have a rash with a marked appearance. There is generalized redness with occasional white scaling of the skin and also raised, wet lesions that may bleed sporadically. There is also the presence of small and large lesions side by side, or satellite lesions.

Infants may be distressed with this infection and may not feed easily. Treatment includes the use of both topical and oral antifungal preparations such as nystatin and fluconazole (Diflucan). When mothers are also infected, treatment must be given to both otherwise there will be an on-going infection which is continually passed from one to the other. There is no need to stop breastfeeding during this time provided that both parties are being treated, unless the mother is experiencing marked discomfort and cannot continue.

If the baby is being bottle-fed, the midwife must ensure that the mother is aware of the importance of washing and effectively sterilizing all of the equipment being used, as a poor technique may lead to thrush infections.

Thrush is also commonly seen among the population of infants being nursed on a neonatal intensive care unit where broad-spectrum antibiotics as well as steroids may be used frequently.

More complex infections

Meningitis

Neonatal meningitis is the condition that perhaps causes the most anxiety among caregivers – parents and professionals alike – because when it strikes the effects can be devastating, causing death or permanent disability.

Meningitis is the inflammation of the membranes or meninges surrounding the brain and spinal cord and usually occurs as part of an existing bacteraemia. It can be caused by a number of infective agents, most commonly GBS (especially early onset), *Escherichia coli* and *Listeria monocytogenes*. The current incidence in England and Wales is thought to be around 0.39 per cent per 1000 births and it is more commonly seen among the preterm population. The infant may present with early as well as late onset infection causing meningitis and because the signs and symptoms can initially be non-specific, as for any other infection (see Table 10.2), its seriousness may not be immediately detected. Once infants develop a high-pitched cry, seizures and a bulging fontanelle, they may already have permanent neurological disability (Dear, 2005).

Death from neonatal meningitis has reduced over the years (Heath *et al.*, 2003; Dear, 2005) though the morbidity remains high, with as many as 30–50 per cent of infants requiring long-term follow-up for cerebral palsy, hearing loss, seizures and blindness (Heath *et al.*, 2003; Dear, 2005). It is therefore important to identify the signs of meningitis as early as possible in order that treatment can be commenced.

Herpes

Neonatal herpes infection is not very common but the results can be devastating if left undetected. Infants most commonly become infected with the herpes simplex virus during birth as vaginal secretions from active lesions in the mother contaminate them. If these are identified prior to delivery a caesarean section may be undertaken to prevent contamination and thus reduce the likelihood of neonatal infection.

Signs and symptoms may be as for any sepsis, with the baby exhibiting some of the signs listed in Table 10.2. They may also develop herpetic lesions, though these may not be identified initially since they can be mistaken for trauma or blistering as a result of instrumental deliveries in association with ventouse chignons and fetal scalp electrode marks. Babies may also develop lesions around the eyes and the mouth. They can also have a central nervous system invasion and infants with this type of herpes infection tend to present with worsening symptoms including seizure activity. These carry the highest mortality and morbidity rates.

Acyclovir is generally the drug of choice to treat both mother and infant.

Human immunodeficiency virus (HIV)

There is still much that is unclear about the transmission of the HIV virus from mother to infant. It is thought that there may be both transplacental transmission as well as intrapartum infection. What is known is that the rate of neonatal infection is markedly reduced with the use of antiretroviral treatment during pregnancy as well as the treatment of the baby with antiretroviral therapy for at least the first four weeks following delivery. Zidovudine is usually given together with the same or similar drugs that the mother has received in the antenatal period; thus the therapy is individualized with the neonatal team working in consultation with the infectious diseases team.

Babies born to mothers who have not disclosed their status or who have not been tested may initially present with no signs or symptoms, making them difficult to identify.

Currently breastfeeding is not recommended in the UK for HIV-positive mothers.

Prevention of infection

While it is true that infection can be acquired congenitally, there are some things that can be done to reduce or prevent the spread of infection to the newborn. The national practice of providing intrapartum antibiotics to mothers who are known to either have a current GBS infection or whose last child was born with a GBS infection is one such practice (Smaill, 1996; Royal College of Obstetricians and Gynaecologists, 2003). This is standard in UK maternity units.

The families of new babies need to observe good practices while they are in contact with healthcare professionals as they are more likely to learn and follow by example. This involves good hand hygiene, especially following nappy care and prior to feeding the baby, being careful around the infant when they have infections themselves, such as colds and flu, and being extra careful about kissing the baby directly when they have weeping cold sores or herpes simplex near the mouth.

Nurses and midwives are in a good position to be able to help parents with direct care and to provide good, clear and consistent information. Issues such as the sterilizing of equipment to be used for the baby as well as advocating and supporting breastfeeding should be within the realm of those caring for the new parents. Professional healthcare staff should also ensure that they provide individualized equipment for each mother and baby and make sure that other

Table 10.3   Current immunization schedule advocated by the UK Department of Health

What diseases are protected against	
Routine scheduled immunizations	
2 months of age	Diphtheria, tetanus, pertussis, polio, *Haemophilus influenzae* type B, pneumococcal infection
3 months of age	Diphtheria, tetanus, pertussis, polio, *Haemophilus influenzae* type B, meningitis C
4 months of age	Diphtheria, tetanus, pertussis, polio, *Haemophilus influenzae* type B, pneumococcal infection, meningitis C
Around 12 months of age	*Haemophilus influenzae* type B, meningitis C
Around 13 months of age	Measles, mumps, rubella, pneumococcal infection
3 years 4 months to 5 years	Diphtheria, tetanus, pertussis, polio, measles, mumps, rubella
13–18 years old	Tetanus, diphtheria, polio
Non-routine immunizations that may also be offered depending on risk factors	
At birth	Tuberculosis (BCG injection)
At birth	Hepatitis B

infected patients are isolated, especially those with chicken pox (varicella zoster) or methicillin-resistant *Staphylococcus aureus* (MRSA) in order to further reduce the likelihood of cross-infection.

Information and advice should not be restricted to within the newborn period. Immunizations are a long-term method of protecting the child against infections. The current schedule advocated by the Department of Health is listed in Table 10.3 and this should also form part of the information given to parents during parentcraft teaching.

Conclusion

Infections in the newborn vary from superficial to life threatening and can have a quick onset or indeed may be insidious in nature. The signs and symptoms are also vague and often difficult to detect. The midwife caring for babies must be vigilant and act swiftly in the detection and investigation of infections having a low threshold for intervention and an inquisitive attitude towards mothers who feel that their child's behaviour has altered. A full maternal history is required as well as a comprehensive assessment of the child in order to ensure that any infections are acknowledged and dealt with quickly and effectively. All measures for the prevention of nosocomial infection should also be in place.

Key Points

- Babies have some protection from infection when they are born but this is limited.
- Preterm infants are more at risk of infection than those born at term.
- Infection can be acquired from the mother or can be acquired after birth from the environment.
- Group B streptococcal disease is particularly hazardous to newborn infants and this is preventable when targeting prophylactic maternal antibiotics during labour.
- The main portals of entry for infection include the umbilical stump, the fingernails, the eyes and the skin where its integrity has been breached.
- Signs of infection may be subtle, so midwives should have a low threshold of suspicion.

References

Boxwell G (2000) Neonatal infection. In: *Neonatal Intensive Care Nursing*. London: Routledge, pp. 259–284.

Cant AJ and Gennery AR (2005) Neonatal infection. In: Rennie JM (ed.) *Roberton's Textbook of Neonatology*, 4th edn. Philadelphia: Elsevier Churchill Livingstone.

Davies EG, Elliman DAC, Hart CA *et al.* (2001) *Manual of Childhood Infections*, 2nd edn. London: WB Saunders.

Dear P (2005) Neonatal infection: infection in the newborn. In: Rennie JM (ed.) *Roberton's Textbook of Neonatology*, 4th edn. Philadelphia: Elsevier Churchill Livingstone.

Fewtrell M and Lucas A (2005) Feeding the full term baby. In: Rennie JM (ed.) *Roberton's Textbook of Neonatology*, 4th edn. Philadelphia: Elsevier Churchill Livingstone.

Health Protection Agency (2007) All new STI episodes seen at GUM clinics in the UK 1998–2007. London. Health Protection Agency. http://www.hpa.org.uk

Heath PT, Nik Yusoff NK and Baker CJ (2002) Neonatal meningitis. *Archive of Disease in Childhood, Fetal and Neonatal Edition* **88**: F173–F178.

Royal College of Obstetricians and Gynaecologists (2003) *Prevention of Early Onset Neonatal Group B Streptococcal Disease*. Guideline number 36. London: RCOG.

Smaill FM (1996) Intrapartum antibiotics for Group B streptococcal colonisation. *Cochrane Database of Systematic Reviews* (**1**): CD000115. DOI: 10.1002/14651858.CD000115.

Further reading

Marieb EN (2006) The lymphatic system and body defences. In: *Essentials of Human Anatomy and Physiology*, 8th edn. San Francisco: Pearson Benjamin Cummings.

Nash P (2001) Common neonatal complications. In: Rice

Simpson K and Creehan PA (eds) *Perinatal Nursing*, 2nd edn. Philadelphia: Lippincott, pp. 575–608.

Percival P (2003) Jaundice and infection. In: Fraser DM and Cooper MA (eds) *Myles Textbook for Midwives*, 14th edn. Edinburgh: Churchill Livingstone.

CHAPTER 11

NEONATAL RESPIRATORY PROBLEMS

Carole England

OVERVIEW

This chapter will explore different common respiratory problems that may present in the hospital labour room or some time later in the postnatal ward. The midwife should be able to recognize signs of respiratory distress, make well-timed appropriate referral and work within the multiprofessional team to effectively manage the condition. The midwife's knowledge of lung development related to respiratory distress and how it affects the baby is crucial in early detection and swift, purposeful intervention. For midwives who work in primary care, midwife colleagues and paramedics constitute the initial team. Assessment, stabilization and safe transfer of the baby into hospital is essential to ensure the best outcome. For midwives in both settings, parental support is an important part of the care provided.

The physiology of lung development in the fetus

According to Blackburn (2007) the fetal lung passes through four main stages of lung development during gestation. At 3–5 weeks a respiratory bud arises from the ventral (front) surface of the oesophagus. At between 6 and 16 weeks the bronchial tree from the trachea to terminal bronchioles is formed. The pulmonary circulation, comprising the arterial and venous systems, develops next. By week 24, distal airways develop and epithelial cells subdivide into type I pneumocytes. These are for gaseous exchange and type II pneumocytes are for the production of surfactant. From 24 weeks to term the terminal sacs, alveolar ducts and finally alveoli form. Surfactant production increases with alveolar growth and development. The lungs of the term baby are about one-fifth of the adult size and alveolar multiplication and maturation continues into early childhood, especially at the first year when the child starts to mobilize.

Respiratory problems are the commonest cause of serious illness and death because neonates are more susceptible to certain diseases that are dictated by their stages of lung development. Their diaphragm and respiratory muscles are more prone to fatigue and their airways are smaller, which generates higher resistance to air flow. Given these susceptibilities, the midwife must anticipate that from each birth any baby could go on to develop a respiratory problem. A thorough knowledge of maternal present and past obstetric and family history is a good starting point to enable the midwife to prepare. Observation of the baby's appearance and behaviour is the first and most important stage of clinical assessment.

Respiratory distress

This is a general term that describes a respiratory problem in the neonate. It is often *mistakenly* thought of as referring to just respiratory distress syndrome (RDS). Respiratory distress is a description of how the neonate is presenting and may be one or a combination of signs. Babies do not present with symptoms although this term is used. Symptoms are what the client verbally complains about, so given that babies cannot speak it is the responsibility of the midwife to look for the signs of respiratory distress in all babies that he or she cares for.

Signs of respiratory distress

Tachypnoea (pronounced tac-ip-near)

This is a respiratory rate when breaths are over 60 per minute. The normal range for a term baby is 30–40 breaths per minute. Preterm babies breathe more quickly compared to term babies. The lower the gestational age, the higher is the metabolic rate. Hypercapnoea, a raised partial pressure of carbon dioxide in the blood (PCO_2), and hypoxaemia, a low partial pressure of oxygen (PO_2) in the blood, lead to stimulation of the medulla oblongata which results in a raised respiratory drive and rate. Over time, tachypnoea is self-limiting as its presence will over-utilize energy resources, one of which is oxygen.

Tachycardia

This is a raised heart rate. A term baby's heart rate will tend to be around 110–140 beats per minute (bpm). Preterm babies have faster heart rates: 140–160 bpm. Tachycardia is a relative term according to gestational age and gives a comparison with what the baby's heart beat is normally, if known. A heart beat over 200 bpm is unacceptably high and constitutes an arrhythmia. The rise in rate is a result of hypoxia (low oxygen level in the extracellular spaces of the tissues) as the heart attempts to circulate the available oxygen to the tissues.

Central cyanosis

This is caused by more severe hypoxia. In all babies, whatever the ethnicity, the tongue and the mucous membranes in the mouth should be immediately inspected to ascertain the level of perfusion to those tissues which will reflect how pink or blue they are. The skin is the most obvious place to make an assessment, but can prove difficult in estimating to what degree the baby is cyanosed. Blue hands and feet (acrocyanosis) can be found in well newborn babies where the tongue and mucous membranes of the mouth are pink and the oxygen saturations normal. It is far easier to place a pulse oximeter onto the baby's left hand or foot to get oxygen saturations, which measure the percentage of oxygen saturation of haemoglobin. The normal level should be 95–100 per cent.

Expiratory grunt

Neonates have the ability, when hypoxic, to raise their oxygen levels by trapping the oxygen that is contained in expiratory air and preserve some internal lung pressure to prevent the airways from collapsing at the end of each breath. As the air reaches the larynx the glottis contracts, which forces the air to do a U-turn over the vocal cords, to return to the trachea and alveoli. This action enables the alveoli to strip the oxygen from the expiratory air, so enhancing oxygenation of the blood, and the back pressure prevents the alveoli from collapsing, thus facilitating gaseous exchange. Each baby will have an individual tone of grunt. It does not sound like a pig grunt, but a noise on every breath. It is a significant sign as it could also indicate that the baby is cooling and that the respiratory distress is part of a changing metabolism as the baby attempts to raise the metabolic rate in order to raise temperature.

Recession

In normal inspiration, a negative pressure is created by the dome-shaped diaphragm which contracts, moves down and flattens out. In effect the height of the thoracic cavity increases. Contraction of the external intercostal muscles results in an elevation of the rib cage and a thrusting forward of the sternum, which expands the thorax both laterally and in the antero-posterior plane. Thus a negative pressure is created which draws atmospheric air into the alveoli. Recession is an abnormal in-drawing of the ribs and sternum in the presence of a strong respiratory drive from the medulla oblongata. The lower the gestational age, the softer and more pliable are the cartilages.

Recession works against the physiology of respiration because as the ribs are drawn in, so a smaller space is created and a lower negative pressure achieved. The type of recession is named in accordance with the affected anatomical landmarks of the baby. Recession of the ribs is called costal recession; of the spaces between the ribs, intercostal recession; and drawing in of the space immediately below the ribs is called subcostal recession. The sternum can also be affected and this is called sternal and substernal recession. Sometimes the breathing has a 'see-saw' pattern as the abdominal movements and the diaphragm work out of unison.

Apnoea

Apnoea is the cessation of breathing for 20 seconds or more and can spontaneously occur in babies that have a respiratory distress. Apnoea in a baby with respiratory distress is an ominous sign and immediate medical assessment and intervention is needed. In a term baby it occurs as the end result of increasing respiratory fatigue. When the level of carbon dioxide rises, a small increase will stimulate the medulla oblongata, but a large amount will depress it. Sometimes the baby will self-stimulate; for others, especially if their condition is generally deteriorating, they will need to be stimulated to breathe by a gentle touch from the midwife. Preterm babies are more prone to apnoea because their more immature medulla oblongata is less responsive to rising levels of carbon dioxide. If the baby fails to re-establish respiration, intermittent positive pressure ventilation (IPPV) by face mask will have to be given to help the baby take in more oxygen and blow off the excess carbon dioxide. Always seek help and follow the guidance of the Resuscitation Council (UK) (2006).

Nasal flaring

This is an attempt to minimize the effect of the airway's resistance by maximizing the diameter of the upper airways.

Common respiratory problems in the newborn

Transient tachypnoea of the newborn

This is usually a disease of term babies but can occur in the preterm. The cause is either increased production of lung fluid or delayed removal via trachea, pulmonary lymphatics and veins. If there is little or no thoracic squeeze created by vaginal compression during birth, the lung fluid remains in the interstitial spaces of the lungs and interferes with gaseous exchange. It takes about 72 hours to resolve (Figure 11.1).

The onset of this disease is between 2–4 hours and the commonest cause is birth by caesarean section. Other predisposing factors include perinatal asphyxia, maternal diabetes, excessive maternal analgesia, precipitant birth and vaginal breech birth. The baby presents with tachypnoea (breaths may be 80–100 per minute), a minimal expiratory grunt and recession. It is important to exclude streptococcal pneumonia so an infection screen and antibiotics may be initiated. The illness is short-lived, with therapeutic oxygen requirements that do not exceed 40 per cent to maintain normal arterial blood gases. In babies who are distressed with a tachypnoea, oral feeding may be delayed with fluids given intravenously.

Meconium aspiration syndrome

This is a disease of mature babies, often post-mature or those having suffered intrauterine growth restriction. For a baby to respond to stress by passing meconium it must have a mature autonomic nervous system. The passage of meconium is rare in preterm babies and a more likely cause is fetal septicaemia caused by *Listeria monocytogenes* or refluxing of bile from intestinal obstruction. When a fetus is stressed the sympathetic nervous system is activated and the

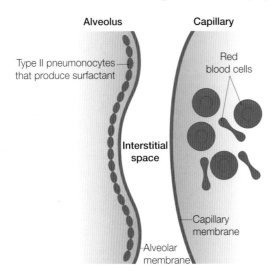

Figure 11.1 The respiratory membrane to show the interstitial space and the site of surfactant production

heart rate is increased, but as oxygen resources diminish, the parasympathetic nervous system reduces the metabolic rate in an effort to preserve what remains available. This system slows the heart rate and can result in bradycardia but also activates the gastrointestinal system. Rectal contraction and anal sphincter relaxation result in the passage of meconium into the liquor amnii.

Meconium can theoretically enter the lungs before or during birth, but how does this happen? The normal gentle breathing movements of a fetus *in utero* are not sufficient to enable the fetus to inhale thick particulate meconium (suspended particles of meconium) in significant quantities. For this to occur the fetus must have been asphyxiated and gasped. It therefore follows that the major determinants of the outcome for the fetus are the circumstances and severity of the asphyxial insult that caused the fetus to gasp, rather than the meconium inhaled as a result of the gasping.

Descriptors of meconium

In about 13 per cent of births, meconium-staining of the liquor occurs and is of less significance if the liquor is brown instead of clear and has no suspended particles of meconium in it. Most babies born through meconium-stained liquor have not inhaled any particulate material into their lower respiratory tract. If they have not done so as a result of anoxic gasping before birth, they are unlikely to do so at birth. This implies that attempting to suck any secretions when the head is on the perineum is of no benefit (Wiswell *et al.*, 2000). Crying babies have an open airway and do not need respiratory assistance.

On the other end of the continuum, if the meconium looks fresh, is tenacious and resembles Marmite, it is thick enough to cause airway obstruction. If the baby is hypotonic (floppy) and makes no spontaneous respiratory effort, the midwife should transfer the baby to the resuscitaire for inspection of the larynx to see whether any meconium has spread beyond the vocal cords. This is a reasonable course of action while awaiting the paediatric team to arrive. The midwife should have received training to use the laryngoscope and inspect the cords under direct vision. Even with wide-bore suction catheters, it is most difficult to evacuate meconium and a Yankeur suction catheter should be used.

The midwife must also ensure that the baby is kept warm by covering the baby. After clearing the airway, if the baby is still not breathing and bradycardic, IPPV is initiated. Help will be needed. Intubation and direct suction to the tube can be performed by the senior paediatrician. In the primary care setting, the midwife needs to alert the paramedics for expedient transfer into hospital and to attempt to evacuate the meconium using postural drainage and manual removal with a cloth or end of a towel. Paper handkerchiefs are not recommended. Thoroughly drying the baby and starting IPPV will then need to follow.

Effects of the aspiration of thick fresh meconium into the lungs

Meconium aspiration syndrome occurs in 4–5 per cent of babies born through meconium-stained liquor. They usually develop respiratory distress in the first hour and deteriorate quickly. Signs of cerebral irritability may coexist. Prolonged asphyxia is thought to cause a continuation of the high pulmonary vascular resistance (vasoconstriction of the pulmonary blood vessels) resulting in persistent fetal circulation, now called persistent pulmonary hypertension of the newborn (PPHN), which can result in pulmonary vascular necrosis and haemorrhage. The lungs receive very little blood supply so the baby has little gaseous exchange and will remain hypoxic and acidotic, and may be hypercapnoeic. These metabolic disturbances will cause inhibition of surfactant, alveolar damage and collapse.

The mechanical effects of the meconium in the airways causes air-trapping. During inspiration the calibre of the airways is enlarged and the meconium is taken deeper into the airway. On expiration, the airway recoils and the air that was taken in on inspiration is now trapped distal to the meconium. On each breath, air is taken into the lungs but cannot escape, so over time air is trapped in the alveoli. The alveoli overexpand and pneumothorax can result. The presence of the meconium in contact with the alveoli tissue is thought to cause a chemical pneumonitis (meconium contains bile salts and is an irritant), which can lead to a secondary pneumonia. Thus the lungs are damaged and, given the accompanying history of asphyxia, the mortality rate is considerable.

In such cases the baby will need to be nursed in the neonatal intensive unit. Parental support is a vital component of the care and the midwife should not always assume that psychological support is being exclusively provided by the neonatal staff.

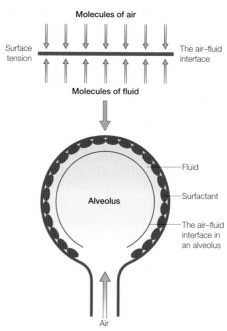

Figure 11.2   To illustrate the air–fluid interface

Respiratory distress syndrome

This disease is caused by surfactant deficiency and the risk of it developing is considerably increased by perinatal hypoxia and acidosis which may, to some degree, damage tissues in the body, including the type II pneumocytes. This can result in inhibition of the production of surfactant just at a time when its production is needed.

How does surfactant work?

Surfactant is a naturally occurring substance comprising 90 per cent fats (lipids) and 10 per cent proteins. It is a powerful antioxidant and synthesized by the type II pneumocytes found in the alveolar walls (see Figure 11.1). Its function is to act as a detergent to lower the tension created when two elements come together, in this case, fluid and air. When the baby takes its first breath, lung fluid drains from each alveolus and air enters. The molecules of air and remnants of the fluid come together and create a platform known as the air–fluid interface (Figure 11.2). In the outside world this platform, or surface tension, supports floating, for example, leaves and ducks float on the surface of the water. Surfactant acts to break up the surface tension into smaller molecules so that the alveoli, once inflated, will remain so on expiration.

Once the alveoli are partly inflated their resistance is lower. When blowing up a party balloon the initial pressures used to 'get it going' are considerable, but once it is half inflated it becomes easier because the balloon walls are thinner and the radius is bigger, according to the Laplace equation. In the presence of surfactant, both large and small alveoli are able to inflate on inspiration. In a baby with little or no surfactant, both large and, to a lesser degree, small alveoli inflate on inspiration, but on expiration the surface tension acts as an opposing force and the small alveoli collapse. Each following breath brings about some inflation, but eventually the baby tires and over time all the alveoli collapse back to their original state (Levene et al., 2008).

The pathophysiology of respiratory distress syndrome

According to Mupanemunda and Watkinson (2005) most babies are born with some surfactant so respiratory distress syndrome is not a disease which directly surrounds birth. The gestational age and degree of asphyxia will affect the production of surfactant and if the gestational age indicates that the surfactant; will be short in supply and not mature, these factors will lead to insufficient amounts of surfactant and in time it will 'start to run out'. This leads to reduced alveolar

Factors that increase the incidence of respiratory distress syndrome

- Gestational age: 80 per cent of babies up to 28 weeks' gestation, 50 per cent up to 32 weeks and below 3 per cent from 33 weeks to term will develop the disease.

- Infants of diabetic mothers are usually term babies but are sometimes preterm, often as a result of a poorly controlled diabetic pregnancy. The baby is macrosomic to different degrees and often large for its gestational age. The type II pneumocytes that produce surfactant are adversely affected by the metabolic alterations caused by hyperglycaemia and hyperinsulinism and although the fetus may be mature by chronological gestation, from a physiological development perspective they tend to respond in a more immature way.

- Black babies have a lower incidence and severity than white babies, matched for age and birthweight.

- Girls have a lower risk, less severe disease and a lower mortality rate than boys.

- In a multiple pregnancy the second twin is more likely to be affected if there is a delay.

- Delivery by caesarean section prior to spontaneous onset of labour increases the risk.

- Asphyxia, acidosis and hypothermia all inhibit surfactant production and its regeneration.

- Familial predisposition: some women are not able to take a pregnancy beyond a certain gestation with a recurring incidence of respiratory distress syndrome.

Factors that decrease the incidence of respiratory distress syndrome

- Stress *in utero*: risk is lower in disorders associated with placental dysfunction that leads to intrauterine growth restriction, but not pre-eclampsia.

- Maternal narcotic addiction, alcohol ingestion, smoking. These factors create chronic stress and enhance the production of fetal endogenous corticosteroids and early maturation of surfactant. However, the baby may have symmetrical growth restriction and be small for its gestational age.

stability, alveolar collapse (atelectasis) and clinical signs of respiratory distress. As the alveoli collapse, the pulmonary arteries and arterioles vasoconstrict. Thus there is inadequate gaseous exchange. Hypoxia and hypercapnoea will follow (O'Callaghan and Stephenson, 2004).

Prolonged hypoxia will result in anaerobic glycolysis (the conversion of glycogen to glucose in the absence of oxygen) to make energy and results in the production of lactic acid. This is a fixed acid and needs to be excreted via the kidneys, which may take up to 48 hours. Its accumulation results in a *metabolic* acidosis.

As the tissues produce carbon dioxide it is converted to carbonic acid to be taken to the lungs for excretion. Poor gaseous exchange results in accumulation of carbonic acid in the blood. This is regarded as a *respiratory* acidosis. In the following expression repesenting this process the symbol $\leftrightarrow$ means it is reversible: in the tissues there is a left to right conversion but in the lungs, right to left.

$$CO_2 + H_2O \leftrightarrow H_2CO_3$$

The body is able to buffer the carbonic acid by removing one hydrogen ion (excreted via the kidneys), converting the acid to bicarbonate, which is a base (alkaline).

The combination of a metabolic and respiratory acidosis reduces the pH (potential hydrogen ions) and renders the baby acidotic. Gradually with increasing alveoli collapse, the lungs are bypassed as the heart reverts to a persistent fetal circulation by shunting blood from right to left through the ductus arteriosus and foramen ovale. The damaged lungs release thromboplastins and form hyaline membranes which can be seen on a post mortem finding. Although midwives use the term respiratory distress syndrome (RDS), the other name for this syndrome is hyaline membrane disease.

Prevention of respiratory distress syndrome

The following two therapies, when combined, constitute a major advance in neonatal care:

- *Antenatal steroids* should be given to all mothers at risk of preterm delivery at 24–34 weeks' gestation, those who have suffered an antepartum haemorrhage, premature rupture of the membranes or any condition requiring elective preterm delivery. Treatment consists of two doses of betamethasone 12 mg intramuscularly, 24 hours apart. This is a synthetic steroid that has a small molecular weight and will pass the placental barrier. It reduces the incidence of respiratory distress syndrome by 60 per cent and mortality by 40 per cent (Lissauer and Fanaroff, 2006). Optimal benefit begins 24 hours after initiation of therapy and lasts at least seven days. The use of repeated courses has not shown significant advantage.

- *The administration of surfactant* after birth, directly into the endotracheal tube, can be given ideally as a prophylactic precaution, before signs of respiratory distress appear, or as a rescue, once the baby has established respiratory distress syndrome. Surfactant stabilizes the alveoli and acts as a powerful antioxidant to offset the effects of high levels of oxygen in the conversion to extrauterine life (Levene *et al.*, 2008).

The midwife's role in the labour room

The midwife should assess any predisposing factors to respiratory distress syndrome, especially gestational age, and arrange for the paediatric team to be ready to act. The baby may be electively intubated to give surfactant treatment or as a supportive measure because of extreme prematurity. Often the baby is well in the first few hours and if the paediatric team agree, skin-to-skin contact and breastfeeding can be initiated. If below 32 weeks the baby will be placed feet first in a plastic bag which is secured at the neck to reduce evaporative heat losses but parental contact is still possible and should be encouraged by the midwife.

The midwife will need to know and understand the plan of care for the baby so that he or she is able to inform and answer any questions the parents may pose. The separation of the baby from the parents should be managed with grace and compassion.

Management principles of respiratory distress syndrome in the neonatal intensive care unit

Respiratory distress syndrome is managed in the neonatal intensive care unit with the application of:

- oxygen therapy (and monitoring to prevent hypoxic encephalopathy and retinopathy of prematurity);
- continuous positive airways pressure (CPAP) or positive end expiratory pressure (PEEP) on a mechanical ventilator to prevent lung collapse;
- intermittent positive pressure ventilation (IPPV) to induce lung expansion; and
- intensive care.

The onset of respiratory distress syndrome is usually within 4 hours of birth. The illness becomes worse over the first 24–72 hours and then 'turns the corner'. From birth, once 8 hours has elapsed, a diagnosis of respiratory distress syndrome is virtually excluded.

Pneumonia

Congenital infections are caused by organisms that affect the fetus and are transmitted transplacentally or when the fetus passes through the birth canal. They usually manifest within the first 72 hours (often within the first 24 hours). Pneumonia in the newborn is usually caused by bacteria. The commonest organism causing congenital pneumonia in the UK is the Gram-positive bacterium group B beta-haemolytic *Streptococcus*. Less commonly, Gram-negative bacilli such as *Escherichia coli*, *Klebsiella* or *Pseudomonas aeruginosa* are responsible. Pneumonia caused by group B beta-haemolytic streptococci mimics respiratory distress syndrome and carries a high mortality rate. That caused by *Listeria monocytogenes* is rare.

Pneumonia as a result of acquired infection occurs after birth and may be caused by *Staphylococcus aureus*, *E. coli* and late onset group B streptococci. It occurs after the first week.

Maternal and birth histories may reveal predisposing factors for neonatal infection. Early clinical signs may be non-specific and may include lethargy, apnoea, bradycardia, temperature instability and intolerance of feeds. The baby may present from birth with respiratory distress or at a later time, which would be more in keeping with a clinical picture of respiratory distress syndrome.

A full infection screen and the commencement of broad-spectrum antibiotics (penicillin and gentamycin) are commenced until the results of the screen are known. For a more detailed account of specific infections, see Chapter 10.

Thoracic air leaks

This term covers respiratory conditions in which air has entered structures of the body outside the thoracic compartment. The alveoli become hyperinflated and rupture.

Pneumothorax is when air escapes into the pleural space (the serous membranes that cover the lungs) and is the commonest form of air leak, occurring in up to 1 per cent of all newborns, although only 0.1 per cent may present with signs of respiratory distress. Pneumothoraces can occur spontaneously at birth or during resuscitation, but thereafter the prevalence is increased in the presence of pulmonary disease such as meconium aspiration syndrome or respiratory distress syndrome. Pneumothorax occurs in babies ventilated for respiratory distress syndrome and is associated with high inspiratory pressures.

Babies that present with large spontaneous tension pneumothoraces suddenly deteriorate with severe respiratory distress. Sometimes a baby who already has respiratory distress from another cause will become pale, with poor peripheral perfusion, bradycardia and hypoxaemia. A specific sign of a unilateral tension pneumothorax is a mediastinal shift, which means the pocket of air in the pleural space has moved the mediastinum out of its normal position. A right-sided pneumothorax will shift the mediastinum and heart towards the left of the thorax. This has implications for the aorta and inferior vena cavae, which are held in position by the diaphragm and can become partially occluded, and accounts for the shock and bradycardia that accompany this condition. Pneumothoraces occur more often on the right side of the chest but are bilateral in 15–20 per cent of cases. In the bilateral presentation, mediastinal shift may not occur.

The baby with pneumothorax will present with reduced breath sounds and chest movement on the affected side. Transillumination of the chest with a fibreoptic light source shows increased illumination as the light passes through air. Confirmation of the pneumothorax is by an anterior–posterior chest X-ray.

A life-threatening tension pneumothorax may be treated by urgent needle (21G butterfly needle with stopcock and syringe) aspiration performed by an experienced paediatrician, and the midwife should have such equipment ready to hand. This will give the senior paediatrician time to insert a chest drain into the second intercostal space in the midclavicular line and connect it to a one-way flutter valve or underwater seal drain. This will gradually release the trapped air.

For non-tension pneumothoraces in term babies, placing them in high concentrations of oxygen will accelerate natural reabsorption of the air.

Congenital abnormalities that cause respiratory problems

Congenital diaphragmatic hernia

Between 4 and 10 per cent of all infant deaths from congenital abnormalities are caused by congenital diaphragmatic hernia. The cause is unknown and the incidence is about 3 per 10 000 births. Other chromosomal anomalies are present in up to 30 per cent of cases, especially heart, gastrointestinal and renal defects.

The hernia is an abnormal passage in the posterolateral aspect of the diaphragm that results from failure of tendon and muscle development in early embryonic life. The defect is on the left side of the diaphragm in 80 per cent of cases and allows abdominal organs to enter the thoracic cavity. The liver covers the right side and tends to plug any defect, but on occasions the liver can herniate through a right-sided defect. The stomach, small and large intestines, liver and spleen can compress the lung on the affected side and shift the mediastinum closer to the unaffected side. If the lung compression starts early in gestational life (<25 weeks) the likelihood of pulmonary hypoplasia in this lung is enhanced. The lung will be generally underdeveloped with fewer bronchioles and alveoli, and have poor vascular development with fewer surfactant cells that are less effective. Maternal betamethasone therapy is recommended.

Predictors of the condition

Many cases are diagnosed by routine ultrasound scan at 17–19 weeks' gestation or following investigations into polyhydramnios, but up to a half may be missed on scans as the hernia develops after the scan has been done. Termination of the pregnancy is an option, especially if there are chromosomal defects such as trisomy 13, 18 or 21 and the presence of major anomalies in other systems. This combination creates a poor prognosis.

The size of the defect and side affected will dictate the presentation at birth. Paediatricians should be present at delivery. Not all babies require assistance at birth but the midwife should be aware that those with large left-sided defects present in the immediate post-natal period with respiratory distress. The midwife may notice the baby has a scaphoid abdomen (con-cave because it is relatively empty) with ectopic heart and bowel sounds in the chest. The paediatric team should start resuscitative measures but mask ventila-tion should be avoided as this will result in some ven-tilation of the gastrointestinal tract, which if in the chest could result in unwanted distension, compro-mising cardiac and respiratory function.

A large-bore orogastric tube should be inserted and the stomach contents in the chest aspirated free of gas and secretions. Intubation of the trachea should be carried out and care should be taken to prevent rupture of the unaffected lung, as the baby is solely dependent on this lung for its respiration. The lowest possible airway pressures should be used to maintain 90 per cent oxygen–haemoglobin saturation. Prophy-lactic surfactant therapy via the endotracheal tube is beneficial.

Persistent pulmonary hypertension of the new-born (PPHN) is a common complication that results in a right-to-left shunt through the ductus arteriosus, bypassing the lungs. The prognosis depends upon the degree of pulmonary hypoplasia and the age at pres-entation. The midwife should be careful not to be too overly optimistic in any expressions of outcome as they may be misguided and not appreciated by the parents in the long term.

Oesophageal atresia and tracheo-oesophageal fistula

Oesophageal atresia occurs in 1 in 4500 live births. An atresia is an interruption of the structure of the oesophagus so that an abnormal blind ending occurs on the upper oesophagus and on the lower oesopha-gus where it recommences again. In between these two blind endings there is a gap. The oesophagus and trachea share a common origin and develop as one in embryonic life. Oesophageal atresia can happen in isolation, but in 85 per cent of cases there is also an abnormal connection between the oesophagus and trachea called a tracheo-oesophageal fistula (TOF). This is extra abnormal tissue that creates a corridor of varying size between the oesophagus and trachea.

There are many different variations of presenta-tion in these conditions. Johnson (2005) notes that early disturbances of organogenesis affect other sys-tems too and the VATER association (vertebral defects, anal atresia, tracheo-oesophageal, [o]esophageal, renal abnormalities) describes coexist-ing anomalies. Also consider the VACTERYL associa-tion (vertebral, anal, cardiac, tracheo-oesophageal, [o]esophageal and radial abnormalities). The CHARGE association stands for colobomata, heart disease, choanal atresia, mental retardation, genital hypoplasia and ear abnormalities. Duodenal atresia is also seen.

There is also a strong link between these abnor-malities and chromosomal abnormalities such as tri-somy 18 and 21. The baby may be preterm (5 times the normal incidence) and small for its gestational age (8 times the normal incidence). Polyhydramnios is present in the mother in 50 per cent of cases. Ultra-sound scanning may detect a small or absent stomach bubble, but generally identification of blind-ending pouches and fistulas are difficult to see, so detection is poor (Johnson, 2005).

The most frequent form of oesophageal atresia is where the oesophagus is divided into an upper proxi-mal blind pouch and a lower distal separated portion that communicates with the stomach in the normal way (Figure 11.3). A fistula connects this lower oesophageal segment with the trachea.

All babies born to mothers with a history of poly-hydramnios must have a nasogastric tube passed soon after birth to exclude tracheo-oesophageal fistula before a feed is given. Diagnosis is usually made early in the postnatal period and given that most babies are offered a feed in the first hour of life this may bring about deterioration in the baby, especially if the baby takes a substantial formula feed. Before a feed is offered, the baby may drool with bubbling saliva, par-ticularly if the proximal oesophageal pouch is small and close to the neck. As the pouch fills, saliva spills into the mouth and may be aspirated into the trachea. Signs of respiratory distress, particularly central cyanosis, may reflect this, alongside choking. The midwife should notice any wetness of the mother when she is in skin-to-skin contact with her baby or if clothing is damp around the mouth area. A thorough examination of the baby may highlight other struc-tural defects. The midwife should not allow the term 'mucousy' to stereotype his or her thinking of other more benign causes.

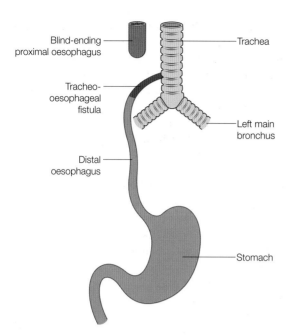

Blind-ending proximal oesophagus

Tracheo-oesophageal fistula

Distal oesophagus

Trachea

Left main bronchus

Stomach

Figure 11.3   The most frequent form of oesophageal atresia with tracheo-oesophageal fistula

If oesophageal atresia is suspected, it is vital that the first feed is delayed and the midwife should call for the passage of a size 10 nasogastric catheter (small catheters can get coiled in the pouch) which on X-ray will illustrate if an atresia exists. If the proximal pouch is long, the initial signs may be later and the baby is more likely to take its first feed. The presence of any degree of respiratory distress associated with feeding should always be noted and referral made immediately.

The baby with an oesophageal atresia and tracheo-oesophageal fistula should be commenced on regular intermittent suction or continuous aspiration of the upper proximal pouch using a double-lumen low-pressure Replogle catheter. The head of the cot should be propped up at 45 degrees to diminish reflux of gastric secretions (secreted even in the absence of a feed) into the fistula then into the lungs. The baby may require initial resuscitation. If respiratory distress is present, ventilation may be warranted, but should be approached as an emergency because the positive pressure can cross the fistula and inflate (even perforate) the stomach. A large stomach will displace the diaphragm upwards and worsen the respiratory distress. The midwife will need to explain to the parents that the baby will be transferred to the neonatal intensive care unit for stabilization and then assessment for surgical repair. This may mean transfer to another hospital for some babies.

A note of communication caution: the abbreviation 'TOF' is also used for Tetralogy of Fallot, a congenital cyanotic disease of the heart.

CASE HISTORY

Tracy, a primigravida was 35 weeks' gestation and had a vaginal birth very quickly. Baby Lee was initially well and had skin-to-skin contact and a breastfeed. On transfer to the postnatal ward, the midwife noticed that his breathing was rapid and on closer inspection he was centrally cyanosed. The midwife informed Tracy of her findings and asked her to hold Lee skin-to-skin to ensure he didn't lose heat. She immediately informed the paediatrician to attend as Lee was now 2 hours old and had a tachypnoea of 70 bpm.

What could be causing Lee's respiratory distress? It is always a good rule of thumb to think of the more common causes before the rare ones. Given the gestational age it is possible but unlikely that he is suffering from respiratory distress syndrome. Surfactant matures around 35 weeks so he should have enough surfactant even though he had a precipitant birth and is male. Pneumonia should always be considered. The presence of group B beta streptococci in a maternal vaginal swab and urine sample is a significant finding. Tachypnoea and central cyanosis are

continued ➤

more suggestive of transient tachypnoea of the newborn and the precipitant nature of his birth tends to support this view. However, when the first feed has been given and a baby becomes cyanosed one cannot rule out congenital abnormality such as oesophageal atresia.

Lee was admitted to the neonatal intensive care unit and a blood gas was taken. He was given 30 per cent therapeutic oxygen via headbox. He was reunited with Tracy three days later. Transient tachypnoea of the newborn was thought to be the respiratory problem.

Conclusion

In any setting, the midwife acts as an informed referral agent when respiratory problems threaten the life of the neonate. Knowledge of significant past pregnancies, events in the present pregnancy and how the labour and birth progressed will help to create a holistic picture of both mother and baby. Maternal disease and gestational age of the baby are strong indicators for some conditions. The timing of onset of the signs of respiratory distress is another factor to consider. The midwife does not make the diagnosis, but can anticipate what may be needed and organize what needs to be done. The care must include parental support. The midwife should be prepared to become advocate to facilitate parental contact with their baby before a needed separation is imposed. In essence, respiratory problems call for the proactive midwife who knows what to do and why.

Key Points

- Recognizing the signs of respiratory distress and their time of onset is vital to differentiating between the causes of neonatal respiratory problems.

- Gestational age, present pregnancy and birth history are important factors in attempting to find a cause.

- Early referral to the multiprofessional team is required so that further investigations and/or transfer to the neonatal unit can be facilitated.

- Parental support, particularly effective communication, is an important part of the midwife's role.

References

Blackburn ST (2007) *Maternal, Fetal and Neonatology Physiology. A clinical perspective*. Washington DC: Saunders.

Johnson PRV (2005) Oesophageal atresia. *Infant* **1**: 163–167.

Levene MI, Trudehope DI and Sunil S (2008) *Essential Neonatal Medicine*. London: Blackwell Publishing.

Lissauer T and Fanaroff AA (2006) *Neonatology at a Glance*. London: Blackwell.

Mupanemunder R and Watkinson M (2005) *Key Topics in Neonatology*. London and New York: Taylor and Francis.

O'Callaghan C and Stephenson T (2004) *Pocket Paediatrics*. London: Churchill Livingstone.

Resuscitation Council (UK) (2006) *Resuscitation at Birth. Newborn life support. Provider Course Manual*. London: Resuscitation Council (UK).

Wiswell TE, Gannon CM, Jacob J *et al.* (2000) Delivery room management of the apparently vigorous meconium-stained neonate: results of the multicenter, international collaborative trial. *Paediatrics* **105**: 1–7.

CHAPTER 12

NEONATAL WITHDRAWAL SYNDROMES

Hilary Lumsden

OVERVIEW

Mothers who take drugs or drink alcohol during pregnancy are potentially putting their developing fetus at risk. In this chapter the various problems associated with this behaviour, such as neonatal abstinence syndrome (NAS) and fetal alcohol spectrum disorders (FASD), are discussed.

Introduction

Problems associated with illicit drug use and substance misuse have multiplied greatly over the past few years and midwives frequently come into contact with women who have drug-related problems during pregnancy. Alcohol and drugs taken antenatally affect babies in different ways and midwives caring for the babies postnatally should be aware of the effects that these substances have on the developing fetus and newly born baby so that the care can be planned in a systematic and coordinated manner.

It should be remembered that for women who have problems associated with drug and alcohol misuse, pregnancy can offer opportunities as well as risks. The challenge for midwives is to maximize the opportunities while minimizing risk. The treatment therefore needs to be as woman- and family-centred as possible. Whittaker (2003) advocates an approach for

the care of substance-misusing women and their babies that is:

- women- and family-centred
- non-judgemental
- pragmatic, with an emphasis on harm reduction
- holistic
- provided by a multidisciplinary and multi-agency team.

Embryology

Any drug administered to the mother during pregnancy can affect the fetus in a number of ways, ranging from no effect to major structural deformity. It is well known that some prescribed drugs can have a harmful effect on the developing fetus, for example some antimicrobials, anticonvulsants and steroids

Table 12.1 Harmful effects of some prescription drugs on the developing fetus

Substance	Trimester affected	PN growth	Learning difficulties	CNS	CV	MS	GU	Eyes & ears
Antibacterials								
Tetracycline	1,2,3					✓	✓	
Streptomycin	1,2,3						✓	
Antineoplastics								
Methotrexate	1,2,3	✓		✓		✓		
Anticonvulsants								
Phenytoin	1,3	✓	✓	✓	✓	✓	✓	✓
Barbiturates	3		✓		✓	✓		✓
Sodium valporate	1,3		✓			✓		
Carbamazepine	1,3			✓		✓		
Steroid hormones								
Androgens	1,2,3						✓	
CNS drugs								
Cocaine	1			✓	✓	✓		
Lithium	1,2,3				✓			
Other								
Warfarin	1,2,3	✓	✓	✓	✓	✓	✓	✓
Alcohol	1,2,3	✓	✓			✓		✓
Tobacco	1,2,3	✓				✓		✓
Vitamin A	1							

Adapted from British National Formulary (2008)

should be avoided during pregnancy because of their teratogenic effect (Table 12.1). A teratogen is any substance, organism, physical agent taken or any deficiency during pregnancy that can interfere with normal embryonic and fetal development causing an abnormal structure or function in the fetus (Tucker Blackburn, 2003). Thalidomide, for example, was recognized as a teratogen in the 1960s because when it was taken for hyperemesis gravidarum in early pregnancy it caused significant malformations of babies' limbs. Other teratogens include radiation; exposure to X-rays during early pregnancy should be avoided.

From 11 weeks to term the fetus becomes more resistant to damage from toxic agents, but in the very early stages of pregnancy exposure to substances that affect fetal development can result in either an incomplete or damaged anatomical structures.

Current trends in drug-taking behaviour

It is estimated that over 70 million adults in Europe have used cannabis at least once, which is over one in five or 22 per cent of all 15–64 year olds (EMCDDA, 2007). In fact, estimates in 2007 suggested that around 23 million European adults used cannabis in the last year, with 12.5 million Europeans using cannabis regularly. This makes cannabis the most used illicit substance. Other drugs include amphetamines, used by between 0.1 and 11.9 per cent of 15–64 year olds, with about 2 million people using this form of drug in 2007, and ecstasy, which has been tried by 9.5 million adults and in 2007 alone was used by 3 million people across Europe (EMCDDA, 2007). There was an increase in the use of both amphetamines and ecstasy during the 1990s and although there are reports that the use of these drugs is stabilizing, it is thought that it is being replaced by cocaine use.

Cocaine remains the second most used drug in Europe, with on average 3.6 per cent of adults having used it at least once. This accounts for 7.5 million people with an estimation that 4 million people used cocaine in 2007. Cocaine use is concentrated mainly in Spain, the UK and, to a lesser extent, Italy, Denmark and Ireland. There is a trend for professional people to use cocaine and certainly its use by celebrities is well reported in the media.

Data relating to opioid use and drug injection are less clear due to the hidden nature of this type of drug use. From the relatively limited data available there is thought to be an estimated average prevalence of problem opioid use in Europe of between 4 and 5 cases per 1000 of the population aged 15–64 years. This could account for 1.5 million users. Although opioid use is less common than that for other illicit drugs, heroin users are the principal clients who seek treatment and injecting drug users are at a higher risk of contracting blood-borne infections such as HIV/AIDS. While many European countries are seeing an increase in this type of drug abuse, the UK has recently reported a stabilization of the problem (EMCDDA, 2007). It is well known that many substance-misusing women take a cocktail of drugs to support their habit and it is not unusual for a woman on heroin to supplement it with cocaine and amphetamines.

In the UK in 2004 nearly one in three adults exceeded the recommended daily benchmark of alcohol on at least one day during the previous week. Men were more likely to exceed the benchmark (38 per cent) than women (23 per cent) (Office of National Statistics, 2006). Tobacco smoking in the UK is estimated at one in four (25 per cent) and the age at which tobacco smoking is at its greatest is between 20 and 49 years, although it is slightly higher in men than in women (Office of National Statistics).

Young people are especially prone to illicit drug use and over the past few years there has been an increase in the number of under 15 year olds who drink alcohol and use cannabis. Statistics from EMCDDA (2007) suggest that figures for children of 13 or younger who report having been drunk are the highest in Denmark, Estonia, Finland and the UK, with a worrying figure of 33–36 per cent. The lowest rates are reported from Cyprus and Turkey, where the rates are 7 per cent and 5 per cent, respectively.

Binge drinking is recognized as a national problem in the UK, not only among the very young but also in older teenagers. In fact, young drinkers aged 11–15 in England doubled their average weekly consumption of alcohol during the 1990s from 5.3 in 1990 to 10.4 units in 2004, with the trend in girls increasing while the trend in boys seems to have stabilized (Office of National Statistics, 2006).

The illicit substance most commonly used by young people under 15 is cannabis. There appears to be a strong increase in the ever-in-lifetime prevalence of cannabis use during the early teenage years. Inhalants such as glue, solvents, gas fuels and aerosols are used by the very young but come second only to cannabis use. While the majority of under-15s have not used illicit substances, and substance dependence is rare, use at an early age must be recognized. The prevalence of daily tobacco smoking (7–14 per cent) and for having been drunk (5–36 per cent) varies in European countries. Families where parents or other family members take psychoactive substances are known to be at higher risk of early drug use in their children. Likewise sibling substance misuse is also highly likely to affect drug-taking behaviour in the family. The risk of early drug use among younger people may occur because of problems in social and psychological family functioning or because of maternal substance use during pregnancy (Bancroft et al., 2004).

Tobacco smoking in the early teenage years was estimated by the Office of National Statistics in 2008 to be around 5 per cent at age 13 increasing to 14 per cent and 25 per cent at the ages 14 and 15 respectively. With the UK having one of the highest teenage pregnancy rates in the developed world, with 56 000 babies born to teenage mothers each year (Brennan, 2002), it is increasingly likely that midwives will encounter teenage pregnancy with an associated illicit drug- or alcohol-related problem.

The fetus is a passive recipient of all substances entering the maternal system. Exposure to some substances in the first few weeks of pregnancy can result in spontaneous abortion. However, those pregnancies that continue and where the fetus is exposed to illicit drugs in the first trimester can result in congenital abnormalities. Babies born to drug-using women are often of low birthweight, with heroin reducing the mean birthweight by 489 g. For women taking either methadone or heroin the reduction can be as much as 557 g, and cocaine users produce babies which are 297 g smaller at birth (Hulse *et al.*, 1997). Mothers who use multiple drugs are known to contribute to the prematurity rate, with Slattery and Morrison (2002) reporting a rate of 25 per cent.

Antenatal care

Substance-abusing pregnant women are at risk of malnourishment, infectious diseases, endocarditis and sexually transmitted infections (STI). It is important to check maternal hepatitis B, hepatitis C and HIV status so that a plan of care can be made. Such women will need sensitive, holistic antenatal care, which, given their erratic and often unpredictable behaviour, is very difficult for the midwife to achieve.

Sometimes a specialist midwife is employed to care solely for drug-abusing women, giving regular antenatal care in conjunction with a drug counsellor for those women who choose to be supported during their pregnancy. It has been found that antenatal care specifically arranged for drug-abusing mothers that is within the community and thus easily accessed is more successful. It is advisable for women to enter into a methadone programme during pregnancy so that care can be coordinated with the giving of prescriptions for methadone. This facilitates compliance with antenatal care.

It is important for the midwife to discuss birth plans with the woman and care of the baby following delivery, and to talk through the possibility of neonatal abstinence syndrome. The mother needs to be aware that neonatal abstinence syndrome can be managed well but that there is also the possibility that the baby may be more severely affected, requiring treatment on the neonatal unit. If the trust has leaflets about neonatal abstinence syndrome it would be useful to give them to the mothers to read before their babies are delivered.

In order for women to cooperate and maintain contact antenatally it is important for midwives to adopt a non-judgemental approach when caring for substance-misusing women. Facilitating care with compassion, encouragement and support will allow care to be maintained. Midwives do need to examine their approach so that a positive pregnancy experience can be created.

Opiate withdrawal

Babies born to substance-misusing women will usually develop a physical dependence to the drugs during fetal life. The term 'dependence' should not be confused with 'addiction'; babies do not demonstrate drug-seeking behaviour and therefore the term 'addiction' should not be used when referring to babies who are drug dependent. Neonatal abstinence syndrome refers to particular withdrawal behaviours, comprising central nervous system hypersensitivity, autonomic dysfunction and gastrointestinal disturbances when babies have been exposed to drug-dependency producing substances *in utero* (Mupanemunda and Watkinson, 2005).

Minor signs of opiate withdrawal

- Jitteriness/tremors
- Irritability
- Shrill cry
- Hyperactivity
- Photophobia
- Poor sleeping/wakefulness
- Excessive sucking/poor feeding/poor weight gain
- Regurgitation
- Diarrhoea/vomiting
- Snuffles, sneezing
- Tachypnoea
- Yawning, hiccoughs
- Sweating, fever
- Stuffy nose, rhinorrhoea
- Excoriation (particularly on the buttocks due to loose stools) but also around the back of the head, shoulders and heels because of excessive rubbing.

Neonatal abstinence syndrome is more common in babies who have been exposed to heroin or methadone than other drugs. The signs are non-specific and are sometimes difficult to identify, and the onset of symptoms and the severity of the disorder will depend on various factors, including:

- the type of drug used
- the rate of elimination from the neonate
- the amount and time of mother's last dose
- duration of mother's dependency
- gestational age of the infant
- type of intrapartum analgesia or anaesthesia
- polydrug use.

Most babies will present with symptoms of drug withdrawal shortly after birth. Heroin withdrawal has a rapid onset whereas withdrawal from methadone can present slightly later, with the peak of withdrawal usually between 24 and 72 hours (in 75 per cent of cases). The withdrawal from methadone can also take longer to complete, lasting up to three weeks (Lall, 2008). Although drug withdrawal can be completed within a few weeks, the effects on growth and on neurobehaviour may last for several months. In the longer term adverse neurodevelopmental outcomes can also occur, with lower verbal and performance IQ and an increased incidence of attention deficit hyperactivity disorder (ADHD) (Jackson, 2006).

Babies with neonatal abstinence syndrome are extremely irritable, suck vigorously but have poor suck/swallow coordination, are very difficult to settle and have a distinctive cry. Hyperphagia is also a symptom of neonatal abstinence syndrome and may result in poor weight gain due to a high metabolic rate (Lall, 2008).

Care of the baby with neonatal abstinence syndrome

The aims of care are to identify withdrawal symptoms following birth and to ensure that the baby is kept as comfortable as possible, to provide adequate nutrition for growth and development and promote bonding. In addition, effective medical treatment should be administered when necessary and to end the baby's physical dependence on drugs. The midwife should also aim to give good parent education in order to facilitate parenting skills.

At delivery

It is vital that the midwife who is conducting the delivery is aware of the mother's drug problem. It is not essential that a paediatrician or advanced neonatal nurse practitioner is present at the delivery and they will only need to attend if the condition of the baby at birth is anticipated to be poor or is poor on assessment. Babies born to heroin/methadone-misusing women who do require resuscitation should not under any circumstances be given naloxone because it will expedite a rapid withdrawal from opiates that could potentially be very dangerous. Skin-to-skin contact should be positively encouraged at birth and normal neonatal care commenced.

The majority of babies born in the UK with neonatal abstinence syndrome are now nursed with the mother for the duration of their withdrawal, as long as there are no child protection concerns (Neonatal Bedside Guidelines, 2007). 'Rooming-in' is now seen to be preferable and withdrawal is completed in a shorter timeframe. Trusts should support the practice of keeping the mother and baby together with the avoidance of prolonged hospitalization, and placement away from the parents should be avoided. Although it can cause a drain on midwifery resources, the overall benefits will outweigh separation of mother and baby and can shorten the overall inpatient stay. This contemporary practice replaces traditional care on the neonatal unit where separation from the mother and long periods of medication to control symptoms was common practice. Some babies with uncontrollable symptoms may have to be admitted to the neonatal unit and this will be discussed later in this chapter.

Postnatal environment

In order to alleviate symptoms that babies with neonatal abstinence syndrome experience they will need to be nursed in a quiet, peaceful environment. On a busy postnatal ward this can be quite difficult to achieve and it may be easier to coordinate the care if the mother and baby are nursed in a side-room or in a bay with other babies with the syndrome. These babies will experience periods of instability, and an aspect of the care is to ensure that the babies' temperature and blood glucose are monitored closely initially and treated when they fall to lower than normal levels. The environment for the care of any baby withdrawing from maternal substance use should be quiet and dimly lit.

Noise

Staff on the ward should be aware that irritable and hyperactive babies need a calm and quiet environment. Educating the mothers and their visitors is important if the babies are to benefit from minimal stimulation. Televisions should be used to a minimum, set on a low volume and when in use with a set time when they can be watched, for example between 09:00 and 21:00 with at least a 2-hour period during the day when televisions are switched off. Use of mobile phones around the bedside should be discouraged; they should be set to silent mode and only used in corridors and dayrooms away from the baby.

Strict adherence to a limit of two visitors at the bedside should be maintained with minimum interchange between visitors.

Ward telephones, doctors' bleeps, radios, banging of bin lids, vacuum cleaners and talking can all contribute to the overall noise level on the ward. Neonatal units have, over the past few years, made great strides in reducing the amount of noise they generate in order to allow sick babies to rest for long periods. The same principles should be applied to wards caring for babies recovering from neonatal abstinence syndrome.

Gentle, soothing background music may be helpful in settling the baby. The music should not be too loud and should be played for short periods rather than continually.

Light

Since photophobia is a symptom of withdrawal, bright light in the postnatal ward should be reduced around babies with neonatal abstinence syndrome. If it is possible, dim the main bay/ward lights, using only a bedside light to keep the brightness of the room to a minimum. If the baby is being cared for in a bay with other mothers and babies, drawing the screens around the bed can reduce light levels from the rest of the room. Blinds or curtains should cover windows during daylight hours, particularly when the sun is shining. Televisions can contribute to the glare of light and mothers should be advised to limit the time they are switched on.

Touch

Too much handling can overstimulate babies with neonatal abstinence syndrome, therefore clustering of care and minimal handling should be promoted. As with any sick infant, the promotion of positive, comforting touch should outweigh negative, invasive touch. The daily plan of care for babies with neonatal abstinence syndrome should include the promotion

---

Examples of negative and positive touch

Negative

- Heel prick blood sampling
- Physical assessment
- Passing nasogastric tube
- Nappy changing
- Cannulation
- Administration of intravenous or intramuscular drugs
- Venepuncture

Positive

- Skin-to-skin contact
- Stroking
- Massage
- Rocking
- Swaddling
- Breastfeeding
- Cuddling.

---

of positive touch, with any episodes of negative touch being planned into the daily routine. Any medical intervention should be kept to a minimum and clustered with other episodes of handling.

The midwife caring for the woman and her baby must adhere to the plan of care and ensure that babies are not disturbed during their rest periods. Passing the baby around visitors should be discouraged. It is acknowledged that when they go home, babies with neonatal abstinence syndrome will be exposed to a chaotic lifestyle and it is likely that the positive environment they have experienced in hospital will not be continued in the home. However, during the recovery phase of neonatal abstinence syndrome it is essential that minimal handling is promoted as much as possible.

Positive aspects of care

The use of supportive therapy has been shown to reduce the effects of withdrawal in infants and should be implemented as soon as possible following birth (Whittaker, 2003). Swaddling the baby in a soft flannelette blanket or sheet will help with tremors and restlessness. A warm bath may help to settle a fractious, irritable baby; plain water with no detergents will be sufficient as discussed in Chapter 7. Meticulous care of the skin is essential, with attention to and appropriate treatment of excoriated areas being paramount. Frequent changes of the baby's nappy may be necessary to prevent excoriation caused by loose stools, however nappy changes should be balanced with the need for rest and clustering of care as discussed above. Strong perfumes and deodorants worn by the mother, visitors or staff should also be avoided, since they can act as a stimulant.

Midwives should monitor the baby's temperature as this can be unstable. Thin layers of clothing are preferable to thicker garments and allow the baby's temperature to be more easily controlled by removing or adding layers as necessary (see Chapter 8).

A dummy or pacifier can be used if the baby is sucking excessively. Care should be taken if the mother is breastfeeding not to introduce a dummy until feeding is well established. Although the use of dummies is contraindicated in the 'Ten steps to successful breastfeeding' (UNICEF/WHO, 2006), an exception is where babies are suffering from neonatal abstinence syndrome and where symptoms such as irritability need to be treated. Babies with neonatal abstinence syndrome should be encouraged to feed regularly, on demand is preferable, and smaller feeds will create less vomiting and prevent dehydration. Where the baby's suck and swallow reflex is poorly coordinated, winding the baby frequently can reduce regurgitation and vomiting.

If the baby's feeding is very poor, tube feeding may be required. Feed the baby 2–3 hourly with expressed breast milk or formula. The amount is based upon the normal feeding regime and using the normal precautions for tube feeding (see Chapter 6).

Breastfeeding

Midwives should give mothers all the information they require to make an informed decision about the method of feeding. Whichever method a mother chooses should be supported.

Unless there are contraindications such as HIV infection, mothers of babies with neonatal abstinence syndrome should be encouraged to breastfeed (Jackson, 2006). Other contraindications to breastfeeding are:

- using large quantities of stimulant drugs such as cocaine, crack or amphetamines;
- drinking heavily (more than 8 units a day); or
- large amounts of benzodiazepines (because of the sedation effects) (Whittaker, 2003, p. 87).

Opiates are excreted in only small amounts in breast milk and therefore breastfeeding may potentially reduce the severity of the withdrawal process. Drugs will not be passed to the baby in breast milk in sufficient quantities to have any major effect. Breastfeeding is best performed immediately before taking medication and should be avoided for up to 2 hours afterwards. Breastfeeding can also help the mother feel that she is actively involved in the care of her baby and that she may be able to settle the baby better, particularly if there are significant withdrawal signs.

Women with hepatitis B or C can also be encouraged to breastfeed. Babies with neonatal abstinence syndrome who are being successfully breastfed may not require pharmacological treatment.

Pharmacological treatment

The paediatric team should review all babies with neonatal abstinence syndrome daily. In babies where there are minor signs, pharmacological treatment should be avoided. However, approximately half of babies exposed to opiates *in utero* will require treatment for neonatal abstinence syndrome (Lall, 2008). Therefore when babies are not responding to conservative methods of treatment, pharmacological treatment may be required. Depending on hospital policy and staffing levels it still may be possible to treat babies with neonatal abstinence syndrome on the postnatal ward, thereby keeping mother and baby together. Where this is not possible and if the baby becomes more difficult to manage, admission to the neonatal unit will be necessary.

The aim of treatment is to reduce distress and control potentially dangerous signs. A scoring chart can be used to assess the level of distress. As with all tools of this nature they can be subjective and open to interpretation. Continuity of carer can help alleviate the problems with subjectivity and getting to know the babies' behaviour and symptoms is a key component of the care. One-off episodes of scoring the baby are

Major signs of opiate withdrawal
• Convulsions (rare – 5 per cent)
• Profuse vomiting
• Watery diarrhoea
• Inability to coordinate sucking, requiring tube feeding
• Baby inconsolable after two consecutive feeds.

Table 12.2   Treatment for symptoms of neonatal abstinence syndrome

Drug	Indication	Dose	Frequency	Comments
Morphine	Maternal opioids	40 µg/kg orally	4 hourly	Increase by 20 µg/kg. If baby feeding well and settled reduce by 10 per cent every 24 hours
Phenobarbital	Seizures	4 mg/kg	Daily	20 mg/kg IV loading dose
Chloral hydrate	Sedation	30 mg/kg orally	6 hourly	As required
Chlorpromazine	Maternal benzodiazepines	1 mg/kg orally	8 hourly	Can reduce seizure threshold

Neonatal bedside guidelines (2007), Northern Neonatal Network (2006).

not helpful and can be misleading, causing the inappropriate administration of treatment.

When the mother has been using opioids, a morphine derivative is usually effective in controlling the baby's symptoms (Table 12.2).

Cocaine

Cocaine is a powerful stimulant and vasoconstrictor and it creates a euphoric effect when taken, which is thought to be a result of the stimulation of dopamine. Vasoconstriction in early pregnancy can cause miscarriage as well as premature delivery. The effects on the fetus can be severe since cocaine is a teratogen, causing defects to the organs and limbs, intrauterine growth restriction and underdevelopment of the brain. Babies born to cocaine-using mothers can have gastrointestinal anomalies, urogenital anomalies and microcephaly. It is also thought that cocaine bingeing can cause fetal brain infarcts. Children of cocaine-using mothers may also have learning difficulties and attention deficit syndromes in childhood.

Following delivery these babies will display symptoms similar to those of opiate-dependent babies. However, the symptoms may be more acute; the babies may not settle well, have long periods of deep or unsettled sleep as well as abnormal sleep patterns and may experience 'panicked awakening'. The principles of care are the same as for neonatal abstinence syndrome.

Amphetamines

According to Whittaker (2003) there is no conclusive evidence that amphetamine use directly affects preg-

nancy outcome. There is inconclusive evidence of the effects on the developing fetus. However, because it is a strong stimulant it can cause vasoconstriction and hypertension in pregnancy and as a result the fetus can become hypoxic and may be small for gestational age.

There is a possibility that the baby of the amphetamine-taking mother will also suffer some withdrawal symptoms following birth and as with other substance-dependent babies will require careful monitoring and individualized treatment.

Benzodiazepines

Taking benzodiazepines during pregnancy is associated with cleft lip and palate in the fetus following prolonged high-dose abuse. The midwife should advise the woman to reduce her benzodiazepine use during pregnancy because of its teratogenic effect. Babies will suffer some withdrawal symptoms which can be severe and may not present until as late as day 12.

Cannabis

Cannabis is the most common drug used in Europe; however, there is very little evidence on its effect in pregnancy. Nevertheless, the half-life is between 36 and 72 hours and withdrawal may be delayed. Babies can be small for gestational age as a result of cannabis being mixed with tobacco and smoked. Symptoms in babies are similar to those of opiate users; babies also do not sleep well, have increased activity and experience jitters. In addition, babies of cannabis-smoking mothers may have problems maintaining their blood glucose following delivery.

Longer term effects include hyperactivity and inattention symptoms up to the age of 10.

Caffeine

High-energy drinks packed with caffeine are popular and readily available in supermarkets. Women who drink these products and/or strong coffee regularly during pregnancy may be putting their baby at risk of withdrawal. The symptoms of withdrawal may last up to five days following delivery and may even last a few weeks. They include feeding difficulties, vomiting, excessive crying, poor sleep patterns and irritability, probably due to headache.

Tobacco

The effect of smoking in pregnancy causing low birth-weight is greater than that from heroin. The effects of nicotine, cyanide and carbon monoxide in cigarette smoking are well noted and smoking cessation services have very good success rates with pregnant women. Other family members should also be advised to stop smoking and can access smoking cessation services free of charge in the UK. Pregnancy is often the catalyst for a woman to stop smoking.

Babies of mothers who smoke during pregnancy may exhibit some withdrawal symptoms such as jitteriness, exaggerated startle reflex, hyperactivity and may be difficult to comfort.

Concealed drug-taking during pregnancy

Some women will conceal the fact they are using illicit substances during pregnancy. As a result their babies when born will demonstrate withdrawal that will be unexpected to the midwife. If the baby is displaying symptoms of withdrawal and the mother denies taking drugs during pregnancy there are investigations that can determine the cause of the baby's symptoms.

- *Urinalysis* can detect recent use of cocaine or its metabolites, amphetamines, cannabis, barbiturates and opiates. However, high levels of false-positive results make the test unreliable.

- *Meconium testing* detects exposure to cocaine and its metabolites. It is more accurate than urine testing since it has a higher sensitivity.

- *Hair analysis* is an effective means of detecting narcotics, cannabis or cocaine/alcohol metabolites. It can detect drug exposure in the last three months of pregnancy and up to 2–3 months postpartum.

Fetal alcohol spectrum disorders

Like many of the substances discussed in this chapter, alcohol is a teratogenic compound that readily crosses the placenta. The most overwhelming effects are the intellectual disabilities associated with the adverse impact of alcohol on fetal brain development and the central nervous system. According to Wattendorf and Muenke (2005), fetal alcohol spectrum disorder (FASD) is an umbrella term for a set of disorders caused by the consumption of alcohol during pregnancy, with fetal alcohol syndrome (FAS) being the most commonly recognizable form. The full presentation of fetal alcohol syndrome involves characteristic facial features as well as growth and neurocognitive deficits (Mukherjee *et al.*, 2006).

Other terms associated with fetal alcohol spectrum disorder are partial fetal alcohol syndrome (PFAS), alcohol-related birth defects (ARBD) and alcohol-related neurodevelopment disorders (ARND).

Pathology

Fetal alcohol spectrum disorder is not a hereditary condition. Even at low concentration levels ethanol (which is a toxin) when taken throughout pregnancy can cause significant damage to the developing fetus. Ethanol inhibits cell molecule adhesion, having subsequent effects on neuronal migration because it alters the cell cycle. Neuronal damage and cell loss in the fetal brain are caused by even small levels of ethanol in the circulation. Ethanol alters glucose utilization and transport which suppresses protein and DNA synthesis. Cell damage and cell death also occurs, which seriously affects the developing brain. In addition, ethanol can cause altered placental function, with hypoxia and ischaemia.

It is interesting to note that there is no particular time during pregnancy when it is safe to drink alcohol.

Wattendorf and Muenke (2005) suggest that central nervous system damage may result at any time, even at around the time of a pregnancy test, which can be very soon after conception. This is of particular relevance to the binge-drinking culture in the UK, particularly when compounded with unprotected sex.

Characteristics

Fetal alcohol syndrome is the most clinically recognized fetal alcohol spectrum disorder (Figure 12.1). The characteristics are multi-faceted and include the following (Mukherjee *et al.*, 2006; British Medical Association, 2007):

- *CNS dysfunction*: This is permanent impairment of brain function which leads to attention deficits, poor social understanding, hyperactivity, developmental and intellectual difficulties, poor coordination, language and memory difficulties, attention deficits, social understanding difficulties and planning difficulties.
- *Pre- and postnatal growth deficiency.* Babies with fetal alcohol syndrome are small and remain small all their lives.
- *Facial dysmorphology*: Fetal alcohol syndrome is associated with abnormal facial features which include short palpebral fissures, thin upper lip vermillion and a flattened philtrum.

Other facial features include microcephaly, flat midface, epicanthal folds, upturned nose with a flat nasal bridge, ptosis of the eyelids and underdeveloped ears. Clindactyly of the fifth finger is also common, as is 'hockey stick' palmer creases.

Antenatal care

Drinking alcohol in pregnancy is still seen to be socially acceptable and there is conflicting advice on safe levels of alcohol consumption during pregnancy. The current advice to women is not to drink alcohol at all during the first three months of pregnancy (NICE, 2008). However, the binge-drinking culture in the UK, particularly among the young, will take many years to change, problematic drinking is still seen and there is a general lack of awareness of the effects of drinking in pregnancy.

Because measures of alcohol in the home are likely to be greater than those in bars and restaurants accurate estimation of alcohol consumption in pregnancy cannot always be made.

Midwives do ask women about their drinking habits at antenatal booking and it is usually documented in the hand-held notes. However, women who drink heavily preconceptually are likely to continue drinking throughout pregnancy. If possible, the midwife should attempt to identify women with problem drinking in early pregnancy, although this may not be easy since many women are able to conceal their addiction. Taylor (2003) recommends the use of 'T-ACE' as a tool for identifying problem drinkers:

- **T** (tolerance) How many drinks does it take to make you feel high? Answer: **3** or more scores 2 points
- **A** (annoyance) Have people annoyed you by criticizing your drinking? Answer: **Yes** scores 1 point
- **C** (cut down) Have you ever felt you need to cut down your drinking? Answer: **Yes** scores 1 point
- **E** (eye opener) Have you ever had a drink first thing in the morning to 'steady your nerves' or to get rid of a hangover? Answer: **Yes** scores 1 point

A total score of greater than or equal to 2 points is considered positive.

Other adverse outcomes of maternal alcohol consumption include:

- infertility
- miscarriage
- preterm delivery and stillbirth.

Management

Prevention of fetal alcohol spectrum disorder is the aim of any preconception or antenatal care. Recognition of the dangers of alcohol consumption during pregnancy is the responsibility of the midwife as well as identifying the signs of alcohol abuse in the pregnant woman, which is very difficult to do unless she is already being treated for alcohol-related problems by another professional. If a hazardous drinking score is obtained using the T-ACE or any other recognized test, the midwife can with the mother's consent refer her to a specialist team, which will include the obstetrician, community psychiatric nurse and local alcohol service for specialist assessment and advice.

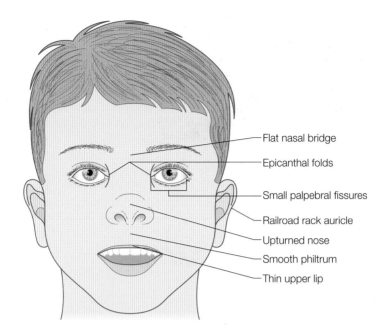

(a)

- Flat nasal bridge
- Epicanthal folds
- Small palpebral fissures
- Railroad rack auricle
- Upturned nose
- Smooth philtrum
- Thin upper lip

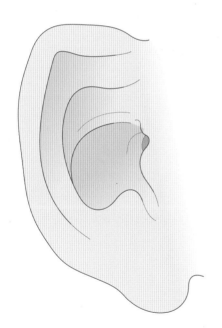

(b)

Figure 12.1 (a) Characteristic facial features in a child with fetal alcohol spectrum disorder include a smooth philtrum, thin upper lip, upturned nose, flat nasal bridge, and midface, epicanthal folds, small palpebral fissures and small head circumference. (b) Characteristic features of an ear of a child with fetal alcohol spectrum disorder. Note the underdeveloped upper part of the ear parallel to the ear crease below. (c) Lip–philtrum guide: The smoothness of the philtrum and the thinness of the upper lip are assessed individually on a scale of 1 to 5 (1 = unaffected, 5 = most severe). The patient must have a relaxed facial expression, because a smile can alter lip thinness and philtrum smoothness. Scores of 4 and 5 in addition to short palpebral fissures, correspond to fetal alcohol syndrome. (Reproduced from Wattendorf and Muenke (2005) with kind permission of the author, Darryl Leja, NHGRI NIH)

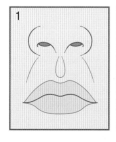  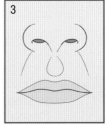 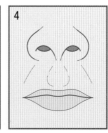 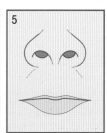

(c)

Detoxification should be considered at any gestation because dependent alcohol use is such a serious risk to the fetus. However, detoxification should only be managed closely with monitoring of the woman and fetus, since sudden cessation of drinking is potentially dangerous. Maternal seizures caused by sudden cessation of drinking can cause fetal distress.

Babies with fetal alcohol spectrum disorders are often misdiagnosed at birth because the facial dysmorphology can be confused with syndromes such as Cornelia de Lange and Williams' syndromes, which have similar clinical characteristics (British Medical Association, 2007). Recognition of fetal alcohol spectrum disorder at birth or in the perinatal period is rare since other characteristics such as developmental delay, hyperactivity and attention deficits will only manifest themselves later in childhood. Nevertheless, formal diagnosis is required at the earliest possible time since specialist services and treatment programmes can be accessed.

In the UK fetal alcohol spectrum disorder is often underdiagnosed because of a lack of a specific diagnostic test, underreporting of alcohol consumption, difficulty in detecting the features of fetal alcohol spectrum disorder and a general lack of knowledge of the disorders among healthcare professionals (British Medical Association, 2007). Ongoing coordinated care of both the woman and her child is required so that they both have access to appropriate resources and services.

Alcohol withdrawal

As with other neonatal dependencies, alcohol withdrawal is likely to occur if the woman has been drinking throughout pregnancy. The level and intensity of withdrawal will depend on the amount of alcohol consumed throughout pregnancy and when the last drink was taken before the onset of labour. The withdrawal effects are similar to neonatal abstinence syndrome and include jitteriness, irritability, hypotonia, exaggerated Moro reflex, poor feeding and seizures. The treatment will depend upon the severity of symptoms and, where possible, non-pharmacological methods should be tried as for neonatal abstinence syndrome before resorting to medication. The regime for medical treatment will be similar to that for neonatal abstinence syndrome.

Child protection

Problem drug and alcohol use either alone or combined in pregnancy and in the postnatal period can have serious negative consequences on the women themselves, their families and the people around them. The misuse of drugs can have an adverse impact on their health and behaviour but can also affect the welfare, development and health of their babies. In spite of many enquiries and the changes to child protection laws and practice, child deaths and neglect still occur.

It should be recognized that the majority of pregnant women with substance misuse problems will provide satisfactory care for their children. However, it is also acknowledged that some babies and children of substance-abusing parents are more at risk of:

- inadequate supervision
- lack of stimulation
- inconsistent caring
- social isolation
- exposure to violence
- emotional and physical neglect and abuse (Whittaker, 2003).

It is essential that the midwife recognizes that there may be consequences from neglect, such as failure to thrive and non-accidental injury. Good communication with other professionals is necessary to avoid catastrophic consequences. The welfare of the baby is paramount and when there is any doubt of the mother's ability to care for her baby appropriately an interagency approach is critical. The midwife should always refer to local guidelines, which should be followed with an urgent referral to social services.

Conclusion

The misuse of drugs is an ever-increasing problem in the UK, with substance abuse starting at earlier ages and crossing all social spectrums. It is likely that most midwives will encounter women with drug or alcohol problems in their professional workload. There are many specialist services available for women who take drugs during their pregnancy but there are less coordinated services for women who drink alcohol during pregnancy. The midwife is in a central position to mobilize services for both the mother and her baby.

Recognition of women who are at risk of having a baby with neonatal abstinence syndrome or fetal alcohol spectrum disorder is an important element of the midwife's role. This will ensure that when the baby is born, appropriate evidence-based care can be managed in a coordinated and organized manner, allowing the baby to be cared for in an environment that is conducive to their withdrawal symptoms.

Key Points

- Healthcare professionals should adopt a non-judgmental approach to the substance-misusing woman during pregnancy, childbirth and the postnatal period.
- Continuous, co-ordinated and collaborative antenatal care can provide a planned, structured framework of care for the woman and her baby.
- The management of the environment is crucial in the early neonatal period for babies withdrawing from maternal substance use.

References

Bancroft A, Wilson S and Burley S (2004) *Parental Drug and Alcohol Misuse: Resilience and transition among young people.* York: Joseph Rowntree Foundation.

Brennan K (2002) Britain is the worst in Europe for teenage pregnancy rates. www.studentbjm.com

British Medical Association (2007) *Fetal Alcohol Spectrum Disorders. A guide for healthcare professionals.* London: BMA. www.bma.org.uk

British National Formulary (2008) www.bnf.org

EMCDDA (European Monitoring Centre for Drugs and Drug Addiction) (2007) Drug use and related problems among very young people (under 15 years old). www.emcdda.eu

Hulse GK, Milne E, English DR and Holman CD (1997) The relationship between maternal use of heroin and methadone and infant birth weight. *Addiction* **92**: 1571–1579.

Jackson L (2006) Handling drug misuse in the neonatal unit. *Infant* **2**: 64–67.

Lall A (2008) Neonatal abstinence syndrome. *British Journal of Midwifery* **16**: 220–223.

Mukherjee RAS, Hollins S and Turk J (2006) Fetal alcohol spectrum disorder: an overview. *Journal of the Royal Society of Medicine* **99**: 298–302.

Mupanemunda R and Watkinson M (2005) *Key Topics in Neonatology*, 2nd edn. London: Taylor and Francis.

Neonatal Bedside Guidelines (2007) The Bedside Clinical Guidelines Partnership in association with Shropshire, Staffordshire and Black Country Neonatal Networks, Stoke-on-Trent, Sherwin Rivers. www.newbornnetworks.org.uk

NICE (National Institute for Health and Clinical Excellence) (2008) Antenatal care. Routine care for the healthy pregnant woman. http://www.nice.org.uk/guidance/index.jsp?action=byID&o=11947 [accessed July 2009].

Northern Neonatal Network (2006) *Neonatal Formulary: Drug use in pregnancy and the first year of life.* London. BMJ Books.

Office of National Statistics (2006) Drinking to excess rising among women. http://www.statistics.gov.uk/cci/nugget.asp?id=922 [accessed July 2009].

Slattery MM and Morrison JJ (2002) Preterm delivery. *Lancet* **360**(9344): 1489–1497.

Taylor DJ (2003) *Alcohol Consumption in Pregnancy.* London: Guidelines and Audit Subcommittee of the Royal College of Obstetricians and Gynaecologists. www.rcog.org.uk

Tucker Blackburn S (2003) *Maternal, Fetal & Neonatal Physiology. A clinical perspective.* St Louis: Saunders.

UNICEF/WHO (2006) *Baby Friendly Hospital Initiative. Revised, updated and expanded for integrated care. Section 1: background and implementation.* New York: UNICEF. http://www.unicef.org/newsline/tensteps.htm [accessed 9 September 2009].

Wattendorf DJ and Muenke M (2005) Fetal alcohol spectrum disorders. *American Family Physician* **72**: 279–285.

Whittaker A (2003) *Substance Misuse in Pregnancy. A resource pack for professional in Lothian.* Edinburgh: NHS Lothian. www.nhslothian.scot.nhs.uk

BIRTH INJURY

Jane Henley

OVERVIEW

The mechanical forces of labour and delivery will sometimes cause birth injury despite skilled midwifery and obstetric care. A risk assessment for each woman and a careful plan for delivery should reduce the incidence but the specific circumstances and progress of each labour may result in an injury to the newborn. In this chapter the risk factors and different types of injuries are discussed.

Introduction

Birth injures are often unavoidable during a complicated vaginal delivery and can be difficult to predict. However, the majority of injuries are minor and will resolve quickly without treatment or long-term complications. They require only careful observation and reassurance for the parents. More serious injuries will be apparent immediately after birth and require attention from the paediatric team. Other injuries may not be apparent until a few hours or days later and will be noted by the parent or the midwife. Some newborns with a birth injury will need close monitoring, observation and follow-up by a paediatric specialist after discharge from midwifery care. The most severe, rare injuries may lead to serious problems for the child and may even be life-threatening.

Risk factors for birth injuries

Many risk factors have been identified and there is often more than one risk factor complicating the labour and delivery. Risk factors include:

- large baby
- breech vaginal delivery
- breech presentation
- instrumental delivery
- cephalopelvic disproportion
- dystocia
- malpresentation
- brow, face presentation
- compound presentation
- unusual progress in labour: prolonged labour, precipitate labour
- fetal distress
- small baby for gestational age
- prematurity
- multiple pregnancy.

Handling of the slippery baby immediately after delivery is also a risk factor

Extracranial and scalp injuries

The commonest birth injuries to the head are caput succedaneum and cephalhaematoma.

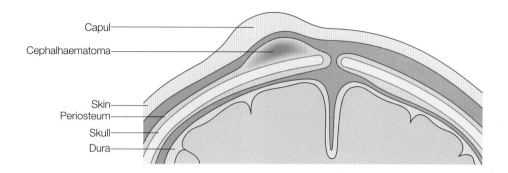

Labels: Capul, Cephalhaematoma, Skin, Periosteum, Skull, Dura

Figure 13.1 Caput and cephalhaematoma

Caput succedaneum

'Caput' is extremely common. A soft, swollen, circular-shaped bruise (ecchymosis) can be seen on the head in the area of the scalp that was the presenting portion during labour. Pressure on that area during labour causes oedema of the superficial soft tissue above the periosteum of the cranial bone. The periosteum is a thick fibrous membrane that covers the surface of bone (Figure 13.1).

The caput feels soft to the touch and will pit with applied fingertip pressure. It may extend over and across the suture lines since the swelling is above the periosteum. Although caput is benign, parents are often concerned about the large bruise on their baby's head. They can be reassured that the bruising is not 'on the brain', that it will improve and resolve over a few days and that no treatment is required.

A similar circular area of oedema and bruising is often caused by the pressure applied during vacuum extraction delivery. This caput-like bruising is referred to as a 'chignon'. Sometimes the skin may also be damaged. As with caput, the chignon will improve over several days. The parents should be advised to keep the area dry if there is skin damage. Infection of the damaged skin is rare.

Cephalhaematoma

Not as common as caput, cephalhaematoma is seen in 1:100 births (Levene *et al.*, 2008). Unlike the softer caput, cephalhaematoma is a firm swelling or bump on the newborn head, often without any visible bruising, formed when blood collects beneath the perios-

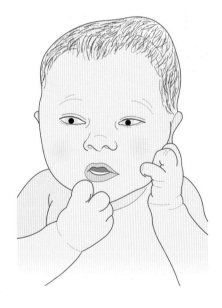

Figure 13.2 Cephalhaematoma

teum of one of the newborn skull bones (see Figure 13.1). Unlike caput, this swelling is limited and confined by the skull bone. It does not cross the suture lines because the periosteum is attached to the margins of the skull bone and so the bleeding is confined within that area. One of the parietal bones is most commonly affected (Figure 13.2).

Cephalhaematoma is caused by rupture or tearing of the blood vessels beneath the periosteum. It results

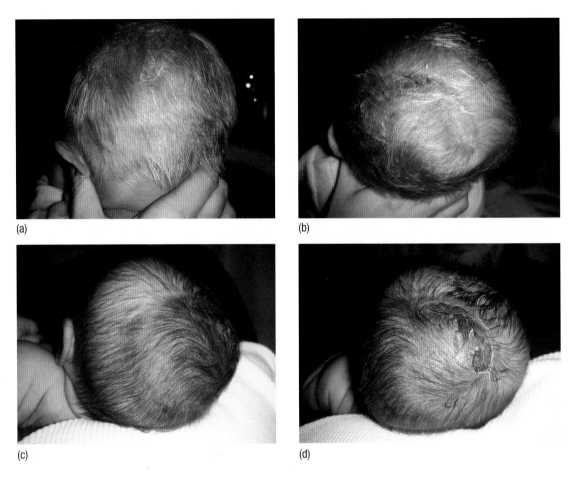

(a)

(b)

(c)

(d)

Figure 13.3   (a) Caput and vacuum extraction chignon. (b) Caput. (c) Vacuum extraction chignon and damaged scalp. (d) Caput and cephalhaematoma

from the mechanical forces of the fetal skull pushing against the maternal ischial spines or against the symphisis during labour. It is commonly associated with prolonged labours and instrumental deliveries.

Sometimes the cephalhaematoma is bilateral and bumps are seen on both sides of the head.

Rarely, newborns with cephalhaematoma may also have a linear fracture of the skull bone. If the newborn head is severely traumatized and there is bruising, abrasions and cephalhaematoma, the paediatric team may arrange an X-ray of the skull to check for fracture.

Because the bleeding beneath the periosteum is usually quite slow the swelling of a cephalhaematoma is rarely seen immediately after birth. It is often first noticed by concerned parents later after the delivery (Figure 13.3). Although no treatment is necessary and

parents can be reassured that the swelling will go down eventually, they should be warned that this could take 6–8 weeks.

The newborn with cephalhaematoma has a higher risk of jaundice due to haemolysis of the blood that has collected beneath the periosteum. It is prudent to warn the parents that their baby is likely to become jaundiced and to require blood tests for monitoring of serum bilirubin. Phototherapy may be used to treat the hyperbilirubinaemia (see Chapter 9).

Subaponeurotic haemorrhage (subgaleal haemorrhage)

Subaponeurotic haemorrhage is rare. It occurs in 1:1250 births (Levene *et al.*, 2008). The galeal aponeurosis is the loose tissue connecting the occipital and frontal muscles of the head. It is a potential space between the scalp and the periosteum. Rupture of the blood vessels within this space will cause a subaponeurotic haemorrhage. A firm but fluctuant 'wobbly' swelling that crosses the suture lines will appear on the newborn head quite soon after birth, usually within 4 hours. The swelling will become much larger as the bleeding continues within the galeal aponeurosis. The head size increases rapidly. Sometimes the swelling mass may extend into the neck and even cause the ears to appear anteriorly displaced.

Subaponeurotic haemorrhage is associated with a prolonged second stage of labour, instrumental delivery, vacuum extraction and with prematurity. The trauma is caused as the fetal head is first compressed and then pulled through the pelvic outlet. It is much more serious than cephalhaematoma since a considerable amount of blood may haemorrhage into the subaponeurotic space. Significant blood loss will lead to hypovolaemic shock and severe anaemia. It can be life-threatening.

The newborn with a wobbly swelling on the head needs immediate referral to the paediatric team. Shock may develop very quickly. The baby will have tachycardia, pallor, delayed capillary refill time, poor tone and signs of respiratory distress. Urgent investigations for haemoglobin and haematocrit monitoring are necessary. There may be an underlying coagulopathy that is contributing to the bleeding, so coagulopathy screening must be performed. A skull X-ray will be arranged to check for fracture.

Severe shock due to blood loss into the subaponeurotic space will need urgent treatment in a neonatal unit. The newborn may require a blood transfusion and transfusions of fresh frozen plasma and coagulation factors. There is an increased risk of jaundice and hyperbilirubinaemia due to haemolysis of the blood that is collecting in the subaponeurotic space so monitoring of serum bilirubin will also be necessary. The swelling may take 2–3 weeks to improve.

Forceps marks and other bruising

Bruising (ecchymosis) and the imprints of forceps blades are often seen on the newborn head following instrumental delivery. Occasionally there may be skin abrasions. Bruises may also be caused by fingers handling the slippery baby at delivery. The parents will be concerned about the bruising. They can be reassured

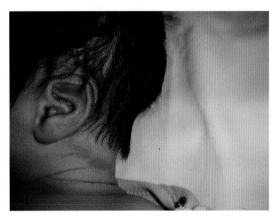

Figure 13.4 Bruise from forceps delivery

that the bruises and forceps marks usually fade and heal rapidly over a few days.

The newborn body and limbs may be bruised by handling during a rapid delivery or an emergency caesarean section delivery. Preterm babies are easily bruised during labour and delivery (Figure 13.4).

Lacerations and abrasions

Lacerations may occur during incision of the uterus during caesarean section, especially in an emergency situation. The blade may nick the face or head. These lacerations are usually small and heal well. They may require Steri-Strip taping to oppose the edges. If suturing is required, the newborn should be referred to a paediatric plastic surgeon for application of specialist suturing techniques.

Abrasions are commonly caused by fetal scalp electrodes and sometimes following artificial rupture of the membranes during labour. They tend to heal quickly.

Traumatic petechiae (traumatic cyanosis)

Petechiae are tiny 'pin-prick' spots that cause a rash-like appearance over the face and head after birth. They are associated with the increase of pressure on the head and chest during delivery and are often seen in newborns whose umbilical cord has been tightly around the neck at birth. Precipitous labour and a very short second stage of labour may also cause traumatic petechiae over the baby's head and neck.

In the majority of newborns there is no cause for concern. The parents can be reassured that the tiny spots will fade after 3–4 days and no treatment is needed. However, similar petechiae are also associated with coagulopathy and serious clotting disorders. Therefore the newborn with traumatic petechiae must always be reviewed by the paediatric team.

Cranial injuries/skull fractures

Fractures of the skull are rare despite the considerable pressure and distortion applied to the fetal skull during labour and delivery. If fractures do occur there may be a predisposing factor such as osteogenesis imperfecta.

Skull fractures of the parietal bones may result from compression forces during application of forceps. They may also be caused by the mechanical forces of the skull pressing against the maternal pelvis during the labour. Occipital fractures may occur during breech vaginal delivery.

Skull fractures are linear or depressed. A linear fracture (commonest form) may be present with cephalhaematoma. However, linear fractures often have no symptoms and they require no treatment. Depressed skull fractures are similar to pressing inwards on a ping-pong ball. The skull bone buckles inward and fractures. The most frequent cause of depressed fracture is application of forceps, although it must be remembered that such fractures are very rare. As with linear fractures, there may be no symptoms although the 'ping pong' fracture may be palpable when the newborn's head is handled. The paediatric team will arrange X-ray of the skull to review the fracture. Many newborn depressed skull fractures resolve without any treatment. Others may require surgery.

Newborns with a skull fracture will be monitored by the paediatric team to assess that healing of the bone is taking place and that there are no further complications. In very rare cases of skull fracture the newborn will be ill and have neurological symptoms. In such cases there may have been direct damage to the cerebrum by the fractured bone. There may be free bone fragments and intracranial bleeding. Specialist paediatric neurosurgical assessment will be required.

Intracranial injuries

Intracranial haemorrhage caused by birth injury is very rare. It should not be confused with the intraventricular haemorrhage that is associated with prematurity. The incidence of major subdural haemorrhage in the newborn is 1:50 000 (Levene *et al.*, 2008).

High and mid-cavity forceps delivery has been linked to intracranial haemorrhage in the past. However, this method of delivery is now rarely used and caesarean section will usually be performed if there is lack of progress in labour. Other risk factors for intracranial haemorrhage are a precipitous delivery, a prolonged second stage of labour, and a large baby. Intracranial haemorrhage has also been linked to maternal aspirin and phenobarbital use.

Intracranial haemorrhage is caused by the traumatic tearing of blood vessels and venous sinuses within the skull. The trauma results from the application of pressure on the head followed by a rapid release of pressure during the labour and delivery. Lacerations of the tentorium, the falx cerebri or the superficial cerebral vein may result from the pressure changes.

Overextension of the head during vaginal breech delivery may cause occipital osteodiastasis. The occipital bone separates and can cause direct trauma to the cerebellum. Intracranial haemorrhage will result.

The newborn with intracranial haemorrhage may be very ill at birth, requiring resuscitation and transfer to a neonatal unit. There may be a fracture of the skull.

Bruises, abrasions and damaged areas of scalp may be visible on the head, particularly if the delivery was instrumental.

In very rare cases massive intracranial haemorrhage will lead to sudden deterioration and death. However, the newborn with intracranial haemorrhage may also initially appear to be normal. As the bleeding continues within the head, the intracranial pressure will increase and the baby will slowly show signs of irritability. There may be signs of respiratory distress; tachypnoea and nasal flaring. Apnoeic episodes can occur as the intracranial pressure rises. Abnormal neurological signs will develop. A tense and possibly bulging anterior fontanelle will be caused by the increased intracranial pressure. In serious cases the newborn may even have eye deviation and unequal pupils. The pupils become fixed and dilated due to the intracranial pressure. The baby will be lethargic and hypotonic. Apnoea and bradycardia, and seizures will occur in severe cases.

The newborn with intracranial haemorrhage needs intensive care in a neonatal unit. An X-ray will be arranged to check for skull fracture. Cranial ultrasound scanning may identify the haemorrhage and an MRI or CT scan may be more sensitive in aiding diagnosis. Even if the baby appears to be well on discharge home, there will be long-term follow-up of neurological development.

Facial injuries

Dislocation of the nasal septum

Pressure on the fetal head and face during labour and delivery may cause dislocation of the cartilaginous nasal septum. This will result in deviation of the nose to one side. The nose looks 'squashed'. The columella (the fleshy portion in front of the nasal septum) will lean to the side opposite the dislocation. The nares appear to be asymmetrical and flattened on the side of the dislocation. The dislocated septum will be more apparent if a fingertip is pressed gently against the tip of the nose (Jeppesen and Windfeld test). Gentle pressure will cause collapse of the nostrils.

There is a risk of airway obstruction and long-term cosmetic deformity. The newborn should be referred to the paediatric team and may require specialist ENT care for manual reduction of the dislocation within the first few days of life.

Eye injuries

Subconjunctival haemorrhages and oedema of the eyelids are common in the newborn. They are caused by pressure on the head during the labour and delivery. Parents are often concerned but they can be reassured that the small red areas in the whites of the eyes and the swelling of the eyelids will improve and need no treatment.

Rarely, an instrumental delivery or the application of a fetal monitoring electrode to a brow presentation may cause lacerations of the eyelid or even more significant damage to the eye. Any injury to the periorbital area requires paediatric assessment. Injuries to the eye itself need specialist ophthalmological referral.

Fractures

Fractures of long bones occur in 1:1000 births (Levene et al., 2008).

Fractured clavicle

The clavicle is the most frequently fractured bone during birth. Risk factors for clavicle fracture are a large baby, a prolonged second stage of labour, shoulder dystocia, instrumental deliveries and vaginal breech deliveries. Very occasionally an audible snap may be heard during the birth. However, a fractured clavicle may also be found in a newborn of normal birthweight following a normal uneventful delivery. Many newborns with fractured clavicle are asymptomatic. The baby shows no signs of distress or discomfort but may have decreased movement of the arm on the side of the fracture. A fractured clavicle may be found in cases of obstetric brachial plexus palsy.

Examination and palpation of the clavicles with the first and second fingers will reveal crepitation or a palpable abnormality in the area. There may be bruising and swelling. The fracture will be confirmed with X-ray. Incomplete fractures require no treatment and heal spontaneously. A callus will form during healing and this can cause quite a large lump in the area. The parents must be warned to expect to feel a lump on the collar bone. Complete fractures are treated by immobilizing the affected arm for approximately one week. The easiest way to immobilize the arm is to tuck it inside the newborn's vest so it is held across the body with the elbow bent at a comfortable right angle. Alternatively the baby can be dressed in a long-sleeved vest and the sleeve taped to the front of the vest.

Fractured humerus

Fracture of the humerus is much less common and the incidence is 1:1000 (Levene et al., 2008). It is associated with difficulty during the delivery and with vaginal breech delivery. An audible snap may be heard during birth. The newborn will have decreased movement of the affected arm. There will be swelling, crepitus and the arm will be obviously deformed. The baby will be in pain especially during handling and may be pyrexial.

The fracture will be confirmed with X-ray. Initially the affected arm should be immobilized by supporting the arm across the body with the elbow bent at a comfortable right angle as described for the care of fractured clavicle. Paracetamol will be prescribed for pain relief. In the longer term binding and strapping of the arm across the body is often necessary to support the limb and reduce pain. A simple backslab splint may be recommended by the orthopaedic specialist and reduction of the fracture could be required if the bone is displaced. The newborn skin underneath the strapping will need care and attention to prevent soreness. Observe the fingers and hand of the affected arm for normal movement, warmth and circulation. The fractured humerus is likely to heal well and long-term damage is rare.

It may be prudent for the paediatric team to rule out other orthopaedic problems and underlying bone disorders such as osteogenesis imperfecta.

Nerve injury

Trauma during labour and delivery may cause nerve injury. The nerves may be stretched or twisted or even torn and separated from their root.

Obstetric brachial plexus palsy

Obstetric brachial plexus palsy can result from a traumatic stretching injury during delivery of the head and neck. The incidence is 1:1000 births (Levene *et al.*, 2008). The brachial plexus is a group of nerves that supply the shoulder, arm and hand. The nerve roots start in the cervical spinal cord: C5, C6, C7, C8. Traction and excessive pulling on the shoulder at the same time as lateral or sideways stretching of the head away from the shoulder may stretch and twist the brachial plexus. If emergency procedures are also performed in order to deliver shoulder dystocia, the stretching is increased because there is simultaneous external suprapubic pressure on the shoulder from the symphysis pubis.

Obstetric brachial plexus palsy is not always associated with shoulder dystocia, however. The stretching injury may occur during vaginal delivery of the head in breech presentation, particularly if there is cephalo-pelvic disproportion. It is also possible that the injury to the brachial plexus may have begun *in utero*. Malposition or pressure on a shoulder from the maternal pelvis during the pregnancy may be contributing factors.

Obstetric brachial plexus palsy can be accompanied by fractures of the clavicle and/or the humerus. Occasionally, there is also facial nerve palsy.

There are four different types of nerve injury:

- stretched – neurapraxia
- stretched and torn – axonotmesis

Factors associated with obstetric brachial plexus palsy

- Large birthweight >3.5 kg
- Shoulder dystocia
- Vaginal breech delivery
- Assisted delivery
- Prolonged second stage
- Precipitous second stage
- Abnormal presentation
- Multiparous mother
- Fetal distress.

- ruptured – neurotmesis
- separated at root – avulsion.

Injuries following neurapraxia and axonotmesis tend to have a better prognosis than those that result from neurotmesis and avulsion. The effects of the latter can be very severe indeed.

Erb's palsy

Ninety per cent of cases of obstetric brachial plexus palsy are classified as Erb's palsy. This injury involves the upper part of the plexus: C5, C6 and sometimes C7. The damage is the result of the nerve roots being stretched (neurapraxia) and oedema and swelling occurs.

The most obvious clinical sign is lack of movement in the newborn arm. One arm will be actively moving but the other arm remains limply at the baby's side. However, the fingers will be seen to move and flex and the grasp reflex is present. Closer examination will show that the arm is adopting a particular appearance, traditionally described as the 'waiter's tip' posture (Figure 13.5). The arm is internally rotated at the shoulder. The elbow is extended and there is pronation of the forearm. The wrist will be flexed. The Moro reflex will be asymmetrical since the baby is unable to lift the affected arm. The clavicle may be fractured.

Klumpke's palsy

This is rare and comprises only about 1 per cent of cases of obstetric brachial plexus palsy. The lower part of the plexus is injured and C7–8 to T1 are the nerves involved. In Klumpke's palsy the affected arm is com-

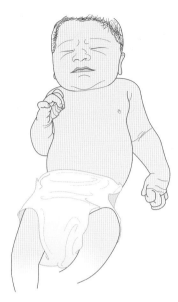

Figure 13.5   Erb's palsy

pletely flaccid as there is paralysis of the shoulder muscles and elbow flexors. The arm lies limply. There may be swelling in the shoulder region and the clavicle may be fractured.

Unlike Erb's palsy, there is weakness of the hand muscles and the grasp reflex is absent. The hand appears to be 'claw-like' since the finger flexors are affected. The baby should be carefully examined since a painful fractured humerus could be the reason for the lack of arm movement rather than Klumpke's palsy.

More severe obstetric brachial plexus palsy

Rarely, obstetric brachial plexus palsy may be accompanied by a phrenic nerve injury. C3, C4 and C5 will be affected, causing paralysis of one side of the diaphragm. In this case the newborn who has lack of movement in one arm will also have signs of respiratory distress. Tachypnoea is the most likely sign but there could also be sternal and intercostal recession, and dusky episodes.

The newborn will require supportive measures to manage the respiratory distress in a neonatal unit. Oxygen will be administered as required and there will be continuous monitoring of oxygen saturation and vital signs. Chest X-ray will show that the diaphragm is elevated. Very rarely the nerves are severed from the spinal cord completely. This is avulsion of the nerve roots. There will be complete paralysis of

the affected shoulder, arm and hand. Involvement of the T1 nerve may cause Horner's syndrome. The newborn will have a dilated pupil and drooping eyelid (ptosis) on the affected side. (Anhydrosis or absence of sweating is a symptom of Horner's syndrome that is not easily observed in the newborn so diagnosis relies on the former signs.)

Examination of the newborn with suspected obstetric brachial plexus palsy

Consider the history of the labour and delivery. A large baby, traumatic delivery and a history of shoulder dystocia increases the risk of obstetric brachial plexus palsy. The newborn who has a limp arm should be examined carefully. The arm should be handled gently to prevent further trauma to the shoulder, elbow and wrist joints. Use the first and second finger to gently palpate the clavicles as there may be a fracture on the affected side. Gently palpate and inspect the arm to assess whether there is a fracture of the humerus. After the examination arrange an X-ray to assess for fracture.

Carefully inspect and examine the other arm and the lower limbs to assess normal movement. Observe the face for any evidence of facial palsy, weakness, drooping eyelid and inability to close the eye. Observe the respiratory pattern and monitor the respiratory rate, bearing in mind the rare risk of a phrenic nerve injury that can cause respiratory distress.

Management of the newborn with obstetric brachial plexus palsy

Support and immobilize the affected arm across the baby's upper abdomen. The easiest way to do this is to tuck the arm inside the vest with the elbow at a comfortable right angle and the forearm across the torso. Alternatively the baby can be dressed in a long-sleeved vest and the sleeve taped to the front of the vest. The aim is to prevent the flaccid arm 'falling' down and causing traction on the shoulder. Keep the arm supported across the newborn torso during feeding. Bathing should be delayed.

Mild cases of Erb's palsy will usually recover within 3–4 days but other cases will need long-term therapy and even surgery. The newborn requires assessment by the paediatric team and by a physiotherapist. Physiotherapy is essential in the management of obstetric brachial plexus palsy. The main aim of therapy is to prevent the development of contractures and to maintain a full range of movement in the developing joints and muscles of both arms while waiting for recovery of the brachial plexus. Recovery could take months.

Passive range of motion exercises for the wrist, elbow, forearm and hand begin immediately. Shoulder exercises may be included in the regime after 48 hours if physiotherapy assessment indicates they are necessary. The parents will be taught how to perform the exercises, how to position the affected arm and to give tactile stimulation to the limb. The exercises and stimulation should be performed several times a day; for example at each nappy change. The importance of these exercises must be made clear to the parents. The baby's joints must remain supple to facilitate normal movement when the nerves recover or if surgery is required.

Regular assessment and therapy will continue during the first three months of life. There will be many hospital appointments for the family to attend. The majority of babies with obstetric brachial plexus palsy will recover by around four months of age. However, if there is no recovery of active elbow flexion by three months the baby will be referred to a specialist centre. Nerve graft surgery is considered if there is failure to recover biceps or wrist function by three months of age and in cases of Horner's syndrome or phrenic nerve injury.

There may be a long period during which there is uncertainty about the degree of nerve injury and permanent damage. Children with a persistent palsy will have a lifelong disability due to their reduced arm function. The family or the young adult with disability due to obstetric brachial plexus palsy may decide to initiate litigation.

Facial nerve palsy

Facial nerve palsy due to birth injury is not common. The incidence is 1:500 (Levene *et al.*, 2008). It is associated with forceps deliveries and with a prolonged second stage of labour. Pressure from the forceps or the prolonged pressure of the maternal ischial spines or maternal sacral promontory causes trauma and swelling around the nerve. This causes weakness of the facial muscles on the affected side. There will often be facial bruising and there may be abrasions from the forceps.

The newborn is unable to close the eye on the affected side. The eye will remain open (widened palpebral fissure) and during crying the mouth will

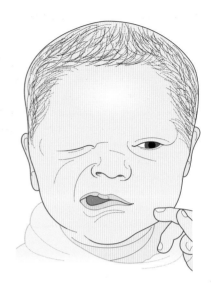

Figure 13.6   Facial palsy

appear to be asymmetrical and drawn away from the affected side (Figure 13.6). The nasolabial folds will appear to be unequal as the fold on the affected side is flattened. Careful examination and assessment by the paediatric team is required to determine that the facial palsy is due to birth injury and not due to a congenital dysmorphic syndrome.

The focus of treatment is to protect the affected eye and prevent corneal damage. An eye pad can be taped in place to keep the eyelid closed. A minimal amount of tape should be used on newborn skin to prevent trauma and epidermal stripping when the tape is removed. Eye drops (1% methylcellulose) may be prescribed and must be administered with attention to infection control procedures.

Most newborns with traumatic facial nerve palsy make a good recovery usually within the first three weeks. It is very rare for permanent facial palsy to occur.

Spinal cord injury

Birth injury to the spinal cord is very rare. High cervical lesions have been associated with traumatic rotating high forceps deliveries or following complicated vaginal breech delivery and hyperextension of the aftercoming head. In both cases excessive traction, stretching and rotation on the cervical spinal cord causes the injury.

The newborn will be ill at birth, requiring resuscitation. If resuscitation is successful, the baby will be hypotonic and have flaccid limbs. A diagnosis of hypoxic ischaemic encephalopathy may lead to delayed diagnosis of spinal cord injury. There will be decreased spontaneous movement below the level of the lesion. Respiratory distress and lack of spontaneous breathing will be seen if the lesion is high. Lower spinal lesions will present with a lack of abdominal movements and an atonic anal sphincter. The bladder will be distended. There are profound implications for the family of the newborn who survives with quadriplegia.

Congenital muscular torticollis ('sternomastoid tumour')

Although birth injury may be implicated, congenital muscular torticollis is not thought to be solely due to trauma during delivery. The sternomastoid 'tumour' is a mass that can be palpated as a soft mobile lump in the side of the newborn neck. It is in or attached to the sternocleidomastoid muscle. The mass is usually apparent after the first week of life and may not be seen until four weeks of age.

It is thought that pressure on the neck while the baby is in the birth canal may cause oedema and necrosis of part of the sternocleidomastoid muscle. Secondary fibrosis will lead to the development of the mass or 'tumour'. Tearing of the muscle during birth may increase the trauma. The sternocleidomastoid muscle contracts and causes torticollis or 'wry neck'. The head becomes tilted towards the affected side. The chin may appear slightly elevated and rotated to the opposite shoulder and the head cannot be moved into a normal position. The mass is felt in the neck as a firm, immobile lump.

The focus of treatment is to reduce the long-term restriction of the baby's range of motion. Parents are taught to perform active and passive stretching movements of the baby's head and neck. Failure to respond to physiotherapy may require corrective surgery.

Intra-abdominal injuries

Injuries to the abdominal organs are very rare. Rupture of the spleen, liver or kidney is a risk during vaginal breech delivery if there is excessive pressure on and handling of the baby's trunk. Dystocia and macrosomia are also risk factors for intra-abdominal injuries.

The newborn will have a distended tender abdomen, pallor, shock and there may be discoloration of the abdominal skin. Immediate attention from the paediatric team is required.

Injuries to the genitalia

Swelling and bruising of the newborn scrotum or labia majora may occur after vaginal breech delivery, particularly if there were repeated vaginal examinations of the breech presentation. It will improve and resolve without treatment, although care should be taken during nappy changing and handling.

Conclusion

The majority of birth injuries are minor and improve quickly during the first few days of life. The commonest injuries involve the newborn head: oedema, swelling, bruising and abrasions. The parents are likely to be alarmed and concerned. The midwife should work in partnership with the parents, supporting them and providing clear explanations for the cause of minor birth injuries. An experienced member of the paediatric team must discuss more serious birth injuries such as obstetric brachial plexus palsy with the parents and the midwife's support will be vital for the family.

Hypoxic–ischaemic encephalopathy (HIE)

Hypoxic–ischaemic encephalopathy is not the result of traumatic injury during birth, it is injury to the newborn brain caused by reduced oxygen supply. The incidence of severe HIE is 1–2:1000 births. The lack of oxygen may have occurred before or during birth because of decreased blood flow to the brain and thus insufficient oxygen is supplied to the neuronal cells. The initial cell damage is followed by secondary cell damage as the brain is reperfused with a blood supply and cerebral oedema develops.

continued ➤

Hypoxic–ischaemic encephalopathy (HIE) *continued*

The newborn with mild HIE may recover well and have no long-term neurological problems. However, babies with severe HIE may develop serious problems such as cerebral palsy and epilepsy. They may have learning difficulties. The most severe cases are fatal since multiple organs are affected.

HIE is almost always seen in babies of term gestational age. The clinical signs tend to be seen at birth or during the first few hours of life. Risk factors include:

- history of fetal distress
- low umbilical arterial blood pH (acidaemia) particularly if the pH is less than 7
- low Apgar scores (0–3) at 5 minutes of age and longer.

The risk may be compounded if the baby is small for gestational age due to intrauterine growth restriction and thus already compromised.

In severe cases the baby will be ill at birth and transferred to the neonatal unit. In milder cases the baby may respond well to resuscitation, if it is needed, and appear to be healthy initially. However, signs of cerebral problems may develop over the first few hours of life. The baby may be hypertonic (have increased muscle tone), irritable, hyperalert and cry excessively. The mother may say that her baby seems to 'jump a lot' at noises and other stimuli; the Moro reflex is exaggerated. Alternatively the baby may feed poorly and be excessively sleepy and lethargic with hypotonia (reduced muscle tone). In such babies, the grasping, sucking and Moro reflexes will be poor.

Babies with increased or reduced muscle tone must be referred to the paediatric team. In more severe cases the lethargic, hypotonic baby may develop seizures or fits. Signs of fits in babies can be very subtle. The baby who is fitting will have rhythmic repetitive movements of one or more limbs. The fit can be distinguished from 'jitteriness' by gently holding the moving limb. The movement will cease if the baby is 'jittery' but will continue if the baby is fitting. The baby's eyes may appear to stare during the fit and the mouth may make repetitive sucking movements.

Abnormal movements and fits are very serious and require immediate paediatric medical care. The baby will be admitted to the neonatal unit.

CASE HISTORY

Karen, a 28-year-old mother, is pregnant for the third time. Her two other children, six and three years old, were spontaneous vaginal deliveries at 37 and 39 weeks' gestation. Their birthweights were 3.6 and 3.9 kg. Karen has no medical history of note and regular antenatal visits have not revealed any problems. Routine ultrasound scan at 20 weeks indicated a biparietal diameter and femoral length equivalent to 22 weeks' gestation. At 36 weeks the symphysis–fundal height was 35 cm.

Spontaneous labour occurs at 41 weeks. She progresses through the first stage in 4 hours. The second stage of labour advances relatively slowly over 1 hour and following delivery of the head, the midwife sees that the baby's chin appears to have difficulty in sweeping the perineum. The midwife performs an episiotomy but there appears to be no external rotation of the head and the midwife is unable to deliver the baby further.

The midwife calls for help, initiating the emergency protocol for shoulder dystocia. Karen is assisted into position for McRoberts manoeuvre and external suprapubic pressure is applied for 30 seconds. The episiotomy is extended. Charlotte is born and her birthweight is 4.0 kg.

Charlotte is blue, floppy and makes no attempt to breathe. She is quickly taken to the waiting paediatrician in the delivery room, dried, the wet towel is removed and she is wrapped in another dry warmed towel. Rapid assessment shows that she is still blue and floppy despite the stimulation of being handled and dried. Auscultation with a stethoscope shows that her heart rate is above 100 bpm.

Her head is placed in a neutral position and as there is still no spontaneous breathing, five inflation breaths are given using a face mask. Chest movement is visible with the third inflation breath and Charlotte begins to breathe spontaneously after the fifth inflation breath. Her heart rate is 130 bpm and she becomes centrally pink. Her tone improves and her legs begin to flex and move. Charlotte cries spontaneously. She is quickly examined by the paediatrician.

Although her tone has improved considerably since birth her left arm is still floppy in comparison to the other limbs which are now well flexed and actively moving. The paediatrician tells Karen and her partner that Charlotte's arm could be temporarily paralysed due to problems during the birth.

continued ➤

CASE HISTORY *continued*

Were there any risk factors for obstetric brachial plexus palsy?

- Postmaturity
- Large birthweight >3.5 kg
- Multiparous
- Relatively prolonged second stage of labour.

What are the immediate needs of the family?

Karen and her partner are shocked and alarmed at the events in the delivery room. Their baby's birth became an emergency and a number of strange health professionals suddenly entered the room giving urgent instructions. They know that the paediatrician was summoned. Charlotte did not cry at birth, was taken to another part of the room and needed resuscitation. The paediatrician has told them that there is something wrong with Charlotte's arm.

It is important to continue with the normal aspects of care. Karen should be encouraged to have skin-to-skin contact with her baby and to initiate breastfeeding as she had planned. She should be advised to gently support Charlotte's left arm; the arm can be held against the baby's chest during feeding and not allowed to 'swing' down as this will 'pull' on the shoulder joint.

Charlotte can be dressed in normal clothing but the arm must be handled carefully and gently to avoid 'pulling' and traction on the shoulder, elbow and wrist. The arm should be supported across the baby's torso in a comfortable position, with the elbow bent. It can be tucked inside the vest or Charlotte can be dressed in a long-sleeved vest and the sleeve taped to the front of the vest.

Karen and her partner need to discuss the events around Charlotte's birth with the midwife and obstetrician. They require a clear explanation of shoulder dystocia so that they understand why emergency procedures were necessary.

Charlotte's diagnosis

Later, the paediatrician examines Charlotte thoroughly. She appears to be well, is active and alert when awake. She has breastfed quite well and passed meconium. She is warm to the touch, pink and appears to be well perfused. Her respiratory rate is 32 bpm and there are no signs of respiratory distress. She has no facial weakness, is closing her eyes appropriately and her nasolabial folds are symmetrical.

Charlotte is not actively moving her left arm. It remains limply at her side and is inwardly rotated at the shoulder. It is very noticeable that the Moro reflex is present only on her right side and her left arm does not move at all. However, the grasp reflex is present in her left hand and the fingers are moving actively. Her right arm and both legs are moving actively and appropriately. There seems to be no fracture of her left clavicle on gentle palpation and there is no obvious deformity of her left arm that could be due to fracture of the humerus. X-ray is arranged and confirms that there are no fractures. The paediatrician diagnoses Erb's palsy.

There is no facial palsy and no evidence of phrenic nerve injury. It seems likely that injury to Charlotte's brachial plexus is caused by neurapraxia or stretching of the nerve roots at the upper part of the plexus – C5 and C6.

Later care and management

The family are told it seems likely that the nerves supplying Charlotte's arm have been stretched and temporarily damaged but that they are likely to improve. Charlotte is referred to the physiotherapist who assesses her range of movement on day 1 and recommends that the supportive care of Charlotte's arm is continued. The physiotherapist performs very gentle movements of Charlotte's wrist and elbow and teaches Karen so that she can do these exercises for her baby. Arrangements are made for outpatient physiotherapy assessment within one week and consultant paediatrician assessment in three weeks.

Key Points

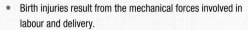
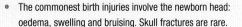

- Birth injuries result from the mechanical forces involved in labour and delivery.
- The majority are minor and recover without treatment or complications.
- Even minor birth injuries cause concern for parents.
- The commonest birth injuries involve the newborn head: oedema, swelling and bruising. Skull fractures are rare.
- Some injuries will require specialist neonatal and paediatric care.
- Very rarely, birth injury is life-threatening.

References

Levene MI, Tudehope DI and Sinha SK (2008) *Essential Neonatal Medicine*, 4th edn. London: Blackwell Publishing.

Rennie JM (2005) *Roberton's Textbook of Neonatology*, 4th edn. Edinburgh: Churchill Livingstone.

Uhing MR (2004) Management of birth injuries. In: Rademacher R and Kliegman R (eds) *Pediatric Clinics of North America: Common issues and concerns in the newborn nursery*, Part 2. Philadelphia: Saunders, pp. 1169–1186.

CHAPTER 14

CULTURAL AND RELIGIOUS ASPECTS OF NEONATAL CARE

Marcia Edwards

OVERVIEW

Over the past 20 years there has been considerable development of interest in the delivering of healthcare to a multicultural society. Much of this awareness has been academic, with few sustained practical initiatives to respond to the cultural and/or religious needs of mothers from minority groups. While we are rarely conscious of our own culture, the culture of others is generally far more obvious to us than our own. When cultural differences are observed, it is common to view these differences as being strange and/or abnormal. As a matter of good practice midwives should familiarize themselves with the cultural and religious beliefs predominating among minority ethnic groups within the community they serve.

How is culture defined?

Culture is the framework that guides and binds life practices. It is not something that is taught, yet almost every experience has a cultural component that is absorbed. It is said by some cultural researchers that cultural understanding is normally established before the age of five years (Stoecklin, 2001). It is a value system of shared norms, values and beliefs. Culture should not be confused with 'race' or ethnic group. Leininger (1970) describes culture as having the following characteristics:

- Culture is a universal experience, yet no two cultures are exactly the same.
- Culture is stable but also dynamic, manifesting continual change.
- Culture fills and largely determines the course of our lives yet people are rarely conscious of it.

Culture therefore, is learned through life experiences after birth and is transmitted from parents to children over successive generations. It originates and develops through the interactions of people through the chief vehicle of language. The elements within a culture tend to form a consistent and integrated system.

We may not understand why people do the things they do but it is patently clear that they behave and act differently to what we are accustomed to. For many people their religious or spiritual belief is central to their lives. Some may describe themselves as belonging to a particular religious group yet may not have any real spiritual belief but strongly uphold ethical and moral values. For example, a mother may describe herself as being a Christian of the Church of England faith. However, she may never go to church but feels strongly that marriages, christenings and funerals should be church events.

Providing culturally competent care includes understanding the dimensions of culture; moving beyond the biophysical to a more holistic approach. Building on the strengths of the woman rather than utilizing a deficit model of healthcare is an essential part of providing such care. The delivery of culturally competent care can make a critical difference in the health and well-being of women and their newborns.

Part of obtaining a mother's booking history is to ascertain her religion. What is the reason for this and how often do practitioners use this information for the true benefit of the client? Asking a mother's religion and knowing something about the beliefs and practices of different religions is an excellent starting point for identifying the potential needs a mother might have for her care during the ante-, intra- and postnatal periods.

Being aware of the mother's cultural background

Today, most mothers have a birth plan. While the birth plan is not always completed in full, most mothers have an idea of how they would like their labour managed. Of course it is impossible to know in advance what experience the mother might have; and more importantly, while a midwife may not always seek out the information, a woman's cultural values and religion are likely to have a significant effect on the way she welcomes her baby into the world. For many women their faith is pivotal in their lives and they need to be empowered to ask questions and challenge information provided by healthcare professionals who may be viewed as authoritarian, thus making mothers reluctant to challenge practices that are unacceptable to them. On the other hand, healthcare professionals often expect mothers to be active participants in their care and to ask questions freely. A body of knowledge supports that mothers from black and minority groups are far less likely than their white counterparts to receive empathy, information and encouragement to participate in decision-making in childbirth (Nápoles-Springer *et al.*, 2005). It is obvious that pregnancy, childbirth and motherhood are significant biological stages in a woman's life, however they are also critical social and cultural experiences.

Ultimately, the goal of the midwife is to obtain the necessary information in order to educate the mother (and her partner) so that a birth plan that suites her cultural values and expectations can be determined. Most midwives, if questioned, would state that they aspire to this goal but how much knowledge of a mother's cultural background would they draw upon

to really 'tailor' or encourage the mother and her immediate family to care for their newborn in a traditional way? The clinical guideline 'Routine postnatal care of mothers and their babies' (NICE, 2006, p. 5) states that:

> Care and information should be appropriate and the woman's cultural practices should be taken into account. All information should be provided in a form that is accessible to women, their partners and families, taking into account any additional needs, such as physical, cognitive or sensory disabilities, and people who do not speak or read English.
>
> Every opportunity should be taken to provide the woman and her partner or other relevant family members with the information and support they need.

The period immediately after the birth of the baby tends to be overshadowed following the huge amount of attention given to pregnancy and the birth itself. Within these highly charged minutes of intense emotion where the mother is making the transition of being pregnant to becoming a mother, the importance of recognizing and allowing symbolic cultural practices to take place may be overlooked or disregarded by the attending midwife.

After Christians, Muslims form the largest religious group in the world. Islam is a universal religion comprising all nationalities of the world and makes no distinction based on colour, 'race' or ethnicity. Islam is the dominant faith in many countries of the Middle East, Africa and Asia and there are minority Muslim communities throughout the rest of the world. The customs followed by Muslim families around the events of childbirth and infant feeding are many, and to the uninitiated they may appear rigid and unnecessary. This is further complicated by the fact that some Muslim cultural traditions differ from those prescribed by religion. However, these traditions still hold deep meaning to their adherents.

A great deal of this chapter focuses on the religious/cultural practices of people with a South Asian heritage as they make up the largest minority ethnic group in the United Kingdom. The birth of a child is a highly emotional and usually joyous experience and a special family event. Childbirth is a life-changing experience within all cultures and ethnic groups. It provokes a wide range of responses that are influenced by a complex interaction of religion, culture, education, social status, economy and the perceived position of women within the society. At the centre of all these powerful forces is a unique individual with her own personality, needs, hopes and fears.

Muslims of Islamic faith

For the 20 000 babies born each year to a population of approximately two million Muslims in the UK, the overwhelming majority of families will respect the rites of passage recommended by Islamic teaching. There are numerous customs and they might seem unnecessarily rigid and prescriptive but to those who are faithful to their culture and traditions, they are deeply symbolic.

Contrary to what is currently practised and encouraged in the UK health system, the placing of the baby on the abdomen of the mother immediately after the birth may be extremely distressful for some Muslim women. They may want the infant washed first to remove any impurities from the birth canal, as vernix and blood are considered unclean substances. It is very important to find out whether the parents will want the baby washed after delivery and whether they will want to carry out any religious or traditional birth ceremonies in the antenatal period.

This practice is in contrast to traditional behaviour in the Chinese community. Some Chinese mothers may be reluctant to bathe the baby until the cord stump has separated for fear of infection. Culturally, they do not bath the newborn baby for at least three days. Some mothers may also fear that the baby will become chilled. Traditionally, both mother and baby should avoid draughts or fresh air for the first month after birth as it is believed that such draughts carry infection. The baby should be kept well wrapped up. For these reasons many Chinese women do not go outside or take their baby outside during the first month (Abuidhail and Fleming, 2007).

The children of Islam have many rights that are clearly articulated in Islamic Law. These rights begin before conception (e.g. they have a right to be born through a legitimate union with full knowledge of their parentage). They also have the right to a 'good name', to be breastfed, educated and above all to be raised in a stable and loving environment.

Immediately after the birth, it is customary for the father or a respected member of the local community to whisper the *Adhan* (ritual call for collective prayer) into the baby's right ear and *Iqamah* (ritual announcement for starting the prayer) in the left ear.

In the world of spirit, man declared his instinctive readiness to accept Allah as his Lord, thus the first sound to reach a baby's ear should be the declaration of Allah's greatness, so that the sound always reverberates in his memory and settles in his soul. It is mentioned in the *Hadith* (a collection of oral traditions about the life of the Prophet Mohammed) that the devil runs away from the sound of the *Adhan*. These words include the name of Allah the Creator immediately followed by the Declaration of Faith: 'There is no deity but Allah; Mohammed is the Messenger of Allah'. It is upon these fundamental declarations that the life of a Muslim rotates, hence their symbolic significance at birth. The entire ceremony takes a few minutes and it would be greatly appreciated if parents were allowed to perform this traditional rite in privacy. Midwives with a lack of knowledge and understanding of these customs and who restrict access to the delivery suite to partners only would affect this practice.

The Adhan (Birth, 2009)

God is Great
I bear witness that there is no God but God
I bear witness that Mohammad is the Prophet of God
Come to prayer
Come to Success
God is great
There is no God but God

Soon after the birth, and preferably before the infant is fed, the *Tahneek* is performed. A small piece of softened date is gently rubbed into the upper palate of the child. Where dates are not easily available, substitutes such as honey may be used so that the child starts her or his life with sweetness. This rite is usually performed by the infant's parent or a respected member of the family in the hope that some of her or his positive attributes will be transmitted to the new family member. *Tahneek* (as the ritual is called) is performed based on the practice of the Holy Prophet. The *Hadith* indicates that the Prophet Mohammed softened dates in his mouth and rubbed them over the soft palates of newborns. It is the taste of the sweetness of the date or similar foods that is sought and not the ingestion of it (Shaikh and Ahmed, 2006).

The wish to perform these traditional acts soon after birth will often clash with maternity unit protocols. The current pressure, as a result of 'Western values', for mothers to have immediate skin-to-skin contact with their babies has unfortunately led to some midwives wrongly assuming that certain mothers are ambivalent and uncaring towards their newborn. Infant feeding protocols in the majority of maternity units may easily cause anxiety in new Muslim parents. Clearly, the understanding of this practice among clinicians caring for the Muslim mother and her family will significantly help in alleviating parental concerns while ensuring the safety of the newborn.

The *taweez* is a black string with a small pouch containing a prayer that is tied around the baby's wrist or neck. This practice is particularly common among Muslims from the Indian subcontinent; it is believed that it protects the baby from ill-health. Clearly, it is of the utmost importance to parents that the *taweez* is handled with respect at all times.

Hinduism

Almost 14 centuries ago, many Hindus converted to Islam and some 600 years ago Sikhism was founded as a variant of Hinduism. As a consequence, Hindu customs have become more and more diluted over the years. Hindu birth customs and ceremonies differ. In some cultures, soon after the birth, a member of the family writes the mystical sign 'Om' or 'Aum' (that represents the Supreme Spirit) on the baby's tongue with honey or ghee. A small dot, often in the shape of Om (Figure 14.1), may be drawn behind the baby's ear using *kajal*, which is a carbon-based substance often used as eye make-up. The person who does this may take on a role similar to that of the Christian godparent. In Britain, this ceremony might be delayed until the mother is at home. The symbol may also be seen on a chain around the baby's neck or indeed be placed in the child's cot. Other families may wish to wrap the baby in a special cloth that has religious significance after the birth. Another traditional practice in some Hindu families is for a married female who is close to the mother to symbolically wash the mother's breasts before offering the baby the first breastfeed. A mixture of cow's milk and water is used and prayers are said.

It is of extreme importance for some Hindu parents to know the exact time of the baby's birth so that they can get an accurate horoscope worked out by the pandit of the temple. This may be referred to later in the child's life for important events (e.g. marriage).

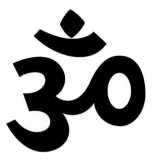

Figure 14.1   The mystical sign of 'Om' or 'Aum'

Astrological influences are often believed to have a strong effect on a person's character, personality and future (Schott and Henley, 2000). Interestingly, the precise date and time of a baby's birth is also an important part of traditional Chinese belief.

The sixth day following birth is considered to be the most propitious in a Hindu's life. On this day, a delicate white cotton thread may be tied ceremoniously around the wrist, ankle or neck of the child. This will fall off spontaneously within a few days. Also on the sixth day a piece of paper and a pen are placed in the baby's cot as it is believed that the goddess of learning charts the baby's future at this time.

Sikhism

There are no particular rituals or religious ceremonies connected with the birth of a child into the Sikh community. Some Sikhs recite the five verses of the Morning Prayer (*Japji Sahib*) into the ears of the newborn child.

A respected, intelligent and favourite member of the family gives a drop of *amrit* (specially prepared honey or sweetened water) to the newborn child as a blessing and to give the child character later in life. As the liquid is also seen to confer a blessing and to have cleansing properties, the mother may drink some of it as well. This is not a ritual and it mostly takes place in the hospital itself.

Similar to the *taweez* within the Islamic faith, health professionals may notice that the newly delivered baby might wear *nazarbattus* (i.e. black thread around the wrist and/or ankle) (Figure 14.2). Some mothers insist that their child wear *nazarbattus* around their necks. This is more deep-rooted superstition than a cultural practice but its purpose is to protect the child from anything untoward such as evil

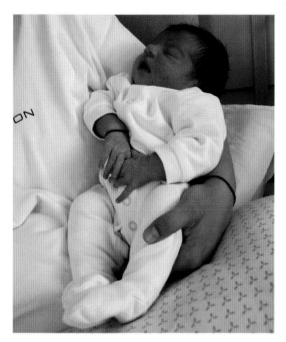

Figure 14.2   Picture of a Sikh mother and her baby (first day postnatal) both wearing wrist *nazarbattus*

spirits or thoughts of envy from others in the days and weeks immediately after birth. Infants are often seen as especially vulnerable during this period, requiring special protection and prayers. Given the high rates of neonatal mortality that still exist in much of the world, such precautions are understandable.

A common question asked by midwives is what the parents intend to name their baby. Within the Sikh community it is traditional to choose a name by opening the *Guru Granth Sahib* (the Sikh Holy Book) at random and choosing a name that begins with the first letter of the first word of the first complete paragraph on the left hand side of the page. Until the formal naming ceremony on the 40th day after birth, the baby may be known by a pet name.

Breastfeeding

Breast feeding within Muslim culture is positively encouraged by religious teachings with the recommendation that it should ideally continue for a period of two years. Similarly, breastfeeding is also positively encouraged within the Sikh community as it is considered to be a completely natural process and the best nourishment for the infant. However, the duration of

breastfeeding within the Sikh community is not prescribed as with Muslims so weaning of the child is entirely a personal choice that is not dictated by religious teaching.

Although many mothers may wish to breastfeed, the insufficient privacy offered by some delivery suite rooms and postnatal wards may be a barrier to doing so. Muslim etiquette demands that women should not expose certain body parts to anyone except their husbands. This includes the breasts, and in order to observe this privacy while in hospital, it is often deemed convenient to bottle feed; this could adversely affect milk production later.

Unnecessary touching between non-related people of the opposite sex should be avoided, which could be a problem with the mother being cared for by male midwives, nurses and doctors. The left hand is considered unclean, so it is preferred that the right hand be used for feeding or administering medications (Gulam, 2003).

Acknowledging these concerns of privacy is important across all cultures and for new Muslim mothers the concern is heightened by religious beliefs. Providing screens and/or covering blankets to facilitate and encourage breastfeeding in a culturally sensitive manner may help Muslim mothers in breastfeeding initiation and continuation.

There is a commonly held belief among some sections of the Muslim community that colostrum is either harmful to the baby or has poor nutritional value. Supplements of honey and water are often used for the first few days of life. Another reason this mixture is given is the belief that it cleans the intestine and makes it soft so that the infant can pass meconium easily. It must be emphasized that this is a cultural practice, not a religious recommendation. Similar views are held by many Hindu, Sikh and Chinese mothers.

Interestingly, these practices are contrary to what is encouraged by the Breast Feeding Initiative worldwide programme of the World Health Organization and UNICEF. The ten steps to successful breastfeeding, especially steps 4, 5 and 6, advise that all breastfeeding mothers should be given their baby to hold with skin-to-skin contact and that no food or drink other than breast milk should be given to the newborn infant unless there is an acceptable clinical reason (UNICEF/WHO, 2009). Nowhere does there seem to be any acknowledgement of the mother's cultural beliefs and how these could be respected within the standards.

In a cross-cultural piece of research undertaken by Holman and Grimes (2003) it was found that there is great variation across cultures in the timing of breast-feeding initiation. After examining 25 separate studies comprising more than 25 000 mother–infant pairs from a variety of countries and cultures, the authors found that some mother–infant pairs initiated breast-feeding within the first few hours while others initiated breastfeeding at approximately 66 hours postpartum, presumably coinciding with the production of 'true' milk. The cultural attitudes regarding the acceptability of colostrum was one important factor that affected a mother's decision about when to start breastfeeding.

Gatrad and Sheikh (2001) and Shaikh and Ahmed (2006) point out that this is an area that offers a very useful window for the development of educational campaigns directed towards Muslim mothers with the support of religious leaders and Muslim organizations. It is unlikely that pressure from outside the cultural group, without support from those respected within the group, will succeed in changing traditional practices. Muslim parents may not be interested or convinced in the scientific arguments that support the value of colostrum for the newborn as it may be interpreted as undervaluing or dismissing cultural beliefs.

Circumcision

The circumcision of male children is a central feature of both Islam and Judaism and is sanctioned in religious law. It is also important in many African cultures. Nevertheless, an increasing number of committed Muslim and Jewish people reject circumcision on ethical grounds, although they are certainly the minority at present and attitudes to circumcision may provoke fierce hostility within families and among communities.

Male circumcision within the Muslim faith is considered important for the purpose of hygiene. When the child grows older and begins offering prayers, then there is no danger that his clothes will become soiled from small amounts of urine held up in the foreskin. This is of extreme importance as soiled garments nullify prayer.

With the difficulty of obtaining circumcision on the National Health Service for religious reasons, parents turn to the private sector for the surgery to be performed. Circumcision is usually performed within

a few weeks of birth. It is prudent that healthcare professionals caring for mothers and babies during the postnatal period are aware of these facts because of the frequency of complications following circumcision by non-professionals. Where babies are jaundiced, circumcision should be delayed because of the potential risk of bleeding. Neither should surgery be performed on babies born with hypospadias or epispadias until a surgical opinion has been sought, as the foreskin may be needed in future surgical repairs.

Where circumcision has been performed during the postnatal period then mothers should be advised that nappies should be changed frequently. Though it is advised that no ointments or creams should be used during the healing process, application of a petroleum-based ointment (e.g. Vaseline/white soft paraffin) for the first few nappy changes may minimize the risks of infection with the associated risks of meatal stenosis and ulceration during wound-healing.

Jewish males are traditionally given their names and circumcised on the eighth day following birth at the ceremony called the *Brit Milah*. It is traditional to keep the child's name secret until this time. If there is the slightest doubt about the child's health then the operation is postponed. The operation is performed by a *mohel* (circumciser) who decides whether the baby is well enough for the circumcision to be performed. Many women are anxious about the physical process of circumcision for their baby and may need extra support and understanding at this time.

Female genital mutilation

Female genital mutilation is one of the most political areas of women's health. Worldwide it is estimated that well over 100 million women have been subjected to it.

Many campaigners, including several Muslim religious leaders, have openly condemned the practice. This does not deter its proponents, however, who maintain that it is their inalienable right to live according to their traditional beliefs and customs. Indeed, some argue that the freedom to carry out female genital mutilation is a fundamental principle of our multicultural society. It is not known when or where the tradition of female genital mutilation originated. However, it is believed that the practice of female circumcision was present before the advent of Islam (Gatrad and Sheikh 2001).

The practice is deeply embedded in local traditional belief systems and a variety of reasons are given for maintaining it. What is important to note is that female genital mutilation is *not* a religious requirement and it carries *no* health benefits. Neither the Bible nor the Koran endorses the practice (Royal College of Midwives, 2005; World Health Organization, 2008).

Female genital mutilation is the term used to describe procedures that involve partial or total removal of the external female genitalia or other injury to the female genital organs whether for cultural or other non-therapeutic reasons (World Health Organization, 2006). Of the millions of girls who undergo the mutilation every year, the majority are under the age of 15 but it is also performed on infant girls under two weeks of age. For this reason, female genital mutilation warrants mention here as the midwife may encounter such a child while caring for the mother and her new baby in the community setting. Alternatively, the neonate may be admitted to hospital with haemorrhage, sepis or other immediate consequences of female genital mutilation.

Female genital mutilation is against the law and has been specifically illegal in the UK since the Prohibition of Female Circumcision Act 1985. However, it was possible to evade the law by having the procedure conducted out of the country. The Female Genital Mutilation Act 2003 came into force in March 2004, replacing the 1985 Act. In the 2003 Act it is made explicitly illegal to take girls abroad for the procedure to be completed. The penalty for committing or aiding female genital mutilation was also increased to 14 years imprisonment.

Female genital mutilation is a human rights issue and a Prohibitive Steps Order (Children Act 1989: section 8) can be sought to prevent parents or carers from carrying out the act without the consent of the Court. Social services may also need to consider whether the circumstances constitute likely significant harm to justify initiating care proceedings or, indeed, emergency protection measures as appropriate.

Shaving the hair

In some communities (Muslims, Hindus, Chinese) scalp hair that has grown *in utero* is removed to symbolize the removing of the uncleanness of birth and also to help the hair grow thickly. Traditionally this is done on the seventh day of life in both boys and girls, but sometimes later. In some communities, oil and saffron are rubbed into the baby's head. An equivalent weight in silver, to that of the hair shaved, is often given to charity.

Stillbirth and neonatal death

Muslims consider that a fetus after the age of 120 days is a viable baby. A spontaneous abortion or an intrauterine death occurring 120 days after conception requires a burial. Therefore fetuses from such events must be given to the parents for a proper burial. Abortion is permitted if the pregnancy threatens the mother's life. Muslims believe in the resurrection of the body after death so they are always buried and never cremated.

In Islam, the body is considered to belong to God and, strictly speaking, no part of the dead body should be cut or harmed. Post-mortems are therefore forbidden unless ordered by the coroner. This should be clearly explained to the family. They may request that organs removed should be returned to the body after examination.

In the Hindu and Sikh traditions adults are cremated but babies and children are buried. For many parents it is simply important to know that their baby's body, at whatever stage of gestation, will be handled and treated respectfully. Some Hindu families may prefer to wash and prepare the baby's body themselves. The family may also wish for a religious ceremony to take place and this could be at the hospital prior to the burial which should take place as soon as possible.

Conclusion

Irrespective of our cultural origins, religious beliefs and practices, we all need to feel that we are respected, accepted, valued and understood. Midwives should consider cultural aspects of newborn care with some knowledge of how ethnic practices may differ from standard hospital/trust practices. It is not safe to assume that hospital protocols will be congruent with a family's cultural practice. Neither is it acceptable to stereotype the behaviour of different ethnic groups by assuming that literature about cultural practices applies to everyone. As an example, British Muslims speak many languages and represent a spectrum of educational backgrounds, social classes and ways of expressing their faith. Stereotypes and misunderstandings can easily affect the care of mothers and their families from these diverse backgrounds.

Cultural beliefs have a great influence on postnatal care practices in different cultures and midwives and other healthcare professionals need to understand the cultural beliefs and practices of women in the postnatal period to provide effective postnatal care that satisfies both the woman's cultural needs and her baby's healthcare needs. Furthermore, midwives need to respect the differences between their culture and that of the woman. It is advisable, therefore, that they gain some basic knowledge of the beliefs and practices of mothers' cultures. As a consequence, the women will have a higher level of acceptance of postnatal care and will comply more readily with postnatal care plans (Abuidhail and Fleming, 2007).

Although it is appreciated that one cannot be expected to have detailed knowledge of every aspect of the multicultural tapestry of present British society, such knowledge is important for midwives and other healthcare professionals to respond to individuals by reflecting on their own culture and recognizing and respecting the differences.

Finally, I would like to end with a quotation from the 'Routine postnatal care of mothers and their babies' guideline (NICE, 2006, p. 5), which succinctly sums up the way in which midwives should care for all women:

Women and their families should always be treated with kindness, respect and dignity. The views, beliefs and values of the woman, her partner and her family in relation to her care and that of her baby should be sought and respected at all times. The woman should be fully involved in planning the timing and content of each postnatal care contact so that care is flexible and tailored to meet her and her baby's needs.

Reflective activity

- What arrangements are in place within your area of work to manage and support a mother with specific cultural needs immediately following the birth of her baby?

- How might your own clinical practice change when caring for a mother from a Muslim background?

- What are some of the assumptions you have heard or hold regarding women from ethnic groups other than your own?

Key Points

- Treat every woman and her family with the dignity and respect you would expect to receive yourself.

- Recognize and guard against your own prejudices; everyone has them.

- Become well-informed/aware of issues that affect people from minority communities.

- Do not assume that treating everyone in the same way is the same thing as treating everyone fairly.

- Some people perceive ethnic minority groups as 'the problem'. However, 'the problem' may lie in these individuals' perceptions of the culture and traditions of minority groups.

- If in doubt, always ask. A polite and well-intentioned inquiry about a particular religious belief will not be offensive when prompted by a genuine desire to do the right thing.

References

Abuidhail J and Fleming V (2007) Beliefs and practices of postpartum infant care: review of different cultures. *British Journal of Midwifery* **15**: 418–421.

Birth (2009) http://re-xs.ucsm.ac.uk/re/passage/birth.htm [accessed 20 March 2009].

Breast Feeding Initiative (2009) Best practice in maternity services. www.babyfriendly.org.uk/page.asp?page=60 [accessed 13 February 2009].

Gatrad AR and Sheikh A (2001) Muslim birth customs. *Archives of Disease in Childhood: Fetal and Neonatal Edition* **84**: F8–F6.

Gulam H (2003) Care of the Muslim patient. *ADF Health* **4**: 81–83.

Holman DJ and Grimes MA (2003) Patterns for the initiation of breastfeeding in humans. *American Journal of Human Biology* **15**: 765–780.

Leininger (1970) cited in Kozier B and Erb G (1987) *Fundamentals of Nursing: concepts and procedures*, 3rd edn. New York: Addison-Wesley.

Nápoles-Springer AM *et al.* (2005) Culture and the medical encounter. *Health Expectations* **8**: 4–17.

NICE (National Institute for Health and Clinical Excellence) (2006) Routine postnatal care of women and their babies: Clinical guideline 37. London: NICE.

Royal College of Midwives (2005) Female Genital Mutilation. Position paper no. 21. London: RCM.

Schott J and Henley A (2000) *Culture, Religion and Childbearing in a Multiracial Society: A handbook for health professionals.* Oxford: Butterworth-Heinemann.

Shaikh U and Ahmed O (2006) Islam and infant feeding. *Breastfeeding Medicine* **1**: 164–167.

Stoecklin VL (2001) Role of culture in designing child care facilities. *Child Care Exchange Information Magazine*, pp. 12–22.

UNICEF/WHO (2006) *Baby Friendly Hospital Initiative. Revised, updated and expanded for integrated care. Section 1: background and implementation.* New York: UNICEF. http://www.unicef.org/newsline/tenstps.htm [accessed 12 February 2009].

World Health Organization (2006) Female genital mutilation and obstetric outcome: WHO collaborative prospective study in six African countries. *Lancet* **367**: 1835–1841.

World Health Organization (2008) Female genital mutilation. Fact sheet no. 241. Geneva: WHO.

CHAPTER 15

TEACHING RESUSCITATION TO PARENTS

Gillian Warwood

OVERVIEW

Although the number of babies dying from sudden infant death syndrome (SIDS) has fallen since 2001, there are still a large number of babies under the age of one year that die unexpectedly and for no apparent reason in the UK. The latest figures from the Office for National Statistics (ONS) showed that 300 babies died in 2005. In addition, there are a great number of babies who experience other life-threatening events requiring emergency help and admission to hospital, such as choking episodes, accidents or convulsions. In the West Midlands alone from July 2006 to 2008 there were 406 calls to the ambulance service for choking episodes and 116 calls for babies who have stopped breathing for other reasons, such as for convulsions, where advice was given over the phone (West Midlands Ambulance Service). Given that these figures may reflect national trends, clear guidelines need to be developed and training standardized so that all parents and carers are offered basic life support training. This would then greatly improve outcome for all infants in the UK.

Evidence has shown that bystander intervention greatly improves outcome. Should all parents therefore be offered basic infant life support (BILS) training at or around the time of their baby's birth? Perhaps it is now time for this to be considered.

Basic infant life support training for parents and carers

There is a paucity of information regarding the teaching of infant resuscitation to parents and carers. Some studies, however, have shown increased levels of parents' confidence after such training. Most people know a little about adult resuscitation but, according to the Resuscitation Council (UK), some children receive no resuscitation because would-be rescuers are afraid of inflicting injury or harm, as they have not received formal training (Resuscitation Council (UK), 2005).

In 2005 the Resuscitation Council (UK) renewed their paediatric basic life support guidelines for lay rescuers. They did so in order to simplify them to assist in teaching and retention and also partly because of new scientific evidence which shows that either doing ventilation alone or chest compressions alone is probably better than doing nothing at all. The previous ratios for babies of five compressions to one breath and 15 compressions to two breaths for children over one year of age have been changed for lay rescuers in order to bring the guidelines in line with adult resuscitation, that is, 30 compressions to two breaths for all casualties regardless of age (Resuscitation Council (UK), 2005).

The British Red Cross runs a 4-hour emergency life support course for children and infants, which includes dealing with choking.

The Foundation for the Study of Infant Deaths

The Foundation for the Study of Infant Deaths issued guidelines for parents to reduce the risks thought to be associated with these unexplained deaths so the emphasis has always been on prevention. Despite this, there are still babies dying so it seems important that we should offer basic infant life support training to all parents to enable them to do at least something rather than nothing at all.

Care of Next Infant (CONI) Programme

The Care of Next Infant (CONI) Programme was set up by the Foundation for the Study of Infant Deaths to offer support and help for parents who have suffered an unexpected death of a baby. It is run in hospitals and community centres and most hospitals have a CONI coordinator. Part of the scheme includes lending apnoea monitors to parents that alert the parents should the baby stop breathing for more than 20 seconds. In some areas the scheme also offers basic infant life support training by health visitors or the CONI coordinator so that parents would know how to respond should the alarm sound because the baby has stopped breathing. The CONI 'plus' scheme is a programme of similar support for families who are anxious about their baby for other reasons, such as if a close relative has had a baby die of cot death or if their baby has suffered life-threatening events.

Health promotion role

The midwife is in an ideal position to teach basic infant life support skills to parents. The midwife is already seen as having a major role in health promotion and indeed, many already include infant resuscitation as part of their parentcraft programme. The

Foundation for the Study of Infant Deaths – Advice to parents

1 Cut smoking in pregnancy – fathers too! Don't allow anyone to smoke in the same room as your baby.

2 Place your baby on the back to sleep (and not on the front or side).

3 Do not let your baby get too hot, and keep your baby's head uncovered.

4 Place your baby with their feet to the foot of the cot, to prevent them wriggling down under the covers.

5 Never sleep with your baby on a sofa or armchair.

6 The safest place for your baby to sleep is in a crib or cot in a room with you for the first six months.

7 It's *especially* dangerous for your baby to sleep in your bed if you (or your partner):

- are a smoker, even if you never smoke in bed or at home
- have been drinking alcohol
- take medication or drugs that make you drowsy
- feel very tired

or if your baby:

- was born before 37 weeks
- weighed less than 2.5 kg at birth
- is less than three months old.

Don't forget, accidents can happen: you might roll over in your sleep and suffocate your baby, or your baby could get caught between the wall and the bed, or could roll out of an adult bed and be injured.

8 Settling your baby to sleep (day and night) with a dummy can reduce the risk of cot death, even if the dummy falls out while your baby is asleep.

9 If your baby is unwell seek medical advice immediately.

10 Breastfeed your baby. Establish breastfeeding before starting to use a dummy.

teaching of cot death prevention is a standard for discharge in most maternity units. The National Institute for Health and Clinical Excellence (NICE) guidance for optimum postnatal care suggests that all parents should be given advice on how to recognize signs of illness in their child.

For many parents, however, the mere contemplation of having to deal with a life-threatening event requiring them to administer life support in the form of mouth-to-mouth resuscitation and/or cardiopulmonary resuscitation (CPR) is frightening. They need to be reassured that the fear is born of simply not knowing what to do and that doing something in such a situation is better than not doing anything at all. Many parents say that they feel more confident to take their baby home after receiving their basic life support training.

Some studies have shown that parents experience increased levels of confidence and reduced levels of anxiety in caring for their newborn baby following such training. With this in mind, parents should be taught how to recognize signs of illness in their baby and be taught how to reduce risks of cot death and how to deal with life-threatening events.

Timing of basic infant life support training

Some parentcraft or antenatal classes include infant resuscitation training for parents in their programme. It is recognized, however, that only a small proportion of expectant couples attend these classes and that the lower socio-economic groups tend not to attend them. The incidence of sudden infant death syndrome is higher amongst these groups. Another group of babies also at greater risk is that of premature babies who have required care in a neonatal unit. As many of these babies are born in the second trimester, their parents miss out on classes, which are usually offered in the last trimester.

The best time to offer the classes then seems to be just after the baby is born because the teaching will be considered relevant to the parent at this time. Also, if done at or around the time of birth it would ensure optimum coverage but, as every midwife knows, with shorter times spent in hospital now and midwifery units being so short-staffed and busy, there is little time to offer the training in the relaxed way that is necessary for effective training of the skill. Furthermore, at the time of the new arrival into the family, probably the last thing parents want to consider is the possibility of such an event happening to them.

The immediate postnatal period may be a better option as the mother may be relaxed enough in a drop-in centre or clinic; even then it would be hard to ensure enough training for everyone in an atmosphere that is free from interruptions and that is conducive to learning.

Provision of training for extended family and carers

Partners, carers, childminders, grandparents and siblings should also be considered for training. The need for some parents to return to work soon after their baby is born means that their baby is likely to be in the care of childminders and grandparents.

There are various ways in which the sessions can be delivered. They can be delivered in group sessions or on a one-to-one basis. In one research study, it was found that some parents do not like being taught in a group and would prefer a one-to-one session (Henley, 1999). This is mainly because they do not like to be questioned or to practise in front of other people. In a group, having more than one mannequin and passing the dolls around the group with the instructor moving among the learners can overcome this problem. However, very young parents might be intimidated if taught on a one-to-one basis. One unit found that younger parents would prefer to be part of a group rather than taught separately as they may perceive being taught by a healthcare professional like being at school. Training can also be delivered in small family groups, particularly if there has been a previous loss or experience that would make the session distressing for parents. A recent study showed that resuscitation training of nurses was equally effective in skills retention and acquisition whether taught in groups or on an individual basis (De Regge et al., 2008).

Neonatal units

One particular group of babies known to be at increased risk of life-threatening events in the first 12 months of life are graduates of neonatal units, particularly premature babies, low birthweight babies and those who have suffered significant respiratory illness in the first few weeks of life. Many neonatal units now offer basic life support training to parents of these babies at or around the time of discharge. However a recent telephone survey in the West Midlands highlighted many inconsistencies in the way training is offered and provided.

The purpose of the survey was to find out how much training is offered in neonatal units and how it is delivered and by whom. Of the 15 units surveyed, only eight units offered training to all parents. The

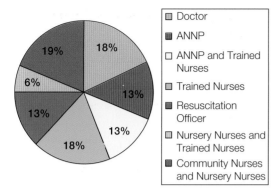

Figure 15.1 Designation of trainer
(ANNP, Advanced Neonatal Nurse Practitioner)

- Doctor
- ANNP
- ANNP and Trained Nurses
- Trained Nurses
- Resuscitation Officer
- Nursery Nurses and Trained Nurses
- Community Nurses and Nursery Nurses

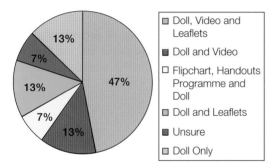

Figure 15.2 Equipment used

- Doll, Video and Leaflets
- Doll and Video
- Flipchart, Handouts Programme and Doll
- Doll and Leaflets
- Unsure
- Doll Only

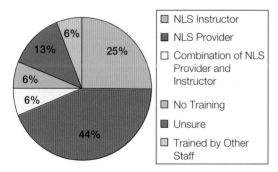

Figure 15.3 Qualifications of trainer
(NLS, Newborn Life Support)

- NLS Instructor
- NLS Provider
- Combination of NLS Provider and Instructor
- No Training
- Unsure
- Trained by Other Staff

There was a mixed bag of health professionals from nursery nurses to consultants providing the training (Figure 15.1) and a variety of teaching equipment in the form of out-of-date videos, which indicated that various different ratios were being used (Figure 15.2). Eleven units offered one-to-one training and four units ran regular group sessions either on a weekly or fortnightly basis. When asked whether the trainers had any particular qualifications to enable them to teach resuscitation, again there was a very mixed response (Figure 15.3).

In order to standardize this training, a working group is looking at an instructor course for those who train parents in basic infant life support skills using a DVD which incorporates the four-stage approach to teaching as described later in the chapter.

Adult learning

Adults are generally responsive to learning if they have a choice about the timing and the direction of their learning. They are more motivated if the content of the teaching is relevant to them and if they know why they need to learn, and their readiness to learn is enhanced if the learning is focused on solving real problems that happen or can happen in everyday life (Knowles *et al.*, 2005). Therefore if parents realize that these events can happen around them, not just to theirs but also to anyone's infant or child, then their motivation to learn would increase.

Preparation

Preparation of the sessions ahead of time is crucial in order to ensure the optimal teaching environment. It is also important to arrange the most appropriate time for the parents in order to be able to deliver the teaching in a session that is free from interruptions and is not rushed. Planning ahead of the session will allow parents to include anyone else who may want to attend, especially family and babysitters or childminders who may be looking after the baby. Evening sessions may be considered, for example, in cases where partners may find daytime classes difficult to attend because of work commitments. It is important that the sessions are structured to include consideration of three components: Set, Dialogue and Closure (Bullock *et al.*, 2008).

other seven units offered training to selected parents only. These parents were selected on the basis of the perceived severity of their child's condition or perceived risk (i.e. any infant who is sent home on oxygen, has had a sibling who has died of sudden infant death syndrome or if the infant itself has suffered any life-threatening events and requires apnoea monitoring at home).

Set

The set includes:

- preparation of room and equipment
- environment
- introductions of self and learners
- establishing an atmosphere
- assessment of prior learning
- stating/setting objectives.

Equipment

Very little equipment is needed to teach basic infant life support. The only essential item is a resuscitation doll (mannequin) to provide visual demonstration. A DVD or video is not essential but can be a powerful training tool. The current guidelines of teaching a ratio of two breaths to 30 compressions are demonstrated in a DVD recently developed by the Council for Professionals as Resuscitation Officers (CPRO) to assist trainers. If using a DVD or video, remember to check that everything is in working order before the session. There is nothing more offputting than finding that the instructor cannot proceed with the session because the equipment fails to work.

Leaflets can be provided for the parents to take away with them after the session, giving a useful reminder of the important points.

It is important that the mannequins are clean and in good working order. They should be cleaned with a medicated cloth between each learner and at the end of each session. Each learner should be provided with a cleaning cloth.

Environment

Whether the training takes place in the clinic, in the home or in a classroom it is important to make sure that there are as few distractions as possible and that the session is not rushed. Attention to the environment is important in order to ensure that it is conducive to learning. The room should be well ventilated and as comfortable as possible. The chairs need to be arranged so that everyone is included equally and so that everyone can see and hear the instructor. Attention should be paid to heating and lighting too.

Introductions/establish atmosphere

If the learners do not already know you, introduce yourself. If in a group, get them to introduce them-

selves. Tell them what you are going to do and what you will expect of them. For example, you may wish to say something like 'First of all, we are going to watch a short DVD then I will go through each of the aspects covered. We will all get a chance to practice etc.' Some people will be afraid that they are going to be singled out to perform in front of others. It is important to make the session as non-threatening as possible while at the same time reaffirming the importance of the session.

Assessment of prior learning

You will need to ascertain any prior learning or other experiences relating to the content of the session. It is possible that your audience might include a resuscitation officer who is used to teaching adult resuscitation or someone may have suffered a cot death or other painful experience. By asking the audience if anyone has any experience of resuscitation, you can then pre-empt any difficult moments that may ensue and pitch the training accordingly.

Dialogue

The dialogue is the actual content of the session. It will consist of teaching prevention in the form of sudden infant death syndrome guidelines and maybe the cause of respiratory arrest in babies. You may also wish to teach parents how to detect signs of illness in their baby such as lethargy, pallor, blueness around the lips, temperature changes or an unwillingness to feed or being particularly unsettled. You need to explain that babies tend to stop breathing first before the heart fails and so it is important to follow the steps in the order that they are taught. You may want to mention that the body takes in oxygen into the lungs and the heart is a pump which pumps the oxygen

---

The four-stage approach to teaching a skill

- Stage One: The instructor runs through the event as though in real time, that is, with little or no dialogue as though it is really happening.

- Stage Two: The demonstration is repeated with discussion of each action along the way.

- Stage Three: The instructor asks the audience to talk through the event.

- Stage Four: The participants demonstrate the skill on their own.

around the body. If the oxygen is not taken in because the baby has stopped breathing then the heart will be unable to work properly. This may seem obvious to healthcare professionals but is not necessarily known by lay people.

The skills should be taught in four stages.

Stage one

Perform this stage as a mock resuscitation in real time as if it is really happening. Sometimes this stage is called the silent run-through. There must be no explanation or interruptions during this stage.

1   Demonstrate (with the dummy) approaching the infant and discovering that the infant is lying pale and not breathing in the cot.

2   Call loudly for help while checking that the area is safe to approach.

3   Pick the infant up and stimulate the infant by calling its name and pressing and squeezing the baby's arm or leg to elicit a response.

4   Open the airway. Place the child on a flat surface and demonstrate putting the head in the neutral position (Figure 15.4).

5   Look, listen and feel for any response (for no longer than 10 seconds) by putting your head near to the baby's mouth while looking at the chest (Figure 15.5).

6   No response is seen so cover the baby's nose and mouth with your mouth to create a seal and breathe gently into the baby's mouth while watching for chest movement.

7   If no chest movement is seen after the first one or two breaths, alter the head position slightly and try again.

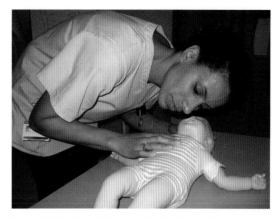

Figure 15.5   Look, listen and feel for signs of life

8   Look, listen and feel again for signs of life. If none, proceed to chest compressions.

9   Choose a place on the child's chest just below the nipple line or just in the centre of the chest. With two fingers (the forefinger and index finger) in upright position, compress the chest approximately one-third of the depth and release to allow for recoil of the chest (Figure 15.6). Do these 30 times at a rate of approximately 100 per minute then give two more breaths. Continue the sequence of two breaths to 30 compressions once or twice more to demonstrate.

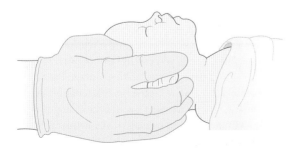

Figure 15.4   Neutral position. (Redrawn from Richmond, 2006, with permission)

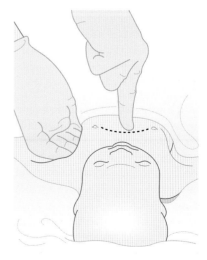

Figure 15.6   Chest compressions using the two-finger technique (Redrawn from Richmond, 2006, with permission)

Stage two

You are now going to repeat the demonstration and discuss each aspect of the demonstration. The learner is more likely to remember if you keep it simple. For example use a simple memory aid such as the three S's (Safety, Shout, Stimulate) and ABC (Airway, Breathing, Circulation).

Safety

Talk about the importance of checking that the area is safe. Talk about safety and why this is important. Stress that it is important to ensure that the area is safe to approach otherwise they might be putting themselves at risk. Point out that they cannot be of any help to the casualty unless they ensure safety for themselves first. Talk about an event possibly occurring while they are driving, for example, or in the middle of an activity such as cooking which may be harmful if the area is not made safe first.

Shout

Discuss calling for help and how one would call for help in different situations. Encourage learners to think about who they would call or who they would ask to go to the phone first. If alone, what would they do first? Tell them to take the baby to the phone with them.

Stimulate

At this point tell them that it is important not to shake the baby but that the stimulation should be such that it would normally waken the baby. For the exercise use an unlikely name. Rather than risking inadvertently using the name of a participant's child, especially if some of them have experienced a previous cot death, it is a good idea to check that none of their babies is called Bertie, for example, and use that name.

Airway

Put the baby on a flat surface and discuss what is meant by the neutral position. Tell them that by putting the head in this position they are opening the airway. Encourage the parent or group to bend down to see that the head is indeed on a level plane with the body, that it is neither flexed nor extended; and while bending down to the baby with an ear directly above the baby's mouth talk about what you are looking, listening and feeling for. 'I'm listening for any signs of life such as breathing, moaning, etc. I'm looking for breathing movements and feeling for breath on my face and with my hand lightly on the baby's abdomen,

am feeling for abdominal movements.' Do this for no longer than 10 seconds. Tell them the importance of not taking too long over this part of the process (i.e. 'because the baby isn't breathing and you need to act quickly' etc.).

It is no longer advised to tell the rescuer to feel for a pulse. Most lay people cannot feel a pulse and it is particularly difficult to feel a baby's pulse.

Breathing

Assuming that no signs of life have been detected, you then demonstrate how to breathe for the baby. 'Take a breath first then by covering the baby's nose and mouth to create a seal, breathe gently into the baby's mouth and watch for chest movements at the same time.' Ensuring that the baby's head is in the neutral position, support the chin with your middle finger, taking care not to press on the soft tissues of the airway in the neck.

Breathe into the baby's mouth up to five times and look for chest movement. If no movement is seen, explain why you need to alter the position of the head slightly in order to open the airway. If the chest is not moving then it is possible that the airway is not open. If no signs of life are evident after five breaths, then proceed to chest compressions.

Circulation

Demonstrate cardiac compressions. Being told to find an exact spot just below the nipple line in the centre of the chest often causes confusion. It is easier to say, 'There's the chest, that's the middle. Put two fingers there.' Continue to demonstrate this and affirm important points, such as that the quality of the compressions is more important than the exact number. State that it is important to continue resuscitation until the child shows signs of life, further help arrives or until you become exhausted.

Stage three

This part of the teaching is when the learner leads the teacher through the process with the teacher providing the actions. Here, you can use this opportunity to ask questions of the learner and encourage the other learners to participate. Practise the resuscitation a step at a time while the learner provides the dialogue and guides you through the process. If the learner forgets any aspect of the practice, you can stress the importance of that part of the action. You can ask questions such as 'Why is it important to spend no longer than 10 seconds when looking, listening and feeling for signs of life?' or 'For how long must you continue with resuscitation?' If in a group, you can elicit responses from other participants.

Stage four

During this stage it is important for the learner to repeat the skill from beginning to end and provide dialogue or justification for the actions demonstrated. This stage can be used to clarify points and to ensure that each individual can perform the skill from beginning to end.

It is important to tell them that they should never practise on a real baby. This is their opportunity to practise and it is important that they complete this stage and 'have a go'. The learners can do this in pairs and practise responding to a choking infant at the same time (Figure 15.7).

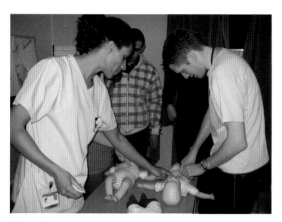

Figure 15.7   Stage four: parents practising in a group

Closure

When closing the session, it is important to allow time for questions. The teacher must also summarize important points. A takeaway message such as 'If you can't remember everything, it is better to do something that nothing at all' may be useful, and memory aids, such as the three S's for Safety, Shout for help and Stimulate or the time-honoured ABC of resuscitation, will make remembering easier.

Leaflets to support the training are very useful as long as they are kept simple. Locally printed leaflets are ideal as long as they are clear and well laid-out and follow the current guidelines. Consideration needs to be given to other languages, particularly in areas that have a diverse ethnic mix. Remember that although leaflets printed in local community languages may be useful, their effectiveness will be limited because they need to be supported by verbal explanation for maximum effect.

Choking

For a demonstration of how to respond to a child who is choking, the same four-stage approach to learning can be used. The stage one demonstration should include the following instructions:

1   Check the area is safe.
2   If the child is coughing, there is no need to do anything but reassure the child and encourage them to cough, but if the coughing is ineffective shout for help immediately.
3   For an infant, sit or kneel with the infant supported, head down in a prone position across your lap. Support the infant's head with your thumb and forefinger under each side of the jaw – this will help to maintain an open airway
4   Give five back blows with the heel of your hand in the middle of the shoulder blades. This may dislodge the foreign body. Check the mouth for signs that the object has dislodged.
5   If back blows fail to dislodge the object give five chest thrusts. These are similar to chest compressions but are slower and sharper.
6   If the child becomes unconscious proceed to cardiopulmonary resuscitation as described previously. It is possible that as the airway relaxes you may be able to breathe a small amount of air past the obstruction
7   Always seek medical advice. Do not leave the child unattended at any stage.

Follow-up

Research has shown that if not practised on a regular basis these skills can only be retained for 4–6 months and so parents should be encouraged to attend future sessions. They may also wish to attend more sessions or bring someone else along that has not been able to attend.

Suggestions for implementing basic infant life support training in your maternity unit/community

- Decide on a room or venue – check to see if a DVD player is available.
- Acquire necessary equipment (i.e. dolls, DVD, etc.).
- Devise your programme, ensuring that you give attention to the set, dialogue and closure. Practise on your colleagues and maybe they will be enthusiastic enough to help you.
- Develop simple leaflets – get a medical illustrator to help you with these. Some excellent leaflets have been printed with pictures incorporating new guidelines and are available from the Association of Paediatric Resuscitation Officers (APRO).
- Decide on a date and advertise your sessions.
- Decide how you are going to follow-up or offer refresher sessions.
- Document that parents have been offered the training and whether or not the training was given/attended.
- Develop simple evaluation forms. You will be surprised at the feedback you get from parents.

Conclusion

Babies dying from sudden infant death syndrome and sustained numbers of emergency calls to the ambulance service are still prevalent despite continued attempts to reduce these figures. The emphasis therefore is on prevention. We know that bystander intervention greatly improves outcome, so the time has come for clear guidelines for a national programme to address the teaching of skills to parents and carers in all corners of the community. The midwife is in a unique position to offer this training, whether in a hospital or community setting, which will help to increase parents' confidence in caring for their baby and hopefully improve outcome for all infants in the UK.

Reflective account

- How are you going to prepare for the session? Think about the optimum time to deliver the training.
- What are the important factors to consider in your preparation of the session? What equipment do you need? Where will you hold the session?
- How are you going to ensure that the learner has understood?

Useful addresses

- Association of Paediatric Resuscitation Officers (APRO) PO Box 39077, London E8 3YF
- Foundation for the Study of Infant Deaths www.fsid.org.uk/cot-death
- British Red Cross www.redcross.org.uk
- British Heart Foundation www.bhf.org.uk
- Council for Professionals as Resuscitation Officers www.cpro.org.uk
- Resuscitation Council (UK) www.resus.org

Key Points

- All parents should be offered basic infant life support training.
- The principles taught should be according to current Resuscitation Council (UK) guidelines.
- Training needs to be structured to include set dialogue closure.
- Teaching a skill should be done using the four-stage approach.
- Training should include other family members and carers.

References

Bullock I, Davis M, Lockley A and Mackway-Jones K (2008) *Pocket Guide to Teaching for Medical Instructors*, 2nd edn. London: BMJ Books, Blackwell Publishing.

De Regge M, Calle PA, De Paepe P and Monsieurs KG (2008) Basic life support refresher training of nurses individual and group training are equally effective. *Resuscitation* **79**: 283–287.

Henley J (1999) Teaching parents in a neonatal unit about sudden infant death syndrome and infant resuscitation. MSc research thesis, University of Birmingham.

Knowles M, Holton E and Swanson R (2005) *The Adult Learner*, 6th edn. San Diego: Elsevier.

NICE (National Institute for Health and Clinical Excellence) (2006) Postnatal care: Routine postnatal care of women and their babies. http://www.nice.org.uk/CG037 [accessed 9 September 2009].

Resuscitation Council (UK) (2005) Paediatric basic life support. http://www.resus.org.uk/pages/pbls.pdf [accessed 9 September 2009].

Richmond S (2006) *Newborn Life Support Manual*. London: Resuscitation Council (UK).

CHAPTER 16

FREQUENTLY ASKED QUESTIONS

Debbie Holmes and Hilary Lumsden

OVERVIEW

This chapter comprises questions that have recently been asked of and by student and qualified midwives. The answers should enable the reader to be prepared and armed with the correct answer should those questions arise in their practice.

Introduction

Since the rise in Internet use parents are more informed than ever before. While the use of Internet sources should be encouraged, it does mean that not all information available to parents is peer reviewed or evidence-based. As a consequence, parents often have questions about their babies that may be difficult to answer. It is essential that healthcare professionals avoid giving misleading or incorrect answers because in order for parents to make any informed decisions about the care or treatment of their baby they should have the correct information. If that information can be supported with a written leaflet in language they understand it will help them reflect upon the answers they have been given and will help them make the informed choice.

Parents may also ask more than one healthcare professional the same question in order to elicit an answer they want to hear. It is helpful before replying to their question to ascertain what they already know about the condition or problem they are asking you about. It may be that their understanding of the answer is not clear. Grandparents and well-meaning friends sometimes give parents advice based on tradition that is wrong or misleading, which can be very confusing. In addition when parents are worried about their baby or are preoccupied with other problems they may repeat the question on several occasions. Patience is required in these instances and repetition of correct information will always be worthwhile.

If you do not know the answer to a parent's question it is always advisable to find someone who can answer it for you rather than try to muddle your way around an unsatisfactory response.

Questions

A dad who has been doing his home work asks: 'Why do you swaddle babies and put hats on them inside the hospital when the books tell us not to do this?'

The transition to extrauterine life includes the maintenance of thermal control. The environmental temperature in hospital is often difficult to regulate and babies become cold very quickly. Making sure that babies are properly dried and wrapped is important so that they do not lose heat by evaporation. Swaddling babies and putting a hat on them is one way of preventing heat loss as well as increasing a relatively low temperature. This does contradict advice given on the prevention of sudden infant death but parents should be reassured that this method of keeping the baby warm is temporary and should only be for the first few hours of life until the core temperature has stabilized. Further information can be found in Chapters 2 and 8.

'Why are you telling us not to use baby wipes and stuff when your care worker has just given us a bottle of baby bath to bath our baby in?'

Many parents like the smell of the chemical-based baby products. The advice is not to use these products until the baby is four weeks old. The free products given out in hospital do contain samples of these baby products. The advice is not to use them on babies' skin because they can cause excema and other drying conditions, but to introduce them gradually when the baby is a month old. The baby should not be immersed in the bath for longer than 5 minutes (see Chapter 7).

A midwife asks: 'When a baby is born following absent end-diastolic flow, they go to the neonatal unit and feeding does not start straight away due its association with necrotizing enterocolitis. I find I can't articulate the answer to parents very well.'

Absent or reversed end-diastolic flow in the umbilical artery is a serious development with a stong correlation with fetal distress and interuterine death. These falling oxygen levels in the fetus result in a redistribution of blood to protect the brain, heart and spleen. This therefore means that the gut is deprived of oxygen during this period. A lack of oxygen to the gut can leave the area vulnerable to cell death and necrosis. If the baby is fed in the early postnatal period it may further compromise the gut, leading to further complications such as necrotizing enterocolitis. In fact many units will start feeds early but will be cautious and increase them more gradually. Feeding with mother's expressed breast milk is preferred to formula milk. Policies of both early milk feeding and late milk feeding are widely used in neonatal units.

A midwife asks: 'The questions I get asked most of the time are really basic and repetitive, but so important to parents, such as: "Why is the baby's skin dry? What should I use?"'

A baby's skin is dry usually because of postmaturity. Vernix caseosa is present on the skin but will be absorbed the more postmature the baby is at birth.

Once born, postmature babies lack the protection that vernix offers and their skin is more vulnerable to irritation and infection if harsh products are used on it. The advice is to use nothing on the skin except plain water and once all the dry skin has peeled away the skin underneath will be undamaged (see Chapter 7).

A parent asks: 'Why, when the cord comes off, is the belly button sticky, and what should I do with it?'

As part of the normal physiology of cord separation small mucoid material may collect around the separating cord. It may sometimes look like pus but it is normal and should not smell offensive. Using products on the skin or around the cord can prolong the separation and make the umbilicus sticky once separated. The advice to parents is to use plain water only in the bath and to pat the umbilicus dry with a dry soft towel. They should also make sure that the nappy does not cover the umbilicus because it can make the umbilicus moist.

A student midwife asks: 'I had to explain talipes to parents, and why massage can help positional talipes, but I'm still not sure if the answer I gave was suitable.'

Positional talipes are a result of malposition *in utero* or oligohydramnios. The feet are unable to move freely *in utero* and as a result an abnormal position of the feet or foot can occur. Positional talipes is treated with massage or stretching exercises that will help the feet regain their natural position. The exercises should be taught by a physiotherapist in the first instance.

A midwife reports that the most frequent questions she gets asked after delivery are 'Why are my baby's hands and feet blue?'

The circulatory changes that take place at birth can take up to seven days to be fully complete, although blueness of the hands and feet should last no longer than two days. Blue hands and feet (acrocyanosis) are perfectly normal and are caused by the instability of the circulatory system. Acrocyanosis should be differentiated from central cyanosis, which is blueness around the mouth and tongue.

And 'Why is my baby sneezing?'

Sneezing is common and normal in the first few hours of life and is a normal reflex to eliminate particles or mucous. It is usually caused by residual fluid in the nasal passages following delivery. The sneezing will stop once all debris has been cleared. It is not necessary to try to clean the nose or use suction to the nares since it can cause damage. Sneezing is also seen in babies with neonatal abstinence syndrome and is a common symptom. Neonatal abstinence syndrome should be ruled out if the sneezing is excessive or prolonged.

Parents often worry about positioning their baby on its back in the cot in case the baby vomits. A midwife admits: 'I have found myself saying "well research shows this reduces SIDS" and not really answering the bit about vomit. I would welcome advice on what others say in this situation.'

If a baby vomits when lying on its back it is unlikely to inhale or choke on the vomit because of the babies' cough reflex, the head will turn to the side and most of the vomit will drain away from the mouth. It is recommended by the Foundation for the Study of Infant Deaths (2009a) that babies sleep in the same room as their parents for the first six months. Any vomiting or problems with breathing will be easily detected.

A midwife says: 'I can explain to parents why they might find blood in their daughter's nappy (i.e. hormonal) but struggle with explaining why what looks like blood in a boy's nappies is actually urates and the cause for this.'

There are two parts to this answer. First, blood in the female baby's nappy is, as you state, due to hormonal imbalances. The blood is per vaginum, is known as pseudo-menstruation and will only last about two days. Second, in the first days postnatally it is expected that the baby will wet his or her nappy at least twice every 24 hours. If you notice that he or she passes tiny orange or pink crystals, these are harmless urates, which react with chemicals in the nappy but can be a sign the baby needs to feed more often and is slightly dehydrated.

A parent asks: 'Why has my baby's poo got seeds in it?'

The stools of breastfed and bottle-fed babies will look very different. Colostrum acts as a laxative, helping to push meconium out of the baby's system. Once the milk becomes established, after about three days, the baby's stools will gradually change to a bright or mustard yellow and be sweet-smelling. They will be loose, but textured, sometimes seeming grainy/seedy or curdled. These 'seeds' are really curds of digested milk.

A midwife asks: 'How do I explain to parents why certain babies are slow to feed and "mucousy" so they are not traumatized when their baby has a big mucousy vomit?'

It can be quite alarming to parents if their baby vomits. They will worry about the milk, why the baby is vomiting and whether he or she will be hungry. Formula-fed babies are more prone to vomiting than breastfed babies, usually due to the amount of air they take in with the teat, and this should be explained to the parents. When babies are 'mucousy', they have usually swallowed liquor at birth and once they have been fed will result in a mucousy vomit. This may happen 2 or 3 times until all the mucus has been cleared from the stomach. Parents needs to be reassured that the vomiting will cease.

A midwife asks: 'According to "Ten steps to successful breastfeeding" it is suggested that breastfed babies must not be given artificial teats or pacifiers but research has shown that dummies reduce the risk of sudden infant death syndrome. So what advice can we give to breastfeeding mothers?'

Dummies are now recommended by the Foundation for the Study of Infant Deaths (2009b) as a way of preventing sudden infant death, but the recommendation is to give the dummy only after one month of successful breastfeeding. Babies on the neonatal unit are often given pacifiers for different reasons, such as when they are on continuous positive airways pressure or in pain. The decision to give non-nutritive sucking to babies on the neonatal unit is usually for medical reasons and not purely on parental request.

A student on the neonatal unit says: 'I have been asked by a parent "Why is breast milk fortifier being added to my breast milk. Is it not good enough? Should I change to artificial feeding?"'

Breast milk is the preferred source of nutrition for all infants (see Chapter 6). However, breast milk may not meet the nutritional needs of preterm babies, in particular energy, protein, sodium, phosphorus, calcium and some vitamins. According to the Institute of Child Health (2007) fortification of expressed breast milk can help to minimize these deficiencies. The other babies for whom fortification of expressed breast milk would be used are those who are fluid restricted, for example those with cardiac problems and those who are failing to thrive because of malabsorption problems. Mothers should be reassured that their expressed breast milk is ideal for their sick baby but that sometimes it is necessary to add vital minerals to help their baby over a critical period of their care. They should continue to express their milk because, even with fortifier it is still preferable to formula milk.

A midwife asks: 'What should I advise the parents of a baby born to a woman with GBS (which may or not have been known at the time)? What is the risk period for the baby? What signs and symptoms should they be alert to? What do they do if they have concerns about the baby's well-being?'

The risk to the baby of early onset group B *Streptococcus* (GBS) is increased significantly if the membranes have been ruptured 18 hours or more and where there is maternal pyrexia in labour or if there is a previous child with GBS infection. The risk period for early onset GBS is from birth to 48 hours, although many will develop signs much earlier at birth or by 6–12 hours. The signs to look for are: tachypnoea, recession and grunting. All babies with these respiratory problems will require full screening and prophylactic treatment.

A student midwife asks about constipation in newborns: 'I have heard that cool boiled water and a teaspoon of orange juice are effective. Is this safe? I don't recommend it as I doubt there is an evidence base.'

Normal healthy babies should be expected to have their bowels open within 24 hours of birth (NICE,

2006). If a baby does not pass meconium within 24 hours of delivery this requires an emergency referral as there might be an anatomical obstruction that will require surgery. It is not common for breastfed babies to become constipated and it is rare for babies under three months of age to become constipated. It is normal for a breastfed baby to pass stools anything from eight times a day to only once in 2 or 3 days, whereas a formula-fed baby will pass stools 4–6 times per day. If the stools are hard in consistency and the baby has difficulty and pain on passing the stool then it is advisable to check that the baby is being fed enough in a 24-hour period and is not dehydrated and that the formula feed is being made up correctly. If the formula is too concentrated it will cause constipation. There is no evidence base for giving orange juice in boiled water, the water alone may be sufficient and the orange juice could cause abdominal pain.

A student asks: 'What is the optimum temperature range for neonates?'

The World Health Organization recommends a neonatal temperature range between 36.5°C and 37.5°C. Hypothermia is classed as a temperature below 36.0°C.

New parents ask: 'Our baby makes a sort of grunting noise. What's causing it and does it mean that something is wrong?'

Grunting is one of the signs of respiratory distress and is often accompanied by tachypnoea and cyanosis. Neonates have the ability to trap air to preserve the pressure in the alveoli and prevent collapse at the end of each breath. The vocal cords close and the baby breathes out against the closed cords, which causes the expiratory sound or grunt.

A midwife asks: 'How can I explain to parents how phototherapy works?'

Exposing as much of the baby's body as possible to a high-intensity light induces rapid photochemical changes to the bilirubin molecule. This enables excretion of isomers from the body via the urine and bile. (An isomer is a compound that has the same molecular formula as another compound, but is not identical to it.) It means that conjugation does not need to take place in the liver and bilirubin can be excreted, lowering the overall blood levels. A photoisomer is water-soluble, unlike unconjugated bilirubin

A mum asks: 'My baby's eyes look "sticky". Are they infected?'

Commonly the eyes of newborn babies become runny and can look 'sticky', which makes the parents suspect that there is an infection present. This occurs in the first day or two after birth and is most often caused by irritation or blockage of lacrimal ducts rather than infection. The eyelashes are stuck together by vernix and this can cause irritation, which in turn makes the eyes wet. No treatment is required other than bathing the eyes with cooled, boiled water when at home, ensuring that the eye is cleaned in one motion, from the inside to the outside, and a new ball of cotton wool is used for each eye. The parents should be told to observe for exudate becoming yellow or green or for any redness or swelling, which may indicate an infection. If this happens the baby may require treatment from the GP.

If the baby remains well, the eyes are not red but there is intermittent wetness and the eyes are sticky with no purulent discharge, a blocked nasolacrimal duct may be the cause. In these cases, the eyes usually settle with little or no intervention by the time the child is around six months of age.

Parents ask: 'Will the cord stump become infected?'

The cord stump does not become infected very easily in the first week of life. What does happen is a process of necrosis or death of the tissue. This can sometimes give off a slight odour and can look moist at times as the dead part of tissue becomes detached. It is important that the parents know about this process, especially if it is their first child. It can also help to ensure that nappies are applied securely and that the penis of boys is pointing downwards to avoid any sprays of urine upwards onto the cord area. The community midwife will be there to advise about any redness or exudate from the cord area in the first few days. Cleansing with plain water will help keep the area clean.

In some instances, the cord will remain moist and fails to heal despite the above treatment. In these cases the child may have a granuloma, which occurs when excess granulation tissue is produced during the inflammation process from cord separation. In these cases the cord may require cauterization.

A new mother asks: 'How will I know if my baby has an infection?'

This is a difficult question to answer since infections can manifest themselves in many ways. However, in the absence of any area which is red or which has any purulent exudate, the baby may exhibit some of the signs discussed in Chapter 10. In general, they will not be hungry so they may not be keen to feed and mothers may notice that they are not sucking or they appear to be sated more quickly than usual. They may not have a high temperature like an adult but rather they can become hot and cold and their temperature may vary. They may also seem a bit more fractious than usual and may not easily settle to go to sleep or be lethargic and sleepy. Changes in behaviour are therefore typical presentations.

Tachypnoea is often the earliest sign of infection in a baby and one further sign, which can sometimes be overlooked, is the infant who fails to thrive or put weight on continually over several weeks. This can be indicative of an undiagnosed urinary tract infection. Again, parents can be given some advice about what to look for and to have a low threshold for seeking advice from the midwife, health visitor or GP.

New parents often ask: 'How long should a newborn baby sleep for?'

It is typical for babies to sleep for between 17 and 18 hours a day in the first few weeks and 15 hours per day thereafter up until the third month of life. However, parents need to be advised that their baby will sleep for periods of 3–4 hours at a time and that sleeping through the night should not be expected until much later on. Feeding and changing through the night should be expected in the newborn period. Some parents try to keep their baby awake in the hope that they will sleep for longer periods through the night. Most babies will only be able to stay awake for about 2 hours and any longer can cause them to be overtired. If babies do become overtired, getting them to settle will be more difficult. Signs that a baby is tired and needs to go to sleep include rubbing the eyes and pulling the ear. Parents should be advised how to recognize tiredness in their baby.

A midwife asks: 'Parents always seem to want to cut their baby's nails. What advice should I be giving them?'

Parents do worry that their babies will scratch themselves if the nails are long. Using mittens can prevent scratching. It is safer to file the nails with a soft nail file than to try to cut them. Cutting can cause the nail to become jagged and sharper than they were. Biting the nails is also not advisable. If the nail is cut too far (into the quick) infection to the nail bed can occur. The parents can use their fingers to gently peel off nails that have already started to come away (see Chapter 7).

When being taught resuscitation, parents often ask if there any chance that they might injure their baby if they blow too hard or press too hard while performing compressions.

There is a small risk that if they press too hard parents could cause injury but a baby's ribs are softer and more flexible than adult ribs. It is better to take that risk than not to perform chest compressions if they are needed.

Parents ask: 'If our baby collapses at home and we're on our own, what should we do first?'

Parents should be advised that if they are on their own it is better to start life support for a minute or so before going to the phone. They may be able to open the airway and get a couple of breaths into the baby. The quicker you can start life support, the better. The baby should never be left alone while you go to the phone. Take the baby with you if necessary.

And 'What if we forget how to do resuscitation?'

People always worry about forgetting what to do but it is better to do something rather than nothing at all. The advice is for them to try to remember ABC. Although it would not harm the baby if things are done in the wrong order, it is important to open the airway first so that when you breathe for the baby air gets into the lungs. This needs to be done first before doing chest compressions, as the heart will not have any oxygen to take around the body.

A student midwife says: 'I'm not sure how to explain why female babies sometimes get swollen breasts.'

Swollen, red, tender breasts or mastitis can be seen in both girls and boys and is a result of maternal oestrogen. Occasionally the breasts become engorged with a milky secretion. This should only last about two weeks at the most. Parents should be reassured that it is normal and that it will subside. They should avoid touching the baby's breasts and the swelling will disappear in time.

Many breastfeeding mothers ask: 'How do I know if my baby is getting enough milk?'

If the breastfed baby is happy, contented and satisfied after feeds, he or she is getting enough milk. The baby should appear healthy and be gaining weight after the tenth postnatal day. The mother's nipples or breasts should not be sore or painful. There should be at least six wet nappies a day and two yellow stools passed each day.

Parents are sometimes worried about Mongolian blue spot. How should this be explained to them?

Hyperpigmented macule or Mongolian blue spot is the most common pigmented lesion in the newborn. It is seen primarily in African Caribbean, Asian and Mediterranean babies although it can be present in white babies as well. They are most commonly seen on the buttocks but can range from the calves to the shoulders. They are caused by melanocytes that infiltrate the dermis. They will fade over the first three years of life. Parents should be reassured that this is not a bruise and the midwife should document that a Mongolian blue spot is present in the child health record so that other health professionals are aware of its existence.

Parents ask: 'When will the "lump" on my baby's head go down?'

When you assess a lump on a baby's head you need to differentiate between caput succedaneum and cephalhaematoma. Caput will cross the suture lines whereas cephalhaematoma will not cross the suture lines. Both types of bumps on the head may look a little unsightly. Parents should be advised that caput will go down in a few days but cephalhaematoma could take 6–8 weeks to go completely.

A midwife asks: 'How can I explain in simple terms what jaundice is?'

This can be difficult to explain and for the full physiology see Chapter 9. However, you can explain to parents that when babies are in the uterus they need more red blood cells to help with the transportation of oxygen. When they are born and are breathing for themselves they do not need the high levels of red cells and the cells start to break down within two days of birth. The red cells are broken down into two parts: one part can be recycled but the other part (bilirubin) needs to be excreted. Some of this goes to the liver. However, where there are higher levels of bilirubin that cannot be transported to the liver they float freely in the circulation and leave the baby's skin looking yellow. In most cases physiological jaundice is harmless but it does need to be monitored in case it reaches a level that requires treatment.

Parents sometimes ask: 'Does it hurt the baby when I touch the cord?'

It should not hurt the baby if the cord is touched, but a hard, drying cord can dig into the skin of the abdomen, which might make the baby's tummy a little sore. It is best to advise parents not to overhandle the cord, to make sure that they wash their hands before they do handle the cord and that they only use plain water to clean it if it becomes soiled, using soft cotton wool.

A new mum asks: 'Can my baby see me?'

According to Siderov (2008) young infants do possess the ability to alter their focusing (not as accurately as older children and adults). In the newborn period the image seen by the baby will be very blurred, improving by four weeks and continuing until six months when their vision is much clearer. Newborns are attracted to faces (Siderov, 2008).

A young mother asks: 'Why has my baby lost weight?'

It is normal for babies to lose weight in the first few days of life and up to 10 per cent can be expected. The weight loss is due to the passage of meconium and fluid from passing urine. The baby will not have taken in a large quanity of food in the first few days and insensible fluid loss from respiration all means that the baby's weight is depleted slightly until feeding is well established. If the birthweight has not been regained by the tenth postnatal day it could be a sign of dehydration, or failure to thrive for other reasons and the cause should be investigated.

A genuine question asked by a new parent: 'Does my baby need feeding in the night?'

Well-meaning people often ask new parents 'Is he/she sleeping through the night yet?' This leaves parents thinking that something is wrong with their parenting skills or with their baby because their baby is not sleeping through the night. It is an unrealistic expectation that babies should sleep throughout the night in the early postnatal period. Midwives should reassure parents that their baby will wake in the night for a feed and with breastfeeding babies it is likely that they will wake more than once. The bonus for breastfeeding mothers is that they do not have to get up and make up the feed in the night. See Chapter 6.

A mum asks: 'What's all the white stuff on my baby?'

Vernix caseosa is a white substance that will give added protection to the skin in the first few days following birth. The thickness of the vernix caseosa will vary depending on the gestational age, with post-term babies having smaller amounts. Vernix caseosa has antimicrobial and antifungal properties and parents should be advised that no attempt should be made to remove it with soap.

And 'Why is my baby's poo black?'

To first-time parents the sight of meconuim can be slightly alarming. Meconium is really very dark green rather than black. It is made up from epithelial cells, mucus, bile and water as well as amniotic fluid that the fetus swallows during intrauterine life. It is a tar-like, sticky substance and is technically sterile. Meconium is passed in the first two days following delivery, with the stools changing after milk feeding is established. It is important that midwives note and document the timing of the first stool since delayed passage can be indicative of Hirschsprung's disease. A meconium plug could indicate cystic fibrosis.

Parents often ask:'Why is my baby crying?'

Babies cry for various reasons, such as hunger, pain, wind, too hot or too cold, they are overstimulated or they just want a cuddle.

Parents become accustomed to their baby's cry quite early in the postnatal period. However, if the crying becomes excessive or the nature of the cry changes a cause should be sought. NICE (2006) guidelines suggest that if a baby is crying inconsolably and excessively, particularly in the evening and if the baby is drawing up the legs and arching the back it could be that the baby has colic. The midwife should urgently assess the feeding, the nature of the stools, the woman's diet if breastfeeding, if there is a family history of allergy and the parent's response to the crying. Parents should be reassured that this is a phase that will pass and to hold their baby throughout the colicky period. Other techniques include a warm bath, swaddling, rocking, and massaging the abdominal area. Crying can be a feature of irritability secondary to an underlying illness and if it is persistent should be investigated.

Conclusion

This compilation of questions and answers has aimed to address some of the common issues that arise in clinical practice every day. Healthcare professionals are used to dealing with questions from parents and it is hoped that this chapter has been able to resolve some of the more common ones. Any advice you give should be evidence-based if you are suggesting healthcare products or services. This should be adhered to when advising parents on products for nappy rash, skin care, colic and constipation, etc. There are a plethora of products available for parents to choose from and ultimately they will choose based on advice given, price and availability.

When responding to questions from parents, always answer them truthfully in language they understand. Try to avoid using medical terminology and jargon and keep answers simple without being condescending. Many parents are well informed, but when their baby is unwell or if there is any deviation from normal, they will be anxious and will need their baby's problem discussing in a way that will help them to understand.

References

Foundation for the Study of Infant Deaths (2009a) Babies sleeping in the same room as parents. www.fsid.org.uk/babycare

Foundation for the Study of Infant Deaths (2009b) Use of dummies in the prevention of sudden infant death. www.fsid.org.uk/babycare

Institute of Child Health (2007) Breast milk fortifier guidelines. www.ich.ucl.ac.uk/clinical_information/ clinical_guidelines/cpg_guideline_00040 [accessed 9 September 2009].

NICE (National Institute for Health and Clinical Excellence) (2006) Postnatal Guidelines. Routine postnatal care of women and their babies. NICE Guideline 37. www.nice.org.uk

Siderov J (2008) The newborn eye: visual function and screening for ocular disorders. In: Davies L and McDonald S (eds) Examination of the Newborn and Neonatal Health. A multidimensional approach. Edinburgh: Churchill Livingstone, chapter 11.

Index